Dyspepsia in Clinical Practice

Dyspepsia in Clinical Practice

Marko Duvnjak

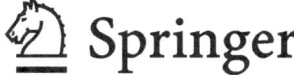 Springer

Editor
Marko Duvnjak
Department of Gastroenterology and Hepatology
University Hospital "Sestre milosrdnice"
Medical School in Zagreb, University of Zagreb
Zagreb
Croatia
marko.duvnjak1@gmail.com

ISBN 978-1-4419-1729-4   e-ISBN 978-1-4419-1730-0
DOI 10.1007/978-1-4419-1730-0
Springer New York Dordrecht Heidelberg London

Library of Congress Control Number: 2011921928

Printed on acid-free paper

Springer is part of Springer Science+Business Media (www.springer.com)

To my family

I dedicate this book to my family, as their love and support are essential for all my work.

Acknowledgments

As the editor of this book, I found myself facing a challenging task having in mind that it was written in an attempt to elucidate this interesting topic from a practical point of view. If the book succeeds in its goal, and I truly believe it will, all the thanks should go to the authors who gave their best to bring in front of you an evidence-based, concise, up-to-date, and practical text on the relevant topic.

I would also like to thank my colleagues who helped me in this enterprise, Marija Gomerči , MD, Sanja Stojsavljevi , MD, Lucija Virovi -Juki , MD, PhD, and Neven Barši , MD, as well as Prof. George Y. Wu, MD, PhD and our publisher Springer Publishing Company, who gave me the idea and the opportunity for this project.

Marko Duvnjak

Contents

ix

Contributors

Lars Aabakken
Department of Gastroenterology, Oslo University
Hospital – Rikshospitalet, Oslo, Norway
larsaa@medisin.uio.no

György Miklós Buzás
Department of Gastroenterology, Ferencváros Health Service
Non-Profit Ltd, Budapest, Hungary
drgybuzas@hotmail.com

Marko Duvnjak
Department of Gastroenterology and Hepatology,
University hospital "Sestre milosrdnice", Medical School in
Zagreb, University of Zagreb, Zagreb, Croatia
marko.duvnjak1@gmail.com

Marija Gomerčić
Division of Gastroenterology and Hepatology,
Department of Medicine, 'Sestre milosrdnice' University Hospital,
Zagreb, Croatia
marijagomercic@yahoo.com

Oleg Jadrešin
Department of Pediatric Gastroenterology and Nutrition,
University Children's Hospital Zagreb, Zagreb, Croatia
oleg.jadresin@yahoo.com

Arne Kandulski
Department of Gastroenterology, Hepatology and Infectious
Diseases, "Otto-von-Guericke" University,
Magdeburg, Germany
Arne.Kandulski@med.ovgu.de

Ivan Lerotić
Division of Gastroenterology and Hepatology,
Department of Medicine, 'Sestre milosrdnice' University Hospital,
Zagreb, Croatia
ilerotic@kbsm.hr

Peter Malfertheiner
Department of Gastroenterology, Hepatology and Infectious Diseases, "Otto-von-Guericke" University, Magdeburg, Germany
peter.malfertheiner@med.ovgu.de

Michael Häfner
Department of Medicince, St. Elisabeth Hospital, Vienna, Austria
Michael.Haefner@elisabethinen-wien.at

Mattijs E. Numans
Professor Innovation & Quality Academic Primary Care,
Amsterdam Free University Medical Center;
and
Coordinator Julius Primary Care Network,
University Medical Centre Utrecht, Utrecht, The Netherlands
m.e.numans@umcutrecht.nl

Roland Pulanić
Department of Gastroenterology and Hepatology,
University Department of Medicine, Zagreb University Hospital,
Zagreb, Croatia
roland.pulanic@gmail.com

Eamonn M. M. Quigley
Department of Medicine, Clinical Sciences Building,
Cork University Hospital, Cork, Ireland
e.quigley@ucc.ie

Alberto Ravelli
GI Pathophysiology and Gastroenterology, University Department of Pediatrics, Children's Hospital, Spedali Civili, Brescia, Italy
alberto_ravelli@yahoo.com

Daniel Schmidt-Martin
Alimentary Pharmabiotic Centre, Department of Medicine,
Clinical Sciences Building, Cork University Hospital,
Cork, Ireland
danscma@yahoo.com

Lea Smirčić-Duvnjak
Vuk Vrhovac University Clinic for Diabetes, Endocrinology and Metabolic Disease, University of Zagreb, School of Medicine,
Dugidol 4a, Zagreb, Croatia
lduvnjak@idb.hr

Sanja Stojsavljević
Department of Gastroenterology and Hepatology,
University hospital "Sestre milosrdnice", Zagreb, Croatia
sanja.stojsavljevic1@gmail.com

Bojan Tepeš
ABAKUS MEDICO d.o.o., Diagnostični center Rogaška,
Rogaška Slatina, Slovenia
bojan.tepes@siol.net

Vedran Tomašić
Division of Gastroenterology and Hepatology, Department
of Medicine, University Hospital "Sestre milosrdnice",
Zagreb, Croatia
vtomasic@globalnet.hr

Marino Venerito
Department of Gastroenterology, Hepatology and Infectious
Diseases, "Otto-von-Guericke" University, Magdeburg, Germany
m.venerito@med.ovgu.de

Introduction

Marko Duvnjak

So simple when we bluntly translate it from its Greek origin "bad digestion," dyspepsia is everything but a simple condition. Even when we try to bind it to a definition that would best suit its characteristics we find ourselves in front of a great brick wall. There are so many aspects that have to be taken into consideration when evaluating, diagnosing, and managing dyspepsia that it is not unusual for physicians to find themselves lost in the sea of conflicting information, clinical tests, and medications that are now available throughout the world. The main reason why we have chosen dyspepsia as the main character in this book is its global presence and large prevalence rate of approximately 25% (range from 13% up to 40%) in the general population from the Far East to the West. Connecting patients from every corner of the world in their adversity, physicians in their struggle to relive the aches of patients, and of course governments in their attempt to control and reduce health care expenditure, dyspepsia has unquestionably become a global health and economic problem.

When presence of dyspepsia leads an individual to seek medical attention, in making the decision on the best approach, physician is often put on a crossroad whether to treat the underlying pathology as benign or life threatening. The final verdict is dependent on many aspects that the physician has to consider and satisfy, on one hand always thinking on the benefit of his patient, and on the other being careful with the expenditure of undertaken procedures. New diagnostic possibilities are enticing but very expensive, whereas unsuitably managed dyspepsia is even more costly, due to impaired quality of life and general dissatisfaction of the patient. This is one of the reasons why many countries have adapted guidelines to steer their physicians to a rightful decision, with the main goal to equilibrate the disbursements and the benefits of diagnostic strategies. However, national guidelines followed by practitioners in different countries vary in diagnostic and therapeutic approach, and because of this there is an evident need for a unique definition worldwide.

This is a very dynamic and growing field, and new researches regarding this topic are being published almost daily. In this book, we sought to summarize all evidence-based information gathered so far and current guidelines to make everyday handling of dyspepsia less complex for physicians. Every chapter chips away a fragment of the challenge that dyspepsia puts in front of us, making its recognition, definite diagnosis, and treatment more simplified. We found that it was of a great importance to give the definition of dyspepsia and its division on the basis of the latest Rome III agreement first, followed by extensive description of individual diseases that lie in the background of dyspepsia, and then to guide the reader through uninvestigated dyspepsia which is irrefutably inherent in primary care, giving highlights on the epidemiology, prognosis, quality of life, economics, and finally treatment of this condition. Because we find that children, elderly, and diabetics are specific groups with their specific needs, we tried to give a perspective from that point of view and elaborate how such patients should be managed.

We made all this possible by gathering a selection of world-class experts on each of the topics previously mentioned and setting before them a challenge how to provide physicians a meaningful and practical manual to answer their questions and guide them through problems associated with the management of this condition on an everyday basis. *Dyspepsia in Clinical Practice* represents a summary of all relevant research data, guidelines, and practical algorithms, and we hope it will become a valuable asset to physicians whenever encountering a patient with dyspepsia symptoms all around the globe.

Chapter 1
The Definition of Dyspepsia

Daniel Schmidt-Martin and Eamonn M.M. Quigley

Keywords: Dyspepsia, Functional dyspepsia, Nonulcer dyspepsia, Gastroesophageal reflux, Irritable bowel syndrome, Peptic ulcer disease, *Helicobacter pylori*, Nonerosive reflux disease, Functional heartburn, Rome Foundation

INTRODUCTION

Dyspepsia, perceived as a very common and sometimes disabling problem, presents a formidable challenge to the clinician and clinical investigator alike. While we all can enumerate a number of symptoms that could be regarded as components of this "syndrome," many, if not all, are nonspecific in terms of organ of origin or underlying pathophysiology. Overlap with other common symptomatic gastrointestinal disorders, such as functional heartburn and irritable bowel syndrome (IBS), is also an issue; where does dyspepsia end and reflux begin? It is in this context that definitions of dyspepsia, which can guide the clinician in diagnosis and therapy and provide the investigator with coherent study populations, must be developed.

WHAT IS "DYSPEPSIA?": AN OVERVIEW

Dyspepsia is not a disease but rather a symptom, or more usually, a symptom complex that is common, affecting up to 29% of people in the community, in some surveys [1]. Dyspepsia has

D. Schmidt-Martin (✉)
Alimentary Pharmabiotic Centre, Department of Medicine,
Clinical Sciences Building, Cork University Hospital, Cork, Ireland
e-mail: danscma@yahoo.com

1

M. Duvnjak (ed.), *Dyspepsia in Clinical Practice*,
DOI 10.1007/978-1-4419-1730-0_1,
© Springer Science+Business Media, LLC 2011

been associated with a variety of personal and environmental risk factors including alcohol, tobacco, and nonsteroidal antiinflammatory medication use and can exert a significant negative impact on the quality of life and incur considerable personal and societal costs [2–5].

One would imagine, therefore, given its frequency and impact that dyspepsia was a readily definable term; in reality, this is far from being the case. Indeed, difficulties with definition have bedeviled this whole area and have generated much confusion and halted progress in research. The term dyspepsia is, of course, a medical term generally arrived at following interpretation of a patient's symptom or symptoms. Inherent to this approach are the hazards of communication and interpretation – factors that are influenced by several variables including ethnicity, culture, age, and above all, language.

The word dyspepsia is derived from the Greek "δυς-" (Dys-) and "πέψη" (Pepse) and can be literally translated as "bad digestion." Dyspepsia can, accordingly, be regarded as synonymous with the lay term "indigestion," so commonly used in the English speaking world. Indeed the term dyspepsia can be and often is used interchangeably with "indigestion" to describe a number of disparate symptoms (from pain to fullness, from heartburn to nausea, from belching to early satiety, etc.), which are considered by the patient or his/her physician to arise in the area of the upper abdomen or lower chest. Only through a careful and thorough interrogation of the patient can an accurate and reproducible interpretation of exactly what is meant by a symptom be reached. Matters become even more complicated as one strays from English; while the term dyspepsia is a feature of many languages of European origin and its interpretation is relatively similar, the same does not hold true elsewhere. Regrettably, there have been few efforts to "translate" this symptom or symptom complex into non-European languages or to understand how a Japanese or Chinese patient, for example, gives voice to his or her upper gastrointestinal symptoms. Further complicating the study of dyspepsia is the relative nonspecificity of its constituent symptoms and the fact that numerous pathological processes may be at play; differentiating between them on the basis of symptoms alone can seem, at times, Quixotic. Over the years, we have learned at our cost that, with the notable exception of heartburn, dyspepsia symptoms are poorly predictive of underlying pathology and, most disappointingly, once heartburn is excluded, even less helpful in indicating likely therapeutic responses.

These difficulties with definition spill over from the clinical into the research arena and render the interpretation of the literature, and, especially that of clinical trials, challenging and frustrating, as investigators provide definitions of dyspepsia, which range from the highly complex to the entirely nebulous.

Dyspepsia has been with us for a long time with the earliest documented instances reported in Scotland in the mid-eighteenth century and in the USA from the late eighteenth century. Interestingly, these recordings of the term dyspepsia occurred in advance of the rise in the incidence of peptic ulcer disease, which is thought to have begun in the late nineteenth century [6]. What precise pathology these early reports of dyspepsia referred to is unknown. From the late nineteenth century until the latter half of the last century two diseases, peptic ulcer disease and gastric carcinoma loomed large in the differential diagnosis of the dyspeptic patient and much effort was exerted into the development of clinical algorithms that could reliably differentiate between these entities as well as between duodenal and gastric ulcers. As these pathologies declined in prevalence in the West, new challenges emerged, such as the definition of functional dyspepsia (FD) and the separation of FD from two, now very prevalent, disorders, gastroesophageal reflux disease (GERD) and IBS.

WHAT SYMPTOMS DOES DYSPEPSIA ENCOMPASS?

In a definition that focused on functional dyspepsia, the Rome process, in its second iteration, Rome II, defined dyspepsia, in a restrictive manner, as "pain or discomfort centered in the upper abdomen" [7]. Does this mean we exclude retrosternal symptoms and focus on the upper abdomen? Does this mean the exclusion of reflux, excessive belching, and heartburn? Equally, if we focus on the upper abdomen, does this mean that we exclude the patient with such additional symptoms as lower abdominal bloating and crampy abdominal pain, which are oft associated with IBS?

These questions go beyond mere semantics as their responses have significant implications for the design of clinical trials; a study that excludes all reflux sufferers will recruit a very different patient population than one which is more inclusive. While it can be argued that the former strategy will provide a more homogenous population, it scarcely takes account of clinical reality: overlap between functional diseases of the esophagus, stomach, and the remainder of the bowel are common and often inseparable! Indeed, between 14 and 27% of patients with either GERD, dyspepsia, or IBS will complain of symptoms suggestive of either one, or both, of the other disorders [8]. Our current understanding of the pathophysiology of functional heartburn, FD, and IBS would also support a more inclusive approach; each has been associated with visceral hypersensitivity and disturbances in the brain gut-axis, for example. Furthermore, while the phenomenon of postinfectious IBS has been well described, new onset functional dyspepsia was, in one study, as likely to occur in the aftermath of salmonella gastroenteritis as IBS [9]. Both postinfective IBS and FD have also been associated with chronic low grade inflammation in the colon and duodenum, respectively [10].

At the other end of the gastrointestinal tract, the margins between GERD and, especially, those individuals with nonerosive reflux disease (NERD) and FD are equally blurred [11]. Characterized by heartburn or reflux in the absence of endoscopic changes, NERD is common and may account for up to 70% of uninvestigated reflux in the community [11]. NERD itself can be further subdivided into three groups depending on the extent of acid exposure and its correlation with symptoms [11]. The first of these exhibits increased acid exposure on prolonged intraesophageal pH testing and may harbor subtle ultrastructural or microscopic changes in esophageal morphology or laboratory evidence of immune activation; this group behaves in terms of therapeutic response in the same manner as GERD, in general. In the second group, while acid exposure is normal, symptoms consistently correlate with episodes of reflux; again a response to acid suppression is to be expected. The third and most challenging group, referred to as functional heartburn, exhibits normal acid exposure and no correlation between symptoms and reflux events – this group is resistant to acid suppression and is associated with an increased incidence of psychopathology [12]. All NERD groups tend to overlap with FD, but this is most evident among those with functional heartburn – a diagnosis that is now regarded as truly "functional" rather than a part of the spectrum of GERD [13].

One is compelled to ask, therefore, whether FD and functional heartburn, on the one hand, or FD and IBS, on the other, are merely different manifestations of the same condition [14].

A WORKING DEFINITION OF DYSPEPSIA

The Canadian dyspepsia working group provided a definition that is quite inclusive: "a symptom complex of epigastric pain or discomfort thought to originate in the upper gastrointestinal tract, and it may include any of the following symptoms: heartburn, acid regurgitation, excessive burping/belching, increased abdominal bloating, nausea, feeling of abnormal or slow digestion, or early satiety" [1]. In our opinion, this approach is most appropriate for clinical practice, providing of course that one remains mindful of the limitations of symptom-based definitions and of the vagaries imposed by language, culture, and ethnicity.

Further complexities lie ahead, however. One issue that is most relevant to the interpretation of clinical trials of such strategies as acid suppression or eradication of *Helicobacter pylori*, for instance, is the degree to which a given population of dyspepsia sufferers has been investigated. In this regard, it is critical, at the outset, to clearly differentiate between study populations that have been investigated (*H. pylori* serology, endoscopy, etc.) and those that have not; the former will have excluded peptic ulceration, gastric cancer, and, in the West in particular, esophagitis, whereas the latter will include some who suffer from these pathologies. Needless to say, a population that still includes subjects with GERD and duodenal ulcers will be much more likely to respond to a proton pump inhibitor or triple therapy.

FUNCTIONAL DYSPEPSIA

As the prevalence of peptic ulcer disease and gastric carcinoma has receded, there has been an increasing appreciation of the prevalence of the unexplained upper gastrointestinal symptoms, leading to the advent of, firstly, nonulcer dyspepsia (NUD) and, secondly, FD. As can be assumed from its very name, NUD, the use of this term is very reflective of an approach to the assessment of the patient with dyspepsia, which first excludes all possible "organic" explanations; in other words, NUD was a diagnosis of exclusion. Cognizant of the unsatisfactory nature of a diagnosis that is based merely on the exclusion of other considerations and of the expense and patient discomfort, which such an approach entails, considerable effort has been exerted in developing clinical criteria or guidelines that might more readily and definitively aid this diagnosis with a minimum of interventions. Chief amongst the advocates of this positive approach has been the Rome Foundation (http://www.theromefoundation.org), an organization dedicated to increasing recognition of functional GI disorders and promoting a scientific approach to their study and management. Accordingly, a number of diagnostic criteria have been developed to aid in the diagnosis and study of functional GI disorders. In developing these criteria, Rome has attempted to differentiate between symptoms of different anatomical origins; in this regard, dyspepsia is seen as a symptom or symptom complex arising in the area of the upper abdomen, while symptoms of reflux, heartburn, and regurgitation come under the heading of functional heartburn. This approach is not without its critics but, nonetheless, has provided a framework for the study of functional diseases of the upper gastrointestinal tract.

In reviewing the history of the Rome approach to FD, the challenges that this concept presents, even to this august organization, are evident. Reference has already been made to the rather restrictive Rome II definition; the recently updated Rome III criteria reflect quite a dramatic shift in emphasis, no doubt based on the many disappointments in both the diagnostic and therapeutic arenas among Rome II-diagnosed FD sufferers over the years [15]. The divisions of FD into those symptoms that were described motility-like, ulcer-like, or reflux-like were abandoned, a testament to two developments; firstly, the failure of symptoms to reliably predict underlying pathophysiology and, secondly, the removal of those with predominant heartburn and other reflux symptoms from the spectrum of FD. Rome III, instead, describes two distinct patterns of dyspepsia depending on whether symptoms are predominantly related to food intake and/or are associated with an inability to finish meals (postprandial distress syndrome) or are less related to food intake and are more dominated by pain (epigastric pain syndrome). While these categories were developed more on the basis of expert opinion than clinical evidence, some data to support clinical relevance for these distinctions is beginning to emerge with one study, for example, indicating that anxiety is associated with the postprandial distress syndrome but not the epigastric pain syndrome and another demonstrating a genetic link for the epigastric pain syndrome and not for the postprandial pain syndrome [16, 17]. On the other hand, it must be stressed that these subgroups are not mutually exclusive; as many as 34% of patients describe symptoms compatible with both. Interestingly, both the overlap and postprandial distress syndrome groups are independently associated with psychopathological factors including psychological stress, somatization, phobia, and depression with those patients with overlap being at the more severe end of the scale for these disorders; factors that could well confound the interpretation of pathophysiological studies and therapeutic interventions in FD [18].

Rome III excludes patients with retrosternal pain and those whose symptoms are associated with bowel action; attempts to differentiate FD from GERD and IBS, respectively; a strategy that may have some appeal to the clinical epidemiologist but little relevance to the clinician [19–22].

CONCLUSIONS

The issue of definition is at the very core of dyspepsia; our struggles with progress in this area are, in large part, based on variations in definition and interpretation of symptoms. Does FD exist or does it represent part of a spectrum of a functional disorder that traverses the gut and encompasses functional heartburn, FD, and IBS? Are the new Rome III subcategories clinically replicable and useful? Can we define populations of dyspepsia sufferers that will predictably exhibit a common underlying pathophysiology or reliably respond to a given therapeutic approach? All of these critical questions remain to be answered; in the interim, the clinician is encouraged to make every effort to fully understand what his or her patient means by their symptoms and to be alert to variations on the definition of dyspepsia in the medical literature.

References

1. Veldhuyzen van Zanten SJ, Flook N, Chiba N, et al. An evidence-based approach to the management of uninvestigated dyspepsia in the era of *Helicobacter pylori*. Canadian Dyspepsia Working Group. CMAJ. 2000;162 Suppl 12:S3–23.
2. Halder SLS, Locke 3rd GR, Schleck CD, Zinsmeister AR, Talley NJ. Influence of alcohol consumption on IBS and dyspepsia. Neurogastroenterol Motil. 2006;18:1001–8.
3. Coppeta L, Pietroiusti A, Magrini A, Somma G, Bergamaschi A. Prevalence and characteristics of functional dyspepsia among workers exposed to cement dust. Scand J Work Environ Health. 2008;34: 396–402.
4. Wildner-Christensen M, Hansen JM, De Muckadell OBS. Risk factors for dyspepsia in a general population: non-steroidal anti-inflammatory drugs, cigarette smoking and unemployment are more important than *Helicobacter pylori* infection. Scand J Gastroenterol. 2006;41:149–54.
5. Kulig M, Leodolter A, Vieth M, et al. Quality of life in relation to symptoms in patients with gastro-oesophageal reflux disease: an analysis based on the ProGERD initiative. Aliment Pharmacol Ther. 2003;18:767–76.
6. Baron JH, Sonnenberg A. Early history of dyspepsia and peptic ulcer in the United States. Am J Gastroenterol. 2009;104:2893–6.
7. Talley NJ, Stanghellini V, Heading RC, Koch KL, Malagelada JR, Tytgat GN. Functional gastroduodenal disorders. Gut. 1999;45 Suppl 2:II37–42.
8. Lee SY, Lee KJ, Kim SJ, Cho SW. Prevalence and risk factors for overlaps between gastroesophageal reflux disease, dyspepsia, and irritable bowel syndrome: a population-based study. Digestion. 2009;79:196–201.
9. Mearin F, Pérez-Oliveras M, Perelló A, et al. Dyspepsia and irritable bowel syndrome after a Salmonella gastroenteritis outbreak: one-year follow-up cohort study. Gastroenterology. 2005;129:98–104.

10. Kindt S, Tertychnyy A, de Hertogh G, Geboes K, Tack J. Intestinal immune activation in presumed post-infectious functional dyspepsia. Neurogastroenterol Motil. 2009;21:832–e56.
11. Quigley EMM. Functional dyspepsia (FD) and non-erosive reflux disease (NERD): overlapping or discrete entities? Best Pract Res Clin Gastroenterol. 2004;18:695–706.
12. Savarino E, Pohl D, Zentilin P, et al. Functional heartburn has more in common with functional dyspepsia than with non-erosive reflux disease. Gut. 2009;58:1185–91.
13. Galmiche JP, Clouse RE, Bálint A, et al. Functional esophageal disorders. Gastroenterology. 2006;130:1459–65.
14. Quigley EMM, Keohane J. Dyspepsia. Curr Opin Gastroenterol. 2008;24:692–7.
15. Tack J, Talley NJ, Camilleri M, et al. Functional gastroduodenal disorders. Gastroenterology. 2006;130:1466–79.
16. Aro P, Talley NJ, Ronkainen J, et al. Anxiety is associated with uninvestigated and functional dyspepsia (Rome III criteria) in a Swedish population-based study. Gastroenterology. 2009;137:94–100.
17. Oshima T, Nakajima S, Yokoyama T, et al. The G-protein beta3 subunit 825 TT genotype is associated with epigastric pain syndrome-like dyspepsia. BMC Med Genet. 2010;11:13.
18. Hsu Y-C, Liou J-M, Liao S-C, et al. Psychopathology and personality trait in subgroups of functional dyspepsia based on Rome III criteria. Am J Gastroenterol. 2009;104:2534–42.
19. Quigley EMM. The "con" case. The Rome process and functional gastrointestinal disorders: the barbarians are at the gate! Neurogastroenterol Motil. 2007;19:793–7.
20. Quigley EMM, Shanahan F. The language of medicine: words as servants and scoundrels. Clin Med. 2009;9:131–5.
21. Talley NJ, Vakil N, Practice Parameters Committee of the American College of Gastroenterology. Guidelines for the management of dyspepsia. Am J Gastroenterol. 2005;100:2324–37.
22. Talley NJ, Vakil NB, Moayyedi P. American gastroenterological association technical review on the evaluation of dyspepsia. Gastroenterology. 2005;129:1756–80.

Chapter 2
Subgroups of Dyspepsia

Bojan Tepeš

Keywords: Dyspepsia, Organic dyspepsia, Functional dyspepsia, Diagnostic criteria, Postprandial distress syndrome, Epigastric pain syndrome

INTRODUCTION

Dyspepsia is a common symptom with an extensive differential diagnosis and a heterogeneous pathophysiology. Its prevalence by itself implies a great health care problem, even though most do not seek medical care [1, 2]. Dyspepsia is responsible for substantial health care costs and considerable time lost from work [3]. The management of dyspepsia represents a major component of clinical practice at the primary care level, and 2% to 5% of family practice consultations are for dyspepsia [4].

The term dyspepsia is derived from the Greek word meaning bad digestion. The condition was described 2,000 years ago. It is a complex of symptoms referable to the upper gastrointestinal tract, but not all clinicians and researches agree on which symptoms should be included in its definition. Guidelines from UK and Canada use the term to mean all symptoms referable to the upper gastrointestinal tract, whereas Rome II definition from 1999 excludes patients with classic heartburn and regurgitation [5–7].

B. Tepeš (✉)
ABAKUS MEDICO d.o.o., Diagnostični center Rogaška,
Rogaška Slatina, Slovenia
e-mail: bojan.tepes@siol.net

9

M. Duvnjak (ed.), *Dyspepsia in Clinical Practice*,
DOI 10.1007/978-1-4419-1730-0_2,
© Springer Science+Business Media, LLC 2011

TABLE 2.1. Structural or biochemical causes of dyspepsia.

Gastroesophageal reflux disease (GERD)

Peptic ulcer disease

Gastric or esophageal cancer

Biliary pain

Medications (including potassium supplements, digitalis, iron, theophylline, oral antibiotics, especially ampicillin and erythromycin, NSAIDs, corticosteroids, niacin, gemfibrozil, narcotics, colchicine, quinidine, estrogens, and levodopa)

Gastroparesis

Pancreatitis

Carbohydrate malabsorption

Infiltrative diseases of the stomach (e.g., Crohn's disease, sarcoidosis)

Metabolic disturbances (hypercalcemia, hyperkalemia)

Hepatoma

Ischemic bowel disease

Systemic disorders (diabetes mellitus, thyroid, and parathyroid disorders, connective tissue disease)

Intestinal parasites (giardia, strongyloides)

Abdominal cancer, especially pancreatic cancer

An international committee of clinical investigators (Rome III Committee) defined dyspepsia as one or more of the following symptoms [1]:

- Postprandial fullness
- Early satiation (meaning inability to finish a normal size meal or postprandial fullness)
- Epigastric pain or burning

Patients with symptoms of dyspepsia who have not undergone any investigations are defined as having uninvestigated dyspepsia. Diagnostic investigation (upper gastrointestinal endoscopy, laboratory, and X-ray) reveals normal findings in 40% to 60% of individuals (functional dyspepsia group), and in the others, organic or structural causes of the symptoms can be found (Table 2.1) [8, 9].

ORGANIC OR STRUCTURAL DYSPEPSIA

In patients with organic or structural dyspepsia, there are three major causes of dyspepsia: gastroesophageal reflux (with or without esophagitis), chronic peptic ulcer disease, and malignancy.

The prevalence of gastroesophageal reflux disease (GERD) is 25% in dyspepsia. Erosive esophagitis is found at endoscopy in 5% to 15% of the cases. The predominant symptom of GERD, heartburn, is not a reliable indicator in differentiation between GERD and dyspepsia. The probability of GERD in the setting of dominant heartburn is 54% [10].

A peptic ulcer is found in approximately 5% to 15% of patients with dyspepsia (see more in Chap. 10) [11].

Gastric or esophageal adenocarcinoma is found in less than 2% of all patients referred to endoscopy to evaluate dyspepsia [12]. Alarm features are used to try and identify patients who need early investigation with endoscopy (see Table 6.1). The sensitivity, specificity, positive, and negative predictive values vary greatly (see Chap. 8) [13].

Other causes of organic dyspepsia are rare. Classic biliary pain can be differentiated from dyspepsia by its clinical picture. It occurs as episodic acute and severe upper abdominal pain, usually in the epigastrium or right upper quadrant, and lasts for at least 1 h (often several hours or more). The pain may radiate to the back or scapula and is often associated with restlessness, sweating, or vomiting. Episodes are typically separated by weeks to months. Gallstones are sometimes implicated as the source of symptoms in patients with dyspepsia. However, such an association should be made cautiously, since gallstones may silently coexist in patients with dyspepsia [14].

Nonsteroidal anti-inflammatory drugs (NSAIDs) can cause dyspepsia. If dyspepsia occurs, their use should be discontinued whenever possible. A meta-analysis found a greater degree of risk reduction in dyspepsia when patients were on proton pump inhibitors [15].

Several other drugs have been implicated as causes of dyspepsia. The use of calcium channel blockers, methylxanthines, alendronate, orlistat, potassium supplements, acarbose, and certain antibiotics, including erythromycin and metronidazole, should also be considered as a potential factor [16].

Gastroparesis results from a range of muscular, neural, or rhythm disorders of the stomach. It is more common in women and in diabetic patients [17].

While chronic pancreatitis, celiac disease, and lactose intolerance may coexist with dyspepsia, they are uncommon causes of the condition [18–20].

Other rare causes of dyspepsia include infiltrative diseases of the stomach (Mb Crohn, eosinophilic gastritis, sarcoidosis), metabolic disturbances (hypercalcemia, hyperkalemia), intestinal angina, intestinal parasites (giardia, strongyloides), hepatoma, and pancreatic cancer [12, 20].

FUNCTIONAL DYSPEPSIA

Functional dyspepsia (FD) is defined as at least a 3-month history of dyspepsia in the absence of any organic, systemic, or metabolic disease that is likely to explain the symptoms [1]. The pathophysiology of FD is unclear. Putative mechanisms include overlapping disorders of upper gastrointestinal motor and sensory function. Approximately 25% to 45% of the patients have delayed gastric emptying, 40% have impaired fundic accommodation, and visceral hypersensitivity occurs in about one third of the patients [21–23]. A specific symptom profile for these subsets of patients does not exist [24]. Psychological distress, including abuse, has been associated with dyspepsia, but a cause-and-effect relationship has not been established [25].

In the past 20 years, several attempts have been made to try to subclassify patients with FD to a subgroup with similar pathophysiological mechanisms and/or symptoms, what would be of help to physicians and researchers.

The Rome I and Rome II consensuses define FD as the presence of pain or discomfort in the upper abdomen in the absence of organic disease. The Rome II definition excluded patients with predominant heartburn and patients with irritable bowel syndrome. Symptoms must be present for at least 12 weeks, which do not need to be consecutive, within the preceding 12 months [7, 26].

The Rome II consensus subdivided patients with dyspepsia in three subgroups:

- Ulcer-like dyspepsia (pain centered in the upper abdomen is the predominant and most bothersome symptom)
- Dysmotility-like dyspepsia (an unpleasant or troublesome non-painful sensation or discomfort centered in the upper abdomen is the predominant symptom; this sensation may be characterized by or associated with upper abdominal fullness, early satiety, bloating, or nausea)
- Unspecified (nonspecific) dyspepsia (symptomatic patients whose symptoms do not fulfill the criteria for ulcer-like or dysmotility-like dyspepsia)

The Rome II subdivision has been criticized because of the difficulty distinguishing pain from discomfort, the lack of an accepted definition of the term predominant, number of patients who do not fit into one of the subgroups, and especially the lack of stability of the predominant symptom even over short time periods [27–29].

The Rome III committee decreased the number of FD symptoms to four specific symptoms that originate from the gastroduodenal region [1]:

- Postprandial fullness
- Early satiety
- Epigastric pain
- Epigastric burning

At least one symptom must be present for at least the last 3 months with an onset of symptoms at least 6 months prior to diagnosis.

Other symptoms may coexist, such as bloating (may be derived from the bowel), nausea (often of central origin), vomiting, belching, and heartburn (esophageal origin).

The Rome III committee subdivided FD into two new diagnostic categories:

- Meal-induced postprandial distress syndrome (PDS), characterized by postprandial fullness and early satiety
- Epigastric pain syndrome (EPS), characterized by epigastric pain and burning

Diagnostic Criteria for PDS (B1a)
Must include one or both of the following:

1. Bothersome postprandial fullness, occurring after ordinary sized meals, at least several times per week
2. Early satiety that prevents finishing a regular meal at least several times per week

Supportive Criteria
1. Upper abdominal bloating or postprandial nausea
2. EPS may coexist

Diagnostic Criteria for EPS (B1b)
1. Pain or burning localized in the epigastrium of at least moderate severity at least once per week.
2. The pain is intermittent.
3. Pain not generalized or located in other abdominal or chest regions.

4. Pain not relieved by defecation or passage of flatus.
5. Not fulfilling criteria for gallbladder and sphincter Oddi disorders.

Supportive Criteria
1. The pain may be of a burning quality but without a retrosternal component.
2. The pain is commonly induced or relieved by ingestion of a meal but may occur while fasting.
3. PDS may coexist.

In the study of Hsu et al., there was a 34.2% overlap between EPS and PDS. Multiple linear regression analysis demonstrated that the diagnosis of PDS was independently associated with higher scores in overall psychopathological stress. In patients with EPS, the diagnosis was not associated with psychopathology [30].

The Rome III subdivision of FD was proposed under the assumption that different underlying pathophysiological mechanisms are present in each of the subgroups and, consequently, that different treatment modalities would be most suitable for each group. The future research will give us the answer weather this assumption is correct [31] (Fig. 2.1).

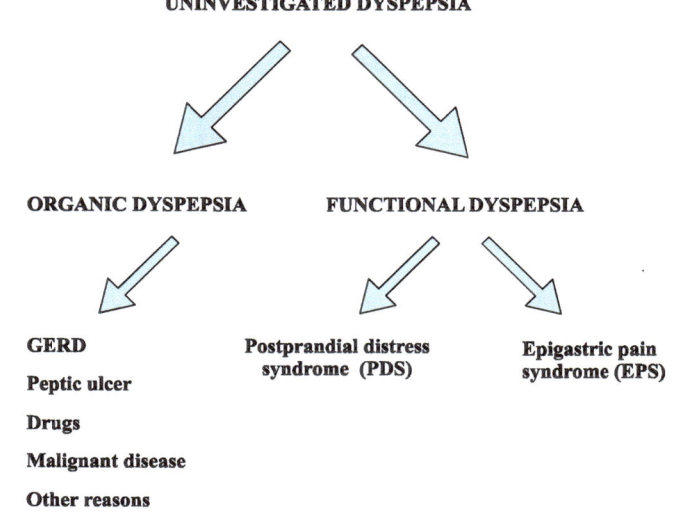

FIG. 2.1 Rome III subgroups of dyspepsia.

CONCLUSIONS

Dyspepsia is a common symptom with an extensive differential diagnosis and a heterogeneous pathophysiology. Its prevalence for itself implies a great health care problem, even though most do not seek medical care. An international committee of clinical investigators (Rome III Committee) defined dyspepsia as one or more of the following symptoms: postprandial fullness; early satiation (meaning inability to finish a normal size meal, or postprandial fullness); epigastric pain or burning with at least a 3-month history in the last year. After diagnostic investigation (upper gastrointestinal endoscopy, laboratory, and X-ray), 40% to 60% of individuals have normal findings (functional dyspepsia group); in the others, organic or structural causes of the symptoms can be found. The Rome II consensus subdivided patients with dyspepsia in three subgroups: ulcer-like dyspepsia; dysmotility-like dyspepsia, and unspecified (nonspecific) dyspepsia. The Rome III committee subdivided functional dyspepsia into two new diagnostic categories: meal-induced PDS, characterized by postprandial fullness and early satiety, and EPS, characterized by epigastric pain and burning.

References

1. Tack J, Talley NJ, Camilleri M, et al. Functional gastroduodenal disorders. Gastroenterology. 2006;130:1466–79.
2. Talley NJ, Weaver A, Zinsmeister AR, Melton III LJ. Onset and disappearance of gastrointestinal symptoms and functional gastrointestinal disorders. Am J Epidemiol. 1992;136:165–77.
3. Kurata JH, Nogawa AN, Everhart JE. A prospective study of dyspepsia in primary care. Dig Dis Sci. 2002;47:797–803.
4. Majumdar SR, Soumerai SB, Farraye FA, et al. Chronic acid-related disorders are commonand underinvestigated. Am J Gastroenterol. 2003;98:2409–14.
5. Dyspepsia: managing adults in primary care. London, England: National Institute of ClinicalExelence; 2004. p. 1–43
6. Veldhuyzen van Zanten SJ, Flook N, Chiba N, et al. An evidence-based approach to the management of uninvestigated dyspepsia in the era of *Helicobacter pylori*. CMAJ. 2000;162:S3–23.
7. Talley NJ, Stanghellini V, Heading RC, Koch KL, Malagelada J, Tytgat GN. Functional gastroduodenal disorders. In: Drossman DA, editor. Rome II: the functional gastrointestinal disorders. McLean, VA: Degnon; 2000. p. 299–350.
8. Lieberman D, Fennerty MB, Morris CD, Holub J, Eisen G, Sonnenberg A. Endoscopic evaluation of patients with dyspepsia: results from the national endoscopic data repository. Gastroenterology. 2004;127:1067–75.
9. Thompson AR, Barkun AN, Armstrong D, et al. The prevalence of clinical significant endoscopic findings in primary care patients with uninvestigated dyspepsia: the Canadian Adult Dyspepsia Empiric

Treatment – Prompt Endoscopy (CADET-PE) study. Aliment Pharmacol Ther. 2003;17:1481–91.

10. Moayyedi P, Axon AT. The usefulness of the likelihood ratio in the diagnosis of dyspepsia and gastroesophageal reflux disease. Am J Gastroenterol. 1999;94:3122–5.

11. Soll AH. Consensus conference. Medical treatment of peptic ulcer disease. Practical guidelines. Practical Parameters of the American College of Gastroenterology. JAMA. 1996;275:622–9.

12. Talley NJ, Silverstein MD, Agréus L, Nyrén O, Sonnenberg A, Holtmann G. AGA technical review: evaluation of dyspepsia. Gastroenterology. 1998;114:582–95.

13. Talley NJ, Vakil NB, Moayyedi P. American gastroenterological association technical review on the evaluation of dyspepsia. Gastroenterology. 2005;129:1756–80.

14. Talley NJ. Gallstones and upper abdominal discomfort. Innocent bystander or a cause of dyspepsia? J Clin Gastroenterol. 1995;20:182–3.

15. Spiegel BM, Farid M, Dulai GS, Gralnek IM, Kanwal F. Comparing rates of dyspepsia with Coxibs vs NSAID+PPI: a meta-analysis. Am J Med. 2006;119:448. e27–36.

16. Hallas J, Bytzer P. Screening for drug related dyspepsia: an analysis of prescription symmetry. Eur J Gastroenterol Hepatol. 1998;10:27–32.

17. Patric A, Epstein AP. Review article: gastroparesis. Aliment Pharmacol Ther. 2008;27:724–40.

18. Sahai AV, Mishra G, Penman ID, et al. EUS to detect evidence of pancreatic disease in patients with persistent or nonspecific dyspepsia. Gastrointest Endosc. 2000;52:153–9.

19. Locke III GR, Murray JA, Zinsmeister AR, Melton III LJ, Talley NJ. Celiac disease serology in irritable bowel syndrome and dyspepsia: a population-based case–control study. Mayo Clin Proc. 2004;79: 476–82.

20. Heikkinen M, Pikkarainen P, Takala J, Rasanen H, Julkunen R. Etiology of dyspepsia: four unselected consecutive patients in general practice. Scand J Gastroenterol. 1995;30:519–23.

21. Quartero AO, de Wit NJ, Lodder AC, Numans ME, Smout AJ, Hoes AW. Disturbed solid-phase gastric emptying in functional dyspepsia: a meta analysis. Dig Dis Sci. 1998;43:2028–33.

22. Caldarella MP, Azpiroz F, Malagelada JR. Antro-fundic dysfunctions in functional dyspepsia. Gastroenterology. 2003;124:1220–9.

23. Tack J, Caenepeel P, Fischler B, Piessevaux H, Janssens J. Symptoms associated with hypersensitivity to gastric distension in functional dyspepsia. Gastroenterology. 2001;121:526–35.

24. Karamanolis G, Caenepeel P, Arts J, Tack J. Association of the predominant symptom with clinical characteristics and pathophysiological mechanisms in functional dyspepsia. Gastroenterology. 2006;130:296–303.

25. Talley NJ, Fett SL, Zinsmeister AR, Melton III LJ. Gastrointestinal tract symptoms and self-reported abuse: a population based study. Gastroenterology. 1994;107:1040–9.

26. Drossman DA, Thompson WG, Talley NJ, Funch-Jensen P, Janssens J, Whitehead WE. Identification of subgroups of functional bowel disorders. Gastroenterol Int. 1990;3:159–72.

27. Talley NJ, Weaver AL, Tesmer DL, Zinsmeister AR. Lack of discriminant value of dyspepsia subgroups in patients referred for upper endoscopy. Gastroenterology. 1993;105:1378–86.

28. Agreus L, Svardsudd K, Nyren O, Tibblin G. Irritable bowel syndrome and dyspepsia in the general population: overlap and lack of stability over time. Gastroenterology. 1995;109:671–80.

29. Laheij RJ, De Koning RW, Horrevorts AM, et al. Predominant symptom behavior in patients with persistent dyspepsia during treatment. J Clin Gastroenterol. 2004;38:490–5.

30. Hsu YC, Liou JM, Liao SC, et al. Psychopathology and personality trait in subgroups of functional dyspepsia based on Rome III criteria. Am J Gastroenterol. 2009;104:2534–42.

31. Geeraerts B, Tack J. Functional dyspepsia: past, present, and future. J Gastroenterol. 2008;43:251–5.

Chapter 3
Epidemiology

Roland Pulanić

Keywords: Dyspepsia, Epidemiology, Overlap syndrome, Uninvestigated dyspepsia

INTRODUCTION

Dyspepsia includes an array of gastrointestinal symptoms present in individuals all over the world, in industrialized countries in particular. A great proportion of individuals visiting primary healthcare offices or gastrointestinal clinics suffer from dyspepsia. However, the true epidemiology of dyspepsia is difficult to assess because of variability in the definition of dyspepsia that would be applicable in all populations, along with variable patient description of dyspeptic symptoms and interpretation of these symptoms by physicians.

PREVALENCE AND INCIDENCE OF DYSPEPSIA

The prevalence of dyspepsia varies considerably among different populations. According to different studies, the prevalence of dyspepsia ranges from 7% to 41%, and it is estimated that about 25% of the general population suffers from dyspeptic symptoms [1, 2]. The most common symptoms are permanent or intermittent pain or discomfort in the upper abdomen, along with flatulence or early satiety. Even if patients with heartburn and nausea without abdominal pain and with irritable bowel syndrome (IBS) are excluded,

R. Pulanić (✉)
Department of Gastroenterology and Hepatology, University
Department of Medicine, Zagreb University Hospital, Zagreb, Croatia
e-mail: roland.pulanic@gmail.com

M. Duvnjak (ed.), *Dyspepsia in Clinical Practice*,
DOI 10.1007/978-1-4419-1730-0_3,
© Springer Science+Business Media, LLC 2011

the prevalence of dyspepsia remains high (10%). The incidence of dyspepsia is even more poorly documented. It is estimated that approximately 9% of individuals free from dyspepsia symptoms in previous years will report new symptoms on follow up. However, those with a history of dyspepsia or peptic ulcer disease were not excluded; thus the rate of onset may be overestimated [3]. Agreus et al. report on the incidence of dyspepsia in Scandinavia to be less than 1% over 3 months [4].

Whatever the incidence, there is a comparable proportion of individuals developing dyspepsia and those that lose the symptoms; thus the prevalence of dyspepsia remains stable.

POPULATION-BASED STUDY AND EPIDEMIOLOGIC FACTORS

Dyspepsia is not a life-threatening disease and is not associated with an increased mortality rate. However, this condition has been shown to have considerable impact on patients and health care services. The quality of life is greatly reduced in patients with dyspepsia. More so, the quality of life in patients with functional dyspepsia (FD) has been shown to be substantially poorer than in patients with chronic liver disease, while comorbid anxiety and depression contribute considerably to the condition (see Chap. 13) [5]. About 20% of people with dyspeptic symptoms and in fear from possible malignancy seek medical help from primary care physicians or hospital specialists. More than 50% of dyspepsia patients were on medicamentous therapy most of the time, while 30% reported taking days off from work or school due to dyspeptic symptoms [6].

In 30% to 60% of dyspeptic patients, objective examinations such as biochemical testing, endoscopic or radiologic studies, and testing for *Helicobacter pylori* (*H. pylori*) infection did not reveal any structural or biochemical cause of their discomforts [7–9]. These patients are classified in the group of nonulcer dyspepsia or FD. However, a structural cause of discomforts is found in some patients pointing to the need of serious psychological and somatic approach in patients with dyspepsia.

Considering the epidemiology of dyspeptic, FD, dyspepsia induced by organic causeses and uninvestigated dyspepsia should be distinguished. Data on uninvestigated dyspepsia vary depending on the dyspepsia definition applied. When individuals with "upper abdominal pain" are included, the prevalence of uninvestigated dyspepsia varies from 7% to 34.2% in different countries worldwide [2, 10–12]. However, if using the definition of dyspepsia as "upper gastrointestinal symptoms," then the prevalence of uninvestigated dyspepsia ranges from 23% to 45% [2, 3, 7, 13, 14]. According to Rome II criteria, the prevalence of uninvestigated dyspepsia is 24% [15].

The prevalence of FD also varies greatly. Shaib and El-Serag from the USA report on the prevalence of FD to be 29.2% and 15% in patients with and without reflux symptoms, respectively [14]. In the UK, the prevalence of FD is 23.8%, and in Norway, 14.7% [16, 17]. These analyses were based on endoscopic or radiologic studies. In Japan, Hirakawa et al. documented a 17% prevalence of FD in adults undergoing a population gastric cancer screening program [18].

Dyspepsia may occur as a sequel of various organic diseases with overt structural damage. Peptic ulcer disease, gastric tumors, biliary and pancreatic diseases, gastroesophageal reflux disease (GERD), and diabetes mellitus are known to lead to dyspepsia [19].

DYSPEPSIA AND OVERLAP SYNDROME

Thorough history and physical examination have a key role in the diagnosis of dyspepsia. Good orientation and analysis of the history and collected physical data are superior to any instrumental or laboratory examination. These data can steer the physician's decision on the diagnostic work-up required. According to Rome III criteria, the diagnosis of FD is based on the lack of evidence for a structural disease. Unlike Rome II criteria, the Rome III criteria use structural instead of organic disease because patients may suffer from altered organ function of unknown origin [9, 20].

Many patients present with two or more functional gastrointestinal discomforts. Within a year of the onset of dyspeptic symptoms, more than one fourth of patients present with a clinical picture of IBS or GERD, whereas 25% of those with IBS develop symptoms of FD or GERD [4].

Precisely defined clinical picture is a prerequisite for an accurate diagnosis of dyspepsia and appropriate therapeutic approach to dyspeptic patient. Dyspepsia per se is not a disease but a symptom or cluster of symptoms [21]. There is considerable overlap of symptoms among patients with FD, GERD, and IBS (Fig. 3.1). Symptom overlap is especially frequent between reflux disease, nonerosive reflux disease (NERD) in particular, and FD. The symptoms of FD and NERD are estimated to overlap in more than 70% of patients with reflux symptoms [22]. However, the true prevalence of FD symptoms and NERD overlap is quite difficult to estimate due to the yet ambiguous definition of overlap. Thus, the prevalence of uninvestigated dyspepsia varies between 10% and 40% if the definition of dyspepsia includes heartburn and regurgitation,

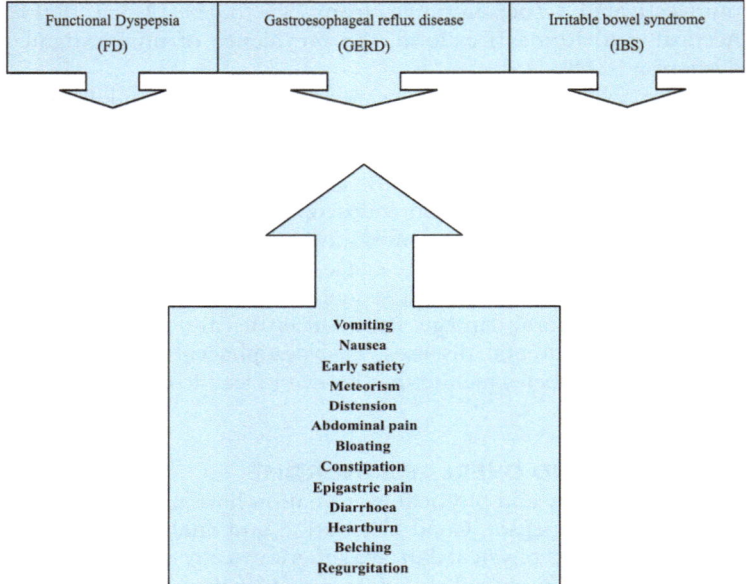

Fig. 3.1 Overlapping symptom complexes of functional dyspepsia, gastroesophageal reflux disease, and irritable bowel syndrome.

but it declines to 5% to 12% if only patients with upper abdominal pain are taken in consideration [3, 23]. The overlap of FD symptoms and IBS is also very common. Constipation retards gastric emptying and is associated with upper gastrointestinal tract symptoms. In contrast, lower gastrointestinal tract, i.e., bowel symptoms, are frequently present in FD. Overlapping of FD symptoms and IBS has been estimated to occur in 40% of patients [24]. Tutega et al. analyzed 1,069 employees integrated in healthcare system in Salt Lake City, UT, USA, and found 70% of IBS patients to suffer from FD, whereas IBS was recorded in 43% of those previously diagnosed with dyspepsia [25].

EPIDEMIOLOGICAL FACTORS
Clinical picture and epidemiologic evaluation of dyspepsia are influenced by culture, age, race, religion, psychological factors, previous experience, and so on [26, 27]. Wigington et al. found in their study investigating ethnic differences that the prevalence of IBS is to be the same in blacks and Caucasians, but variation was

recorded according to socioeconomic factors. Black individuals with IBS and diarrhea had a significantly lower income as compared to Caucasians that tended to have higher income. There were no between-group differences according to age, sex, and level of education [28].

In their epidemiologic study, Minocha et al. compared the prevalence of IBS, uninvestigated dyspepsia, and overlap syndrome between Afro-Americans and American Caucasians. The prevalence of IBS, uninvestigated dyspepsia, and overlap syndrome was 0.6, 17, and 7.3% in Afro-Americans, and 0, 13, and 13% in American Caucasians, respectively. In the group of subjects with uninvestigated dyspepsia, overlap syndrome was detected in 30% of Afro-Americans and 50% of American Caucasians. Study results indicated that Afro-Americans with uninvestigated dyspepsia are to be of younger age. Unlike Afro-Americans, marital status, level of education, and socioeconomic status had no impact on the onset of dyspepsia in American Caucasians. Uninvestigated dyspepsia was more common than overlap syndrome in Afro-Americans of lower socioeconomic status (22% vs. 10%), while overlap syndrome was more common among married American Caucasians of lower educational level and living in urban setting. The authors conclude that the overlap syndrome is more common in American Caucasians than in Afro-Americans [26].

A study by Locke et al. conducted in the general population of the Olmsted County, Minnesota, USA, showed the overlap syndrome to be a rule rather than an exception in this community sample. This applied to IBS with constipation and IBS with diarrhea in terms of overlap with upper gastrointestinal symptoms [13].

Analysis of a multiracial population in Singapore, South East Asia, indicated the ethnic-adjusted prevalence of uninvestigated dyspepsia to be 8.1, 7.3, and 7.5% in the Chinese, Malays, and Indians, respectively [12].

When analyzing dyspepsia from the epidemiologic viewpoint, other factors influencing its prevalence should also be mentioned. These include age, sex, alcohol consumption, cigarette smoking, use of nonsteroidal anti-inflammatory drugs (NSAIDs), *H. pylori* infection, and obesity [29–31]. Many of these factors, along with the severity and frequency of dyspeptic symptoms, will influence its prevalence and patient decision to seek medical help.

Although epidemiologic data suggest that there is no association of dyspepsia with any particular age and that dyspepsia is not predicted by age, a certain trend appears to exist. In a Japanese study, reflux-like symptoms were more common in middle-aged adults, dysmotility-like symptoms in those aged <59, and ulcer-like predominant symptoms in those aged <39 [18]. In the surveys conducted in the British, Taiwanese, and Danish populations, the prevalence of uninvestigated dyspepsia appeared to decrease with increasing age [12, 16, 32].

Female individuals appear to be more prone to dyspepsia than male ones [14, 32, 33]. In a population-based study in Australia, female adults significantly outnumbered males in most functional gastrointestinal disorders including FD [33].

There is no definitive evidence on alcohol consumption and cigarette smoking to be predictors of dyspepsia. However, regular cigarette smoking has been identified as a risk factor in patients with uninvestigated dyspepsia from the USA, Canada, and UK, and alcohol consumption in patients with uninvestigated dyspepsia from India and New Zealand [7, 11, 14, 34]. These findings may be explained by the proportion of organic diseases among subjects with uninvestigated dyspepsia.

Upper gastrointestinal tract symptoms are common in the elderly, and NSAIDs are believed to be important risk factors. Talley et al. performed a population-based study to evaluate the association of NSAIDs with dyspepsia and heartburn in an age- and sex-stratified random sample consisting of Caucasian aged 65, residents of the Olmsted County, Minnesota. The authors concluded that aspirin and non-aspirin NSAIDs were associated with an almost twofold higher risk of upper gastrointestinal tract symptoms in the elderly, while smoking and alcohol were not found to be significant risk factors [35]. In a British study, NSAID usage was identified as an independent risk factor for uninvestigated dyspepsia and was thought to be responsible for 4% of dyspepsia cases in the community [7].

The same authors analyzed the association of *H. pylori* infection and dyspepsia [7]. Dyspeptic symptoms were more common in those harboring *H. pylori* infection than in *H. pylori*-negative subjects (44 vs. 36%). The authors concluded that *H. pylori* status to be predictive of uninvestigated dyspepsia. *H. pylori* infection had a 5% population attributable risk for dyspepsia assuming causal association. The association of *H. pylori* and FD is less clear. Results of a study conducted in Croatia assessing the seroprevalence of *H. pylori* infection in subjects with dyspepsia indicated a higher prevalence of this bacterial infection in dyspeptic patients as compared with blood donors in all age groups. In the patient group, *H. pylori* seroprevalence was not age dependent [36]. However, according to Wildner-Christensen et al., NSAIDs, cigarette smoking, and unemployment are more important risk factors for dyspepsia in general population than *H. pylori* infection [30].

Obesity has been associated with an increased rate of reporting gastrointestinal symptoms. Cremonini et al. assessed the association between changes in body weight and changes in upper gastrointestinal symptoms. It was a prospective cohort study including a random sample of Olmsted County, Minnesota residents, assessed for distinct upper gastrointestinal symptom complexes, GERD, chest pain, dyspepsia-pain predominant, and dyspepsia–dysmotility. Baseline body weight was associated with GERD, chest pain, and dyspepsia-pain predominant symptom complexes. An increase in body weight >10 lb between surveys was associated with new onset of dyspepsia–dysmotility. There was no association between weight loss >10 lb and upper gastrointestinal symptom complexes [31]. Moderate body weight gain and loss is not associated with upper gastrointestinal symptom changes over time in the general population.

CONCLUSIONS

At the time when the incidence of peptic ulcer disease and gastric carcinoma is on a decline, dyspepsia is becoming an ever more challenging entity that captures interest from both scientific and medicosocial aspects. Data published to date indicate that dyspepsia is common in most populations all over the world. Yet, variable data on the prevalence and incidence of dyspepsia, even in similar geographical locations, result from differences in the definition of dyspepsia, interpretation of dyspeptic symptoms, and description of symptoms by dyspepsia patients. The accurate epidemiology of dyspepsia is additionally masked by the overlap syndrome and difficulties in excluding organic diseases in a large number of individuals.

References
1. Locke III GR. Prevalence, incidence and natural history of dyspepsia and functional dyspepsia. Baillières Clin Gastroenterol. 1998;12:435–42.
2. Talley NJ, Zinsmeister AR, Schleck CD, Melton III LJ. Dyspepsia and dyspepsia subgroups: a population-based study. Gastroenterology. 1992;102:1259–68.
3. Talley NJ, Weaver AL, Zinsmeister AR, Melton III LJ. Onset and disappearance of gastrointestinal symptoms and functional gastrointestinal disorders. Am J Epidemiol. 1992;136:165–77.
4. Agreus L, Svardsudd K, Nyren O, Tibblin G. Irritable bowel syndrome and dyspepsia in the general population: overlap and lack of stability over time. Gastroenterology. 1995;109:671–80.
5. Haag S, Senf W, Häuser W, et al. Impairment of health-related quality of life in functional dyspepsia and chronic liver disease: the influence of depression and anxiety. Aliment Pharmacol Ther. 2008;27:561–71.

6. Haycox A, Einarson T, Eggleston A. The health economic impact of upper gastrointestinal symptoms in the general population: results from the Domestic/International Gastroenterology Surveillance Study (DIGEST). Scand J Gastroenterol Suppl. 1999;231:38–47.

7. Moayyedi P, Forman D, Braunholtz D, et al. The proportion of upper gastrointestinal symptoms in the community associated with *Helicobacter pylori*, lifestyle factors, and nonsteroidal anti-inflammatory drugs. Leeds HELP Study Group. Am J Gastroenterol. 2000;95:1448–55.

8. Johnsen R, Bernersen B, Straume B, Forde OH, Bostad L, Burhol PG. Prevalences of endoscopic and histological findings in subjects with and without dyspepsia. BMJ. 1991;302:749–52.

9. Talley NJ, Stanghellini V, Heading RC, Koch KL, Malagelada JR, Tygat GN. Functional gastroduodenal disorders. Gut. 1999;45 Suppl 2: II37–42.

10. Kay L, Jorgensen T. Epidemiology of upper dyspepsia in a random population. Prevalence, incidence, natural history, and risk factors. Scand J Gastroenterol. 1994;29:2–6.

11. Haque M, Wyeth JW, Stace NH, Talley NJ, Green R. Prevalence, severity and associated features of gastro-oesophageal reflux and dyspepsia: a population-based study. N Z Med J. 2000;113:178–81.

12. Ho KY, Kang JY, Seow A. Prevalence of gastrointestinal symptoms in a multiracial Asian population, with particular reference to reflux-type symptoms. Am J Gastroenterol. 1998;93:1816–22.

13. Locke III GR, Zinsmeister AR, Melton III LJ, Talley NJ. Overlap of gastrointestinal symptom complexes in the community. Am J Gastroenterol. 2003;98:S273.

14. Shaib Y, El-Serag HB. The prevalence and risk factors of functional dyspepsia in a multiethnic population in the United States. Am J Gastroenterol. 2004;99:2210–6.

15. Westbrook JI, Talley NJ. Empiric clustering of dyspepsia into symptom subgroups: a population-based study. Scand J Gastroenterol. 2002;37:917–23.

16. Jones RH, Lydeard SE, Hobbs FD, et al. Dyspepsia in England and Scotland. Gut. 1990;31:401–5.

17. Bernersen B, Johnsen R, Straume B. Non-ulcer dyspepsia and peptic ulcer: the distribution in a population and their relation to risk factors. Gut. 1996;38:822–5.

18. Hirakawa K, Adachi K, Amano K, et al. Prevalence of non-ulcer dyspepsia in the Japanese population. J Gastroenterol Hepatol. 1999;14:1083–7.

19. Jurčić D, Bilić A. Rational approach to the patient with dyspepsia. Medicus. 2006;15:15–23.

20. Tack J, Talley NJ, Camilleri M, et al. Functional gastroduodenal disorders. Gastroenterology. 2006;130:1466–79.

21. Quigley EM, Koehane J. Dyspepsia. Curr Opin Gastroenterol. 2008;24:692–7.

22. Keohane J, Quigley EM. Functional dyspepsia and nonerosive reflux disease: clinical interactions and their implications. MedGenMed. 2007;9:31.

23. El-Serag HB, Talley NJ. Systemic review: the prevalence and clinical course of functional dyspepsia. Aliment Pharmacol Ther. 2004;19: 643–54.

24. Halder SL, Locke III GR, Schleck CD, Zinsmeister AR, Melton III LJ, Talley NJ. Natural history of functional gastrointestinal disorders: a 12-year longitudinal population-based study. Gastroenterology. 2007;133:799–807.

25. Tutega AK, Talley NJ, Joos SK, Hickam DH. Overlap of functional dyspepsia and irritable bowel syndrome in a community sample. Am J Gastroenterol. 2003;98:S272.

26. Minocha A, Chad W, Do W, Johnson WD. Racial differences in epide-miology of irritable syndrome alone, un-ivestigated dyspepsia alone, and "overlap syndrome" among african americans compared to Caucasians: a population-based study. Dig Dis Sci. 2006;51:218–26.

27. Geeraerts B, Vandenberghe J, Van Oudenhove L, et al. Influence of experimentally induced anxiety on gastric sensorimotor function in humans. Gastroenterology. 2005;129:1437–44.

28. Wigington WC, Johnson W, Cosman C, et al. Comprehensive descrip-tion of irritable bowel syndrome by subtypes in African-Americans versus Caucasians. Am J Gastroenterol. 2003;98:S267.

29. Halder SL, Locke III GR, Schleck CD, Zinsmeister AR, Talley NJ. Influence of alcohol consumption on IBS and dyspepsia. Neurogas-troenterol Motil. 2006;18:1001–8.

30. Wildner-Christensen M, Hansen JM, De Muckadell OB. Risk factors for dyspepsia in a general population: non-steroidal anti-infammatory drugs, cigarette smoking and unemployment are more important than *Helicobacter pylori* infection. Scand J Gastroenterol. 2006;41:149–54.

31. Cremonini F, Locke III GR, Schleck CD, Zinsmeister AR, Talley NJ. Relationship between upper gastrointestinal symptoms and changes in body weight in a population-based cohort. Neurogastroenterol Motil. 2006;18:987–94.

32. Lu CL, Lang HC, Chang FY, et al. Prevalence and health/social impacts of functional dyspepsia in Taiwan: a study based on the Rome criteria questionnaire survey assisted by endoscopic exclusion among a physical check-up population. Scand J Gastroenterol. 2005;40:402–11.

33. Koloski NA, Talley NJ, Boyce PM. Epidemiology and health care seeking in the functional GI disorders: a population-based study. Am J Gastroenterol. 2002;97:2290–9.

34. Tougas G, Chen Y, Hwang P, Liu MM, Eggleston A. Prevalence and impact of upper gastrointestinal symptoms in the Canadian population: findings from the DIGEST study. Domestic/International Gastroenterology Surveillance Study. Am J Gastroenterol. 1999;94: 2845–54.

35. Talley NJ, Evans JM, Fleming KC, Harmsen WS, Zinsmeister AR, Melton III LJ. Nonsteroidal antiinflammatory drugs and dyspepsia in the elderly. Dig Dis Sci. 1995;40:1345–50.

36. Marušić M, Presečki V, Katičić M, Bilić A, Jurčić D, Schwarz D. Seroprevalence of *Helicobacter pylori* infection in dyspeptic patients. Coll Antropol. 2008;32:1149–53.

Chapter 4
Structural Causes of Dyspepsia

Daniel Schmidt-Martin and Eamonn M.M. Quigley

Keywords: Dyspepsia, Gastroesophageal reflux disease, Nonerosive reflux disease, Barrett's esophagus, Peptic ulcer disease, *Helicobacter pylori*, Gastric carcinoma, Gallstones, Celiac disease, Gastric metastasis, Gastroparesis, Functional dyspepsia

INTRODUCTION

The definition of dyspepsia and its interpretation, as previously discussed in Chap. 1, are challenging. Encompassing a constellation of symptoms located in the retrosternal area, as well as in the upper abdomen, and potentially indicative of a number of different pathological processes, dyspepsia may have many and, in some cases, a number of causes. Although certain symptoms may seem, at first sight, more suggestive of the underlying pathology, efforts to identify which symptoms correlate with particular disease processes have been largely unsuccessful. In a seminal paper, Crean and colleagues attempted to define such clinico–pathological correlations and found that most supposed predictive symptoms did not hold up when critically examined. The most striking feature of this study, perhaps, was the uncertainty exhibited by clinicians when attempting to diagnose functional dyspepsia (FD), despite adequate investigation. This contrasted markedly with clinician certainty in diagnosing irritable bowel syndrome (IBS) [1].

D. Schmidt-Martin (✉)
Alimentary Pharmabiotic Centre, Department of Medicine,
Clinical Sciences Building, Cork University Hospital,
Cork, Ireland
e-mail: danscma@yahoo.com

M. Duvnjak (ed.), *Dyspepsia in Clinical Practice*,
DOI 10.1007/978-1-4419-1730-0_4,
© Springer Science+Business Media, LLC 2011

Structural causes of dyspepsia are many, with the most common being gastroesophageal reflux disease (GERD) and peptic ulcer disease (PUD). Although the latter is on the decline in the West, it still comprises 10% of all instances of dyspepsia. The discovery of Helicobacter pylori (*H. pylori*) as the etiological agent in the majority of cases of PUD has resulted in a sea change in both our understanding and management of the condition and should eliminate, for the most part, the occurrence of chronic PUD-related symptoms. Other less common structural causes of dyspepsia include gallstone disease, celiac disease, and malignancy, both primary and metastatic, though the latter is rare. On the surface, gastroparesis would appear to be a common cause of dyspepsia; however, the boundary between what might be described by some as gastroparesis and what would be considered by others as no more than an instance of FD with a mild, and probably clinically irrelevant, delay in gastric emptying remains blurred. In any event, caution is advised in interpreting gastric emptying studies among those with FD.

Table 4.1 lists the more common causes of dyspepsia. It should be emphasized that this listing is based on a Western population and does not allow for variations in demographics, ethnicity, or geography. For example, in an older population, malignancy will be a more important consideration, whereas in a younger patient in Europe or North America, *H. pylori* has become an uncommon finding. Time of study is also a factor; among over 1,500 patients with dyspepsia studied in Scotland in the early 1990s, Crean and colleagues found that the final diagnosis was a peptic ulcer in 26%, a proportion that would be much lower nowadays [1].

TABLE 4.1.   Common causes of dyspepsia.

Common causes of dyspepsia
Gastroesophageal reflux disease
H. pylori
Peptic ulcer disease
Gastric cancer and other tumors
Cholelithiasis
Celiac disease
Medications, e.g., NSAIDs
Gastroparesis

GASTROESOPHAGEAL REFLUX DISEASE

Defined as a condition that develops when the reflux of gastric contents into the esophagus causes troublesome symptoms and/ or complications, GERD is thought to account for 30% of all cases of dyspepsia. Heartburn, other reflux symptoms, and complications of GERD have been shown to be significant causes of morbidity [2]. Estimates of prevalence suggest that reflux disease affects between 14% and 40% of the general population in Western Europe and North America [3, 4]. This wide range in estimated prevalence is likely due to variations in the reporting of symptoms and the fact that some patients with esophagitis and even complications of GERD are asymptomatic. Chronic GERD may lead to the development of Barrett's esophagus (BE), a condition that predisposes to esophageal adenocarcinoma. GERD, previously uncommon in Asia, is now beginning to emerge in countries like Japan and China though complicated GERD and Barrett's esophagus, in particular, remain rare in these parts of the world.

The diagnosis of GERD is usually made on the basis of symptoms alone; in contrast to many of the other symptoms which constitute dyspepsia, heartburn is unusual in its specificity for GERD; so much so that, in the absence of alarm symptoms, further investigation is often not necessary. The most common presenting symptoms of GERD are heartburn and/or regurgitation, but patients may complain of a number of other symptoms including dysphagia, chest pain, or, less commonly, odynophagia, water brash, nausea, chronic cough, and/or hoarseness. GERD has also been associated with a host of other extra-esophageal manifestations including asthma, laryngitis, sinusitis, and erosion of the dental enamel. In some instances, these associations rest on fairly firm ground, whereas in others, initial enthusiasm for a link with GERD has waned in the face of high-quality prospective studies. Patients with suspected GERD who present complaining of dysphagia, weight loss, or chest pain should be considered for urgent further investigation [5].

Treatment of GERD is mainly symptomatic with acid suppression being the cornerstone of modern therapeutic approaches; when symptomatic improvement does not ensue, endoscopy and esophageal pH studies may prove valuable in defining whether the symptoms are truly related to acid exposure or are functional in origin [6].

Monozygotic twin studies indicate a genetic component in GERD. Recent work has identified a single nucleotide polymorphism which seems to alter visceral sensitivity and is associated with an increased risk of GERD [7].

GERD is caused by the recurrent reflux of acidic fluid into the lower esophagus, which, in certain individuals, and for reasons that remain obscure, results in the development of erosions and ulcers. This may be further complicated by the development of hemorrhage, stricture, or columnar metaplasia (Barrett's esophagus); a potentially premalignant condition. Factors associated with more advanced manifestations of GERD include: the presence of a hiatus hernia, lower esophageal sphincter hypotension, loss of esophageal peristaltic function, abdominal obesity, gastric hypersecretion, delayed gastric emptying, overeating, the use of certain medications, and smoking [8].

Patients with GERD symptoms but who also manifest dysphagia, an epigastric mass, persistent vomiting, gastrointestinal bleeding, progressive unintentional weight loss, and iron deficiency anemia should undergo early endoscopic evaluation. When investigating a patient with suspected GERD where the main symptom is chest pain, it is essential that the physician consider coronary artery disease before diagnosing GERD. In patients with typical symptoms (heartburn and acid regurgitation) and in the absence of alarm symptoms (as described above), endoscopy should be reserved for ones in whom symptoms persist despite adequate medical management [5].

There is a poor correlation between the nature or severity of symptoms and endoscopic findings; as few as 25% of patients who have symptoms suggestive of GERD have either endoscopic or histological evidence of esophagitis. Furthermore, in one study, 37% of those who harbored esophagitis were asymptomatic and 40% of those who had Barrett's esophagus had no symptoms [4].

The application of endoscopy and prolonged recordings of intraesophageal pH to large populations of individuals with GERD-type symptoms have made it clear that GERD is not a single discrete entity, but rather a heterogeneous disorder which includes subgroups that can be subdivided, in the first instance, on the basis of endoscopic findings into three groups [9]:

1. Negative endoscopy (or nonerosive) reflux disease (NERD), which is characterized by grossly normal endoscopic appearances in the absence of prior acid suppressive therapy
2. Erosive esophagitis and related complications (ulceration and stricture)
3. Barrett's esophagus

It has become evident, from a number of community and other broad-based surveys, that NERD is common and may account for up to 70% of uninvestigated reflux in the community [2]. NERD, though not associated with the same complications as GERD (stricture, Barrett's esophagus, esophageal adenocarcinoma), has been shown to be a significant cause of morbidity with two recent studies indicating that both its impact on quality of life and symptom severity are similar to GERD, in general [10, 11]. NERD has been shown to respond to acid suppression, but not in all cases [12].

NERD itself can be further subdivided into three groups based on patterns of acid exposure (as defined by acid exposure time (AET), on prolonged intraesophageal pH monitoring) and correlations between acid exposure and symptoms, as follows:

Group 1: Increased acid exposure, AET positive NERD, possibly associated with subtle microscopic or ultra-structural changes or evidence of immune activation. These individuals are likely to respond to acid suppression.

Group 2: Normal acid exposure time but symptoms correlate with episodes of reflux. In the past, these individuals may have been referred to as the "sensitive esophagus." Again a response to acid suppressive therapy is to be expected.

Group 3: In these individuals, not only are acid exposure times within the normal range, but symptoms and reflux events do not correlate. This group, referred to as functional heartburn is resistant to acid suppression, is associated with an increased incidence of psychopathology and no longer regarded as part of the spectrum of GERD and looked upon as a true functional disorder akin to FD or IBS [6].

The relationship between GERD and *H. pylori* is complex. Co-existent *H. pylori* infection could, in theory, either worsen or improve the symptoms of GERD depending on the location of the infection and its consequent effect of either increasing or decreasing acid production. As a result, its eradication may not necessarily result in an improvement in GERD symptoms. In those instances where a relapse of GERD symptoms does accompany eradication therapy for *H. pylori*, symptomatic remission can usually be readily accomplished by acid suppressive therapy. These issues notwithstanding, *H. pylori* eradication, triggered by a positive urease breath test, continues to be recommended in view of the strong association of this bacterium with both peptic ulceration and gastric carcinoma [13].

BARRETT'S ESOPHAGUS

Characterized by the presence of columnar metaplasia proximal to the gastroesophageal junction, BE has the potential to act as a

premalignant condition. Estimations of the true prevalence of BE
are few and far between, with prior estimates being compromised
by issues such as the selection bias that is inherently associated
with the use of data based on endoscopic series. The best data to
date on the true prevalence of BE comes from a study in northern Scandinavia where endoscopy was performed on a randomly
selected population. BE was documented in 1.6% of cases [14]. Of
importance to the design and interpretation of studies of GERD
and BE was the observation that a significant proportion of this
patient population will not return for follow-up. Although these
patients with BE often presented with typical reflux symptoms, a
proportion of patients were asymptomatic. Between 10% and 15%
of patients undergoing evaluation for suspected GERD will have
BE on endoscopy. BE is associated with long duration of symptoms, male sex, Caucasian ethnicity, increasing age, and increasing
central obesity. Alcohol and smoking are also contributory factors
and *H. pylori* infection seems protective. The rate of transformation
to adenocarcinoma has been estimated at 0.5% per annum and the
benefits of either acid suppressive medication or anti-reflux surgery in preventing this progression remain to be proven [15].

PEPTIC ULCER DISEASE

First described in the USA as recently as the late nineteenth century, PUD went on to reach almost epidemic proportions through
the mid twentieth century before declining in prevalence over
the last 25 years. Previously thought to arise as a result of an
abnormality in gastric acid secretion, our understanding of the
pathophysiology of PUD was revolutionized with the discovery
of *H. pylori* in 1982; therapy has changed drastically as a consequence, from a former emphasis on acid suppression to the current antibacterial regimes.

PUD encompasses both gastric and duodenal ulcers. Patients
often present with epigastric pain, dyspepsia, nausea, early satiety,
bloating, and heartburn but may also be asymptomatic. The pain of
duodenal ulcers was traditionally described as nocturnal or prominent in the fasted state. In the seminal study by Crean and colleagues,
nocturnal pain, pain while fasting, and relief by eating were equally
common among gastric and duodenal ulcer patients, however [1]. In
PUD, in general, relief with antacids and acid suppression are more
accurate predictors of pathology. Although the discovery and treatment of *H. pylori* have resulted in a reduction in the overall prevalence of PUD, we are now seeing increasing numbers of patients with
PUD as a result of long-term nonsteroidal anti-inflammatory drugs

(NSAIDs) and low-dose aspirin use. Bleeding is the most common complication of PUD occurring in 50–70 per 100,000 cases. The optimal approach to the treatment of those dyspeptic individuals whose sole endoscopic finding is *H. pylori*-related gastritis has been the subject of some controversy, though most authorities would recommend *H. pylori* eradication to eliminate gastric cancer risk while acknowledging that the impact on symptoms will be modest, at best [16].

H. pylori Infection

The discovery of *H. pylori* prompted a significant change in the approach to the investigation and management of what to that point had been termed PUD. More common in the Far East and on the decline worldwide, the factors responsible for diminishing prevalence of *H. pylori* remain somewhat of a mystery. In the presence of ulceration or other overt pathologies, the benefits of eradication have been proven beyond doubt. It is, however, the question of the benefits of eradication in the absence of these pathological features that most vexes clinicians today; the use of the term "gastritis" to explain symptoms in dyspepsia is time-honored but based on little or no evidence and should be discouraged unless very specific pathologies are defined. Evidence favoring symptomatic improvement in FD following eradication is extremely limited though there is some suggestion that this is race dependent. In Western populations, *H. pylori* eradication in patients with FD significantly reduces acid exposure but does not result in an improvement in quality-of-life scores [17]. This contrasts with the experience among Asian populations where *H. pylori* rates are much higher, where a recent study demonstrated a marked improvement in dyspeptic symptoms following eradication [18]. An early recurrence of symptoms following successful eradication seems ominously predictive of long-term outcome; accordingly, patients with *H. pylori*-related FD are more likely to seek pharmacological therapy [19].

GASTRIC CARCINOMA

The last quarter of a century has seen a significant reduction in the incidence of gastric adenocarcinoma, the most common primary gastric carcinoma. As a consequence, this disorder is now rare in the Western world though rates remain higher in Asia. Nevertheless, it remains the fourth highest cause of cancer-related death in Europe. With a male preponderance (1.5:1), being rare in patients under the age of 50 and with a peak incidence in the seventh decade, gastric cancer is often detected at an advanced stage at the time of diagnosis. Associations include cigarette smoking, heavy alcohol intake, *H. pylori* infection, atrophic gastritis, prior partial gastrectomy, and inherited syndromes such as hereditary nonpolyposis colorectal cancer, familial adenomatous polyposis, and Peutz–Jeghers syndrome. Epigastric pain, nausea, vomiting, and early satiety are common features; the presence of persistent vomiting, unexplained weight loss, or dysphagia and/or the detection of an epigastric mass should prompt early endoscopy though this may prove negative in some cases [20].

Overall, an underlying malignancy will be found in as few as 1% of cases of dyspepsia [21]. Other primary gastric tumors include lymphoma, leiomyosarcoma, and carcinoid syndrome. Linitis plastica, a form of diffusely infiltrative gastric carcinoma, which results in gross thickening and associated contraction of the gastric wall, a feature which has become known as "leather bottle stomach," is a rare form of gastric carcinoma [22]. It may also occur in association with metastases to the ovary when it is known as a Krukenberg tumor.

METASTASES TO THE STOMACH

The metastasis of tumors to the stomach is rare and it occurs in as few as 1% to 2% of patients with any form of cancer in one study. The most common tumors to metastasize to the stomach are breast, lung, or melanoma. Metastases most commonly present as melena, epigastric pain, or anemia [23]. Other primary tumors that may also metastasize to the stomach include ovary, cervical, pancreatic, and hepatocellular [22].

GALL STONES

Identified as the cause of dyspepsia in as many as 4% of patients, cholelithiasis, or gallstone disease, is an important consideration when evaluating a patient with dyspepsia. With a female preponderance, this is a disease of middle age [24]. Patients will often describe epigastric pain that is worse postprandially but may also describe right hypochondrial pain, bloating, reflux, nausea, or vomiting. The term gallstone dyspepsia is not without its critics and some argue that, though gallstones are undeniably a cause of episodic acute upper abdominal pain, there is little overlap between this and "typical" dyspepsia. At least one meta-analysis has provided reasonable evidence to suggest that one should be cautious in ascribing dyspeptic symptoms to gall stones identified on one or other modality of abdominal imaging [25].

Data such as this would encourage a more conservative approach to gall stones in the absence of more classical symptoms or complications. Not surprisingly, though the usual approach to the dyspeptic patient in whom gallstones are identified ultrasonographically is to recommend cholecystectomy, symptoms have been reported to resolve in as few as 46% of cases following surgery.

While the relationship between gallstones and chronic dyspepsia may continue to generate some controversy, there is no support for abnormalities in gallbladder emptying (detected by scintigraphic studies) as a cause of dyspepsia [26].

CELIAC DISEASE

The advent and availability of sensitive and specific serological tests has significantly altered our understanding of celiac disease and has resulted in a radical reassessment of the "typical" celiac phenotype [27]. Classically described as a condition of malnutrition with associated steatorrhoea, the increasing recognition of clinically silent celiac disease has resulted in a revision of worldwide prevalence rates suggesting it to be as common as 1:200–1:100 in many countries and ethnic groups. With prevalence rates of this order, coincident occurrence of celiac disease among patients with a variety of symptoms is to be expected. It affects males and females equally; it is an autoimmune condition characterized by sensitivity to the gluten component of wheat. The exclusion of gluten from the diet results in symptomatic cure in most cases. Diagnosis, though highly suggested by positive anti-tissue *trans*-glutaminase antibodies or antiendomysial antibodies, is supported by the endoscopic features which include scalloping or atrophy of duodenal mucosa and then confirmed on histology. Several studies have suggested that the prevalence of celiac disease is increased among patients who complain of dyspepsia, though a recent meta-analysis found that this association was not statistically significant [28]. Nonetheless, the widespread availability and relative lack of expense mean that serological testing should be, at the very least, considered prior to diagnosing FD.

GASTROPARESIS

Characterized by delayed gastric emptying in the absence of mechanical obstruction, gastroparesis affects up to five million people in the USA with a female-to-male ratio of 4:1. The three main causes of gastroparesis are diabetes, prior gastric surgery, and idiopathic. Patients complain of postprandial fullness, nausea, vomiting, and early satiety. Pain has been reported as a prominent feature of gastroparesis in some series [29–31]. Dyspepsia related to gastroparesis may affect 5% to 12% of diabetics, typically occurs in the context of multiple target organ complications such as retinopathy, neuropathy, or nephropathy, and can have a significant effect on glycemic control, as well as nutritional status.

The pathophysiology of gastroparesis is multifactorial and complex. The gastric response to a meal is complex and includes fundic relaxation to accommodate the meal, tonic contraction of the fundus and upper corpus to effect liquid emptying, antral trituration to grind down solid particles, and coordinated antro-pyloro-duodenal motor activity to ensure appropriately timed and efficient delivery of nutrients to the small intestine. The net result should be a tightly regulated delivery of calories in a readily digested format to the absorptive surfaces of the intestine. Control over each of these activities may be exerted centrally (mediated predominantly by vagal sensory and motor input), locally (through the enteric nervous system), and hormonally (both endocrine and paracrine). A host of phenomena ranging from acute stress to degenerative diseases of the autonomic nervous system, enteric neuropathies and myopathies, and neurological disease may disrupt gastric emptying at one or multiple levels and cause the clinical syndrome of gastroparesis [32].

Modalities used to diagnose gastroparesis include scintigraphy (still the gold standard) where the time taken to empty a solid radiolabeled test meal is measured. Optimum results are obtained if scintigraphy is extended to at least 4 h postprandially. Regional gastric emptying can be used to assess fundic and antral function. Dual-labeled scintigraphy can offer insights into the differential handling of liquids and solids by the stomach. Based on its ability to identify transit into the duodenum by a sudden and profound change in pH, the wireless motility capsule is able to estimate the rate of gastric emptying and provide estimates of gastric and colonic motor function in the absence of radiation exposure, though availability remains limited and cost prohibitive for many [33]. Other modalities, under evaluation for use in the diagnosis and research of gastroparesis, include the octanoic acid breath test, functional MRI, and both 2D and 3D ultrasonography [34].

Though gastroparesis may cause dyspepsia, the significant overlap between it and FD means that the finding of delayed gastric emptying in a patient with dyspeptic symptoms, in the absence of either more classical symptoms of gastroparesis or an underlying disease process, known to result in a pathological delay in gastric emptying rate, should be interpreted with caution [32]. Delayed gastric emptying has been reported in anywhere from 25 to 40% of patients with FD. Correlations with symptoms and responses to prokinetic agents have, however, been most disappointing [32, 35].

MEDICATION- AND DRUG-INDUCED DYSPEPSIA

A host of agents have been reported to result in iatrogenic dyspepsia and range from alcohol, through a variety of "recreational" drugs to over-the-counter and prescription NSAIDs to the powerfully emetogenic cancer chemotherapeutic agents [1, 36–38]. While a complete list of all agents that may induce dyepeptic symptoms is beyond the scope of this review, it stands to reason that a thorough assessment of intake of all potentially gastro-toxic compounds should be an essential component of the investigation of a patient with dyspepsia. The physician must remain ever vigilant for the use of alcohol and NSAIDs, in particular, in this context.

CONCLUSIONS

Reflecting the myriad of symptoms that may be included within the broad umbrella that is dyspepsia, the list of disorders and pathological processes that may cause dyspepsia is virtually endless. Based largely on geographic and temporal variations in the prevalence of *H. pylori,* the relative contributions of common entities such as PUD and gastric cancer to dyspepsia can vary dramatically. In the West, and to an increasing extent elsewhere, GERD has emerged as the dominant pathology, and the contribution of dysmotility, as manifested by gastroparesis, for example, is less clear-cut.

References

1. Crean GP, Holden RJ, Knill-Jones RP, et al. A database on dyspepsia. Gut. 1994;35:191–202.
2. Vakil N, van Zanten SV, Kahrilas P, Dent J, Jones R, Global Consensus Group. The Montreal definition and classification of gastroesophageal reflux disease: a global evidence-based consensus. Am J Gastroenterol. 2006;101:1900–20. quiz 1943.
3. Camilleri M, Dubois D, Coulie B, et al. Prevalence and socioeconomic impact of upper gastrointestinal disorders in the United States: results of the US Upper Gastrointestinal Study. Clin Gastroenterol Hepatol. 2005;3:543–52.
4. Ronkainen J, Aro P, Storskrubb T, et al. Gastro-oesophageal reflux symptoms and health-related quality of life in the adult general population – the Kalixanda study. Aliment Pharmacol Ther. 2006;23:1725–33.

5. Kahrilas PJ, Shaheen NJ, Vaezi MF, American Gastroenterological Association Institute; Clinical Practice and Quality Management Committee. American Gastroenterological Association Institute technical review on the management of gastroesophageal reflux disease. Gastroenterology. 2008;135:1392–413.

6. Quigley EM. Functional dyspepsia (FD) and non-erosive reflux disease (NERD): overlapping or discrete entities? Best Pract Res Clin Gastroenterol. 2004;18:695–706.

7. de Vries DR, ter Linde JJM, van Herwaarden MA, Smout AJPM, Samsom M. Gastroesophageal reflux disease is associated with the C825T polymorphism in the G-protein beta3 subunit gene (GNB3). Am J Gastroenterol. 2009;104:281–5.

8. Kahrilas PJ. Clinical practice. Gastroesophageal reflux disease. N Engl J Med. 2008;359:1700–7.

9. Quigley EM. Gastro-oesophageal reflux disease-spectrum or continuum? QJM. 1997;90:75–8.

10. Kulig M, Leodolter A, Vieth M, et al. Quality of life in relation to symptoms in patients with gastro-oesophageal reflux disease – an analysis based on the ProGERD initiative. Aliment Pharmacol Ther. 2003;18:767–76.

11. Fennerty MB, Johnson DA. Heartburn severity does not predict disease severity in patients with erosive esophagitis. MedGenMed. 2006;8:6.

12. Talley NJ, Armstrong D, Junghard O, Wiklund I. Predictors of treatment response in patients with non-erosive reflux disease. Aliment Pharmacol Ther. 2006;24:371–6.

13. Schwizer W, Thumshirn M, Dent J, et al. *Helicobacter pylori* and symptomatic relapse of gastro-oesophageal reflux disease: a randomised controlled trial. Lancet. 2001;357:1738–42.

14. Ronkainen J, Aro P, Storskrubb T, et al. Prevalence of Barrett's esophagus in the general population: an endoscopic study. Gastroenterology. 2005;129:1825–31.

15. Belhocine K, Galmiche J-P. Epidemiology of the complications of gastroesophageal reflux disease. Dig Dis. 2009;27:7–13.

16. Malfertheiner P, Chan FK, McColl KE. Peptic ulcer disease. Lancet. 2009;374:1449–61.

17. Bektas M, Soykan I, Altan M, Alkan M, Ozden A. The effect of *Helicobacter pylori* eradication on dyspeptic symptoms, acid reflux and quality of life in patients with functional dyspepsia. Eur J Intern Med. 2009;20:419–23.

18. Gwee KA, Teng L, Wong RK, Ho KY, Sutedja DS, Yeoh KG. The response of Asian patients with functional dyspepsia to eradication of *Helicobacter pylori* infection. Eur J Gastroenterol Hepatol. 2009;21:417–24.

19. Maconi G, Sainaghi M, Molteni M, et al. Predictors of long-term outcome of functional dyspepsia and duodenal ulcer after successful *Helicobacter pylori* eradication – a 7-year follow-up study. Eur J Gastroenterol Hepatol. 2009;21:387–93.

20. Talley NJ, Vakil NB, Moayyedi P. American gastroenterological association technical review on the evaluation of dyspepsia. Gastroenterology. 2005;129:1756–80.

21. Solaymani-Dodaran M, Logan RF, West J, Card T. Mortality associated with Barrett's esophagus and gastroesophageal reflux disease diagnoses – a population-based cohort study. Am J Gastroenterol. 2005;100:2616–21.

22. Lawrence Jr W. Gastric cancer. CA Cancer J Clin. 1986;36:216–36.

23. Menuck LS, Amberg JR. Metastatic disease involving the stomach. Am J Dig Dis. 1975;20:903–13.

24. Johnson AG. Cholecystectomy and gallstone dyspepsia. Clinical and physiological study of a symptom complex. Ann R Coll Surg Engl. 1975;56:69–80.

25. Kraag N, Thijs C, Knipschild P. Dyspepsia – how noisy are gallstones? A meta-analysis of epidemiologic studies of biliary pain, dyspeptic symptoms, and food intolerance. Scand J Gastroenterol. 1995;30:411–21.

26. DiBaise JK, Oleynikov D. Does gallbladder ejection fraction predict outcome after cholecystectomy for suspected chronic acalculous gallbladder dysfunction? A systematic review. Am J Gastroenterol. 2003;98:2605–11.

27. Dickey W. Joint BAPEN and British Society of Gastroenterology Symposium on 'Coeliac disease: basics and controversies'. Coeliac disease in the twenty-first century. Proc Nutr Soc. 2009;68:234–41.

28. Ford AC, Ching E, Moayyedi P. Meta-analysis: yield of diagnostic tests for coeliac disease in dyspepsia. Aliment Pharmacol Ther. 2009;30:28–36.

29. Khayyam U, Sachdeva P, Gomez J, et al. Assessment of symptoms during gastric emptying scintigraphy to correlate symptoms to delayed gastric emptying. Neurogastroenterol Motil. 2010;22:539–45.

30. Friedenberg FK, Parkman HP. Persistent nausea and abdominal pain in a patient with delayed gastric emptying. Clin Gastroenterol Hepatol. 2008;6:1309–14.

31. Hoogerwerf WA, Pasricha PJ, Kalloo AN, Schuster MM. Pain: the overlooked symptom in gastroparesis. Am J Gastroenterol. 1999;94:1029–33.

32. Quigley EMM. Review article: gastric emptying in functional gastrointestinal disorders. Aliment Pharmacol Ther. 2004;20 Suppl 7:56–60.

33. Rao SS, Kuo B, McCallum RW, et al. Investigation of colonic and whole-gut transit with wireless motility capsule and radiopaque markers in constipation. Clin Gastroenterol Hepatol. 2009;7:537–44.

34. Parkman HP, Camilleri M, Farrugia G, et al. Gastroparesis and functional dyspepsia: excerpts from the AGA/ANMS meeting. Neurogastroenterol Motil. 2010;22:113–33.

35. Quigley EM, Keohane J. Dyspepsia. Curr Opin Gastroenterol. 2008;24:692–7.

36. Leong RW, Chan FK. Drug-induced side effects affecting the gastrointestinal tract. Expert Opin Drug Saf. 2006;5:585–92.

37. Lanza FL, Chan FK. Practice Parameters Committee of the American College of Gastroenterology. Guidelines for prevention of NSAID-related ulcer complications. Am J Gastroenterol. 2009;104:728–38.

38. Quigley EM, Hasler WL, Parkman HP. AGA technical review on nausea and vomiting. Gastroenterology. 2001;120:263–86.

Chapter 5
Functional (Nonulcer) Dyspepsia

Marino Venerito, Arne Kandulski, and Peter Malfertheiner

Keywords: Functional dyspepsia, Postprandial distress syndrome, Epigastric pain syndrome

INTRODUCTION

The term dyspepsia describes a heterogeneous group of symptoms originating from the epigastric region (stomach and duodenum). Dyspeptic symptoms include postprandial fullness, early satiation, epigastric pain, and epigastric burning (Table 5.1). Structural causes responsible for dyspeptic symptoms are discussed in Chap. 4. According to the Rome III consensus conference (2006), functional dyspepsia (FD) is defined as the presence of dyspeptic symptoms thought to generate in the gastroduodenal region, in the absence of organic, systemic, or metabolic disease that is likely to explain the symptoms [1]. Symptoms originating from the esophagus such as heartburn or regurgitation are not included in the current definition. For diagnosis of FD, the presence of one or more dyspeptic symptoms for the last 3 months with symptoms onset at least 6 months before diagnosis is required. Particularly for pathophysiological and therapeutic research purposes, the Rome III consensus conference defined two subentities of FD:

1. The postprandial distress syndrome (PDS), which is meal-induced and includes postprandial fullness and early satiation.
2. Epigastric pain syndrome (EPS), which is not meal-induced and includes epigastric pain and epigastric burning.

M. Venerito (✉)
Department of Gastroenterology, Hepatology and Infectious Diseases, "Otto-von-Guericke" University, Magdeburg, Germany
e-mail: m.venerito@med.ovgu.de

M. Duvnjak (ed.), *Dyspepsia in Clinical Practice*,
DOI 10.1007/978-1-4419-1730-0_5,
© Springer Science+Business Media, LLC 2011

TABLE 5.1. Dyspeptic symptoms as defined by the Rome III committee [1].

Symptoms	Definition
Epigastric pain	Epigastric refers to the region between the umbilicus and lower end of the sternum and marked by the mid-clavicular lines. Pain refers to a subjective, unpleasant sensation; some patients may feel that tissue damage is occurring. Other symptoms may be extremely bothersome without being interpreted by the patient as pain.
Epigastric burning	Epigastric refers to the region between the umbilicus and lower end of the sternum and marked by the midclavicular lines. Burning refers to an unpleasant subjective sensation of heat.
Postprandial fullness	An unpleasant sensation like the prolonged persistence of food in the stomach.
Early satiation	A feeling that the stomach is overfilled soon after starting to eat, out of proportion to the size of the meal being eaten, so that the meal cannot be finished. Previously, the term "early satiety" was used, but satiation is the correct term for the disappearance of the sensation of appetite during food ingestion.

EPIDEMIOLOGY

Considering epidemiological data, it is important to distinguish the subjects with dyspeptic symptoms who received a diagnostic label after they have been investigated (with or without an identified cause for the underlying symptoms) from patients who have not been investigated. Prevalence rates of dyspepsia depend on how dyspepsia is defined. Indeed, previous definitions of dyspepsia included symptoms of gastroesophageal reflux disease (GERD) such as heartburn and regurgitation. The definition of dyspepsia used in this book is the one proposed by the Rome III consensus conference [1]. Epidemiological studies taking into account the current criteria for the diagnosis of dyspepsia are limited. In a systematic review published in 2004, after excluding patients with heartburn or regurgitation, the prevalence rate of dyspepsia was 5% to 12% [2]. Similar results were found in a population-based endoscopic study conducted in Italy where the prevalence of FD was found to be 11% [3]. Prevalence of dyspeptic symptoms is slightly higher in women than in men and appears to decline with age. The incidence of dyspepsia (number of new cases in a population at risk) is poorly documented. In a Scandinavian study conducted on a period of 3 months, the incidence of dyspepsia was lower than 1% [4]. Longitudinal studies suggest that symptoms improve or disappear over the time in less than half of the patients [2, 5]. The probability of remission is lower in patients with a longer history of dyspeptic symptoms, lower educational level, or psychosocial stress.

Most patients have symptoms that overlap with those of other functional disorders of the gastrointestinal tract, such as functional heartburn and irritable bowel syndrome (IBS). Indeed, up to 2/3 of patients with IBS have dyspepsia and up to 2/3 of patients with dyspepsia have symptoms of IBS [6–8]. Furthermore, patients with functional disorders of the gastrointestinal tract often have extraintestinal symptoms such as migraine headache, fibromyalgia, and urinary or gynecologic complaints [5]. The management of patients with dyspepsia is one of the major problems in clinical praxis. Indeed, although less than half of the patients with dyspeptic symptoms seek medical attention, 2% to 5% of medical consultations are for dyspepsia [9]. Factors inducing patients to seek medical consultation include the severity or frequency of symptoms, fear of underlying disease (especially cancer), lower social class, advancing age, anxiety, psychological stress, and lack of adequate psychosocial support [10, 11].

ETIOPATHOGENETIC FACTORS

A number of pathophysiological mechanisms that may contribute to the generation of dyspeptic symptoms have been described (Fig. 5.1) [12]. Like other functional gastrointestinal disorders,

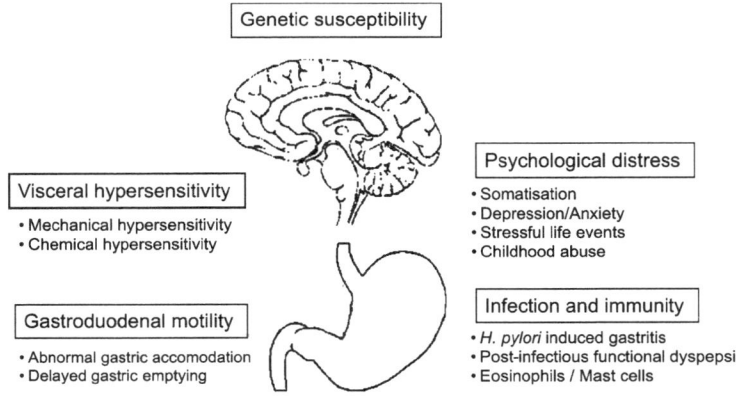

FIG. 5.1   Putative mechanisms linked to functional dyspepsia. Modified from Talley et al. [12].

FD may be best understood in the context of the biopsychosocial model of illness in which symptoms arise out of a complex interaction between abnormal gastrointestinal physiology and psychological factors that affect how a person perceives, interprets, and responds to altered gastrointestinal physiology [5]. Persons with abnormal gastrointestinal physiology but no psychological abnormalities, a stable social support, and good coping mechanisms either may not seek medical care or may respond readily to reassurance, whereas patients with both abnormal gastrointestinal physiology and psychological problems, increased life stress, or poor social support may be more likely to seek medical attention [5].

Genetic Predisposition

Recent evidence suggests that genetic factors may be involved in the pathogenesis of FD. In a nested case–control study, a positive family history of abdominal pain was shown to be an independent risk factor for FD (OR = 4.7, 95% CI = 1.5–14.9) [13]. In a case–control study by Holtmann et al. aiming to assess the association of specific G-protein beta 3 (GNβ3) subunit gene polymorphisms with FD, the homozygous GNβ3 825C carrier status was associated with an increased risk of developing FD (OR = 2.2, 95% CI = 1.4–3.3) [14]. Polymorphisms of other candidate genes including alpha adrenergic receptors, serotonin receptors, the serotonin reuptake transponder, and CCK receptors were not associated with FD [15].

Alterations of the Gastroduodenal Motility

Disorders of the gastroduodenal motility are present in as many as 20% to 50% of patients with FD and include impaired gastric accommodation to a meal and delayed gastric emptying.

Gastric accommodation to a meal. Accommodation of the stomach to a meal is a vagal mediated reflex that occurs postprandially and consists of a relaxation of the proximal stomach, providing the meal with a reservoir: it enables the stomach to handle increases in gastric volumes without proportional increases of intragastric pressures [16, 17]. Studies including ultrasonography, scintigraphy, magnetic resonance imaging, intragastric barostat, single photon emission computed tomography (SPECT), or noninvasive surrogate markers (satiation drinking test) demonstrated that accommodation of the proximal stomach is abnormal in up to 40% of patients with FD [18–22]. Insufficient accommodation of the proximal stomach during and after the ingestion of a meal may be accompanied by increased intragastric pressure and activation of mechanoreceptors in the gastric wall, thus inducing symptoms.

Delayed gastric emptying. In a meta-analysis of 17 studies involving 868 dyspeptic patients and 397 controls, significant delay of solid gastric emptying was present in almost 40% of patients with FD [23]. However, attempts to link specific dyspeptic symptoms (i.e., postprandial fullness) and delayed gastric emptying have met mixed results [24]. Furthermore, therapeutic trials have shown a poor correlation between improvement in symptoms and changes in the rate of gastric emptying, casting doubt on the importance of delayed gastric emptying in causing symptoms [25, 26].

Visceral Hypersensitivity
The majority of stimuli from the gastrointestinal tract (i.e., accommodation, distention, contraction, or gastric emptying) are not perceived consciously. However, the perception threshold to visceral physiological or minor noxious stimuli is lower in subjects with FD. Studies with intragastric barostat demonstrated hypersensitivity to balloon distension of the proximal stomach in 40% of patients with FD [27]. Hypersensitivity does not appear to be related to abnormalities in gastric acid secretion, gastric accommodation, compliance, or emptying; however, patients with hypersensitivity are hypothesized to be more likely to experience discomfort or pain when these pathophysiologic abnormalities are present [26]. In a study with intragastric barostat, visceral hypersensitivity was associated with the meal-related subgroup of FD [28]. At present, no tests for visceral hypersensitivity are available outside a clinical research setting [29].

Infections
Infections may be involved in the pathogenesis of FD. A large retrospective, tertiary referral center study showed that a subset of dyspeptic patients had a history suggestive of postinfectious dyspepsia [30]. Compared with patients with unspecified onset-dyspepsia, patients with presumed postinfectious dyspepsia had more prevalent symptoms of early satiety, weight loss, nausea, and vomiting, and had a significantly higher prevalence of impaired accommodation of the proximal stomach, but no differences were found in the prevalence of delayed gastric emptying or hypersensitivity to gastric distension. Based on additional pharmacological studies of nitrergic gastric function using sumatriptan and amylnitrate, the authors suggested that impaired accommodation in patients with presumed postinfectious FD is attributable to a dysfunction at the level of gastric nitrergic neurons [31]. In a prospective cohort questionnaire-based study, the development of dyspepsia was found to be fivefold increased at one year after acute *Salmonella* gastroenteritis, compared with controls

without baseline infection [30]. Further studies are needed to identify risk factors and long-term prognosis of postinfectious dyspepsia.

Helicobacter pylori Infection

Many studies have tried to establish a relationship between *Helicobacter pylori* (*H. pylori*) infection and FD. However, no consistent differences in the prevalence and severity of dyspeptic symptoms have been found between *H. pylori*-positive and *H. pylori*-negative subjects [32, 33]. Moreover, large-scale studies failed to find a relationship between *H. pylori* infection and an increased gastric sensitivity, impaired accommodation, or delayed gastric emptying in patients with FD [34–36]. On the other hand, in a meta-analysis eradication therapy for *H. pylori* infection compared with controls induced at 12 months a small but statistically significant reduction in the frequency of dyspeptic symptoms [37]. The clinical significance of these findings are unclear because the effect occurs only late and is relatively small, with a number needed to treat of 15 (95% CI: 10–28) *H. pylori*-positive patients to achieve one cure. The main reason for *H. pylori* eradication in patients with FD may relate more to prevention strategies (peptic ulcers, gastric malignancies) than to improvement of dyspeptic symptoms.

Immunity (Allergy)

In a recent study, an increased prevalence of gastrointestinal symptoms was observed in patients with allergic disease (asthma or allergic rhinitis) compared to a nonasthmatic population [38]. These findings suggest that activated mast cells and eosinophils my play a role in the pathogenesis of dyspeptic symptoms. Animal studies on guinea pigs have shown that mediators released by activated mast cells increase the excitability of enteric neurons, leading to abnormal sensory and motor function [39, 40]. In an endoscopic study on pediatric patients with dyspepsia, 71% were diagnosed with abnormal duodenal eosinophilia, and therapy with histamine receptor antagonists reduced both eosinophilia and dyspeptic symptoms [41]. Noteworthy, in a crossover study, the therapy with montelukast or placebo in dyspeptic children with eosinophilia induced a positive clinical response in 62% and 32%, respectively [42]. The association of FD with duodenal eosinophilia has been confirmed also in an adult population after adjusting for age, sex, and *H. pylori* status [43]. In particular, the prevalence of duodenal eosinophilia has been shown to be significantly higher in the subgroup of dyspeptic patients with postprandial distress syndrome than in controls (47.3%, $p < 0.04$) [44]. The observation that dyspeptic symptoms are associated with duodenal eosinophilia may result in a change of the current management of FD.

Psychological Factors

In patients with FD, the frequency of psychosocial disorders, including anxiety, depression, and somatization, is higher than in normal subjects [9]. Furthermore, a health-seeking behavior and alterations in illness behavior and coping styles have been described [45–47]. Recent population-based surveys of community subjects suggest that baseline psychosocial distress is predictive of chronic abdominal pain but independent of health care-seeking behavior [9, 11, 48]. Compared with healthy asymptomatic community subjects, patients with dyspepsia report an increased number of stressful or threatening life events (e.g., death in family, unemployment, serious illness, divorce) within the prior 6 months [48]. Prior life events, such as an unhappy childhood, physical or sexual abuse, or positive reinforcement for abdominal symptoms (parental attention, excuse from school) also may affect illness behavior [11]. These psychosocial factors are probably influenced by and influence upper gastrointestinal symptoms, and the bidirectional flow is presumably mediated through the brain-gut axis [49]. To date, studies on the efficacy of psychological therapies in FD remain inconclusive [50].

CONCLUSIONS

FD is still a poorly understood entity but appears to be a highly heterogeneous disorder. Contributors to the pathogenesis of FD include genetic, environmental, pathological, and psychological factors. Progress in the understanding of the underlying pathogenetic mechanisms may result in a better management of these patients.

References

1. Tack J, Talley NJ, Camilleri M, et al. Functional gastroduodenal disorders. Gastroenterology. 2006;130:1466–79.
2. El-Serag HB, Talley NJ. Systemic review: the prevalence and clinical course of functional dyspepsia. Aliment Pharmacol Ther. 2004;19:643–54.
3. Zagari RM, Law GR, Fuccio L, et al. Epidemiology of functional dyspepsia and subgroups in the Italian general population: an endoscopic study. Gastroenterology. 2010;138:1302–11.
4. Agréus L, Svärdsudd K, Nyrén O, Tibblin G. Irritable bowel syndrome and dyspepsia in the general population: overlap and lack of stability over time. Gastroenterology. 1995;109:671–80.

5. McQuaid KR. Dyspepsia. In: Feldman M, Friedman LS, Brandt LJ, editors. Sleisenger & Fordtran's gastrointestinal and liver disease. 8th ed. Philadelphia: Saunders Elsevier; 2009. p. 121–42.

6. Talley N, Dennis EH, Schettler-Duncan VA, Olden LBE, KW CMD. Overlapping upper and lower gastrointestinal symptoms in irritable bowel syndrome patients with constipation or diarrhea. Am J Gastroenterol. 2003;98:2454–9.

7. Corsetti M, Caenepeel P, Fischler B, Janssens J, Tack J. Impact of coexisting irritable bowel syndrome on symptoms and pathophysiological mechanisms in functional dyspepsia. Am J Gastroenterol. 2004;99:1152–9.

8. Stanghellini V, Tosetti C, Barbara G, et al. Dyspeptic symptoms and gastric emptying in the irritable bowel syndrome. Am J Gastroenterol. 2002;97:2738–43.

9. Koloski NA, Talley NJ, Huskic SS, Boyce PM. Predictors of conventional and alternative health care seeking for irritable bowel syndrome and functional dyspepsia. Aliment Pharmacol Ther. 2003;17: 841–51.

10. Quadri A, Vakil N. Health-related anxiety and the effect of open-access endoscopy in US patients with dyspepsia. Aliment Pharmacol Ther. 2003;17:835–40.

11. Koloski NA, Talley NJ, Boyce PM. Predictors of health care seeking for irritable bowel syndrome and nonulcer dyspepsia: a critical review of the literature on symptom and psychosocial factors. Am J Gastroenterol. 2001;96:1340–9.

12. Talley NJ, Choung RS. Whither dyspepsia? A historical perspective of functional dyspepsia, and concepts of pathogenesis and therapy in 2009. J Gastroenterol Hepatol. 2009;24 Suppl 3:S20–8.

13. Gathaiya N, Locke 3rd GR, Camilleri M, Schleck CD, Zinsmeister AR, Talley NJ. Novel associations with dyspepsia: a community-based study of familial aggregation, sleep dysfunction and somatization. Neurogastroenterol Motil. 2009;21:922–e69.

14. Holtmann G, Siffert W, Haag S, et al. G-protein beta 3 subunit 825 CC genotype is associated with unexplained (functional) dyspepsia. Gastroenterology. 2004;126:971–9.

15. Camilleri CE, Carlson PJ, Camilleri M, et al. A study of candidate genotypes associated with dyspepsia in a U.S. community. Am J Gastroenterol. 2006;101:581–92.

16. Kindt S, Tack J. Impaired gastric accommodation and its role in dyspepsia. Gut. 2006;55:1685–91.

17. Azpiroz F, Malagelada JR. Gastric tone measured by an electronic barostat in health and postsurgical gastroparesis. Gastroenterology. 1987;92:934–43.

18. Tack J, Piessevaux H, Coulie B, Caenepeel P, Janssens J. Role of impaired gastric accommodation to a meal in functional dyspepsia. Gastroenterology. 1998;115:1346–52.

19. Troncon LE, Bennett RJ, Ahluwalia NK, Thompson DG. Abnormal intragastric distribution of food during gastric emptying in functional dyspepsia patients. Gut. 1994;35:327–32.

20. Kim DY, Delgado-Aros S, Camilleri M, et al. Noninvasive measurement of gastric accommodation in patients with idiopathic nonulcer dyspepsia. Am J Gastroenterol. 2001;96:3099–105.
21. Mearin F, Cucala M, Azpiroz F, Malagelada JR. The origin of symptoms in the brain-gut axis in functional dyspepsia. Gastroenterology. 1991;101:999–1006.
22. Sarnelli G, Vos R, Cuomo R, Janssens J, Tack J. Reproducibility of gastric barostat studies in healthy controls and in dyspeptic patients. Am J Gastroenterol. 2001;96:1047–53.
23. Perri F, Clemente R, Festa V, et al. Patterns of symptoms in functional dyspepsia: role of *Helicobacter pylori* infection and delayed gastric emptying. Am J Gastroenterol. 1998;93:2082–8.
24. Tack J, Bisschops R, Sarnelli G. Pathophysiology and treatment of functional dyspepsia. Gastroenterology. 2004;127:1239–55.
25. Feinle-Bisset C, Vozzo R, Horowitz M, Talley NJ. Diet, food intake, and disturbed physiology in the pathogenesis of symptoms in functional dyspepsia. Am J Gastroenterol. 2004;99:170–81.
26. Timmons S, Liston R, Moriarty KJ. Functional dyspepsia: motor abnormalities, sensory dysfunction, and therapeutic options. Am J Gastroenterol. 2004;99:739–49.
27. Mertz H. Review article: visceral hypersensitivity. Aliment Pharmacol Ther. 2003;17:623–33.
28. Tack J, Caenepeel P, Fischler B, Piessevaux H, Janssens J. Symptoms associated with hypersensitivity to gastric distention in functional dyspepsia. Gastroenterology. 2001;121:526–35.
29. Camilleri M, Coulie B, Tack J. Visceral hypersensitivity: facts, speculations, and challenges. Gut. 2001;48:125–31.
30. Mearin F, Pérez-Oliveras M, Perelló A, et al. Dyspepsia and irritable bowel syndrome after a Salmonella gastroenteritis outbreak: one-year follow-up cohort study. Gastroenterology. 2005;129:98–104.
31. Tack J, Demedts I, Dehondt G, et al. Clinical and pathophysiological characteristics of acute-onset functional dyspepsia. Gastroenterology. 2002;122:1738–47.
32. Saslow SB, Thumshirn M, Camilleri M, et al. Influence of *H. pylori* infection on gastric motor and sensory function in asymptomatic volunteers. Dig Dis Sci. 1998;43:258–64.
33. Tucci A, Corinaldesi R, Stanghellini V, et al. *Helicobacter pylori* infection and gastric function in patients with chronic idiopathic dyspepsia. Gastroenterology. 1992;103:768–74.
34. Thumshirn M, Camilleri M, Saslow SB, Williams DE, Burton DD, Hanson RB. Gastric accommodation in non-ulcer dyspepsia and the roles of *Helicobacter pylori* infection and vagal function. Gut. 1999;44:55–64.
35. Rhee PL, Kim YH, Son HJ, et al. Lack of association of *Helicobacter pylori* infection with gastric hypersensitivity or delayed gastric emptying in functional dyspepsia. Am J Gastroenterol. 1999;94:3165–9.
36. Sarnelli G, Cuomo R, Janssens J, Tack J. Symptom patterns and pathophysiological mechanisms in dyspeptic patients with and without *Helicobacter pylori*. Dig Dis Sci. 2003;48:2229–36.

37. Moayyedi P, Deeks J, Talley NJ, Delaney B, Forman D. An update of the Cochrane systematic review of *Helicobacter pylori* therapy for nonulcer dyspepsia: resolving the discrepancy between systematic reviews. Am J Gastroenterol. 2003;98:2621–6.
38. Powell N, Huntley B, Beech T, Knight W, Knight H, Corrigan CJ. Increased prevalence of gastrointestinal symptoms in patients with allergic disease. Postgrad Med J. 2007;83:182–6.
39. Liu S, Hu HZ, Gao N, et al. Neuroimmune interactions in guinea pig stomach and small intestine. Am J Physiol Gastrointest Liver Physiol. 2003;284:G154–64.
40. Reed DE, Barajas-Lopez C, Cottrell G, et al. Mast cell tryptase and proteinase-activated receptor 2 induce hyperexcitability of guinea-pig submucosal neurons. J Physiol. 2003;547:531–42.
41. Friesen CA, Sandridge L, Andre L, Roberts CC, Abdel-Rahman SM. Mucosal eosinophilia and response to H1/H2 antagonist and cromolyn therapy in pediatric dyspepsia. Clin Pediatr (Phila). 2006;45:143–7.
42. Friesen CA, Kearns GL, Andre L, Neustrom M, Roberts CC, Abdel-Rahman SM. Clinical efficacy and pharmacokinetics of montelukast in dyspeptic children with duodenal eosinophilia. J Pediatr Gastroenterol Nutr. 2004;38:343–51.
43. Talley NJ, Walker MM, Aro P, et al. Non-ulcer dyspepsia and duodenal eosinophilia: an adult endoscopic population-based case–control study. Clin Gastroenterol Hepatol. 2007;5:1175–83.
44. Walker MM, Salehian SS, Murray CE, et al. Implications of eosinophilia in the normal duodenal biopsy – an association with allergy and functional dyspepsia. Aliment Pharmacol Ther. [published online ahead of print March 4, 2010].
45. Drossman DA, Creed FH, Olden KW, Svedlund J, Toner BB, Whitehead WE. Psychosocial aspects of the functional gastrointestinal disorders. Gut. 1999;45 Suppl 2:II25–30.
46. Talley NJ, Phillips SF, Bruce B, Twomey CK, Zinsmeister AR, Melton LJ. Relation among personality and symptoms in non-ulcer dyspepsia and the irritable bowel syndrome. Gastroenterology. 1990;99:327–33.
47. Tanum L, Malt UF. Personality and physical symptoms in nonpsychiatric patients with functional gastrointestinal disorder. J Psychosom Res. 2001;50:139–46.
48. Locke 3rd GR, Weaver AL, Melton 3rd LJ, Talley NJ. Psychosocial factors are linked to functional gastrointestinal disorders: a population based nested case–control study. Am J Gastroenterol. 2004;99:350–7.
49. Mayer EA, Gebhart GF. Basic and clinical aspects of visceral hyperalgesia. Gastroenterology. 1994;107:271–93.
50. Soo S, Moayyedi P, Deeks J, Delaney B, Lewis M, Forman D. Psychological interventions for non-ulcer dyspepsia. Cochrane Database Syst Rev. 2005:CD002301.

Chapter 6
How to Diagnose Dyspepsia

Lars Aabakken

Keywords: Dyspepsia, Diagnostics, Upper endoscopy, Clinical diagnosis, Acid suppressive therapy, *Helicobacter pylori*

INTRODUCTION

Dyspepsia is a somewhat vaguely defined symptomatic entity that spans a range of clinical conditions. The majority of patients presenting this symptom will eventually be found to suffer from "functional dyspepsia," effectively an exclusion diagnosis. However, a number of serious and/or treatable conditions may present in a similar fashion, and some degree of workup is mandatory, to avoid missing important diagnoses with an acceptable certainty.

The diagnostic workup of dyspepsia includes making a selection of diagnostic maneuvers that make sense in relation to the individual patient. Because of the large number of patients presenting with variants of dyspepsia, a reasonable trade-off between diagnostic accuracy and an adequate use of time and resources is the goal, but it is often a challenging goal to achieve. This chapter describes the diagnostic modalities relevant for the dyspeptic patient and aims to define their respective roles related to specific patient features.

L. Aabakken (✉)
Department of Gastroenterology, Oslo University
Hospital – Rikshospitalet, Oslo, Norway
e-mail: larsaa@medisin.uio.no

M. Duvnjak (ed.), *Dyspepsia in Clinical Practice*,
DOI 10.1007/978-1-4419-1730-0_6,
© Springer Science+Business Media, LLC 2011

SYMPTOMS AND SIGNS

In the clinical setting, a practicable definition of dyspepsia is "any episodic or persistent symptom or combinations of symptoms, which are thought by the physician to be referable to the upper gastrointestinal (GI) tract" [1]. Before contemplating any additional diagnostic workup, the physician's main challenge is to determine if dyspepsia is indeed present and to what extent red flag symptoms or signs exist (Table 6.1). Thus, once the red flags occur, the diagnostic ambition changes and certain aspects of the workup become imperative. While the patient history is vital in the workup, the clinical investigation is frequently unremarkable in the setting of classic dyspepsia – clinical findings are more likely present in the context of one or more alarm symptoms, even if their predictive value has been disappointing in clinical studies [2, 3].

Without the red flags, symptom-based diagnostic strategies have been suggested to differentiate the potential diagnoses through symptom profiles. Unfortunately, the subgroup overlap is substantial, and none of these strategies have been shown to predictably coin a correct diagnosis [5, 6]. Moreover, the clinical value of subgrouping functional dyspepsia (ulcer-like, reflux-like, and dysmotility-like dyspepsia) remains speculative, e.g., in the selection of tailored therapy.

EMPIRICAL PROTON-PUMP INHIBITOR THERAPY

A short course of potent acid suppression [usually proton-pump inhibitor (PPI) in full therapeutic doses] with subsequent minute evaluation of the clinical effect is an attractive approach, being easy, pragmatic, noninvasive, and possibly offering the patient rapid

TABLE 6.1. Alarm symptoms and signs (adapted) [4].

Age over 55 with new onset symptoms
Family history of gastric cancer
Unintended weight loss
Gastrointestinal bleeding
Progressive dysphagia
Odynophagia
Unexplained iron deficiency anemia
Persistent vomiting
Palpable mass or lymphadenopathy
Jaundice
Lymphadenopathy
Palpable abdominal mass

symptom relief. However, the test has no value in differentiating between the various potential causes of the dyspeptic symptoms. Moreover, the symptomatic effect is most prominent in patients with gastroesophageal reflux disease (GERD) or peptic ulcer, and the strategy may result in an inadvertent selection of endoscopy-negative patients (those without effect) for endoscopy, while, for example, *Helicobacter pylori* (*H. pylori*)-positive ulcer patients remain infected with recurrent disease. In many cases, the patient or the doctor will eventually opt for an upper endoscopy; in that case, the trial therapy is equally futile. On the other hand, symptomatic relief of GERD is associated with endoscopic healing as well; thus, empiric trial therapy may be adequate for long-term relief. However, if *H. pylori*-associated ulcer disease is temporarily healed with PPI trial therapy, the trial therapy only adds to the cost and duration of the workup. Studies on the value of trial therapy differ in their conclusions, likely because of variable assumptions in the models [7, 8]. However, some of the studies indicate a cost-effectiveness benefit with trial therapy, mostly by avoiding endoscopies, at least in the short term. A number of recent guidelines recommend empirical PPI therapy as first line intervention in low *H. pylori* prevalence areas, which presently includes the US and most of Europe.

If acid suppression is chosen as a trial therapy, then proactive evaluation of the effect is pivotal. This is particularly important in children, where the symptom profile may be less classical. If after 6–8 weeks of full dose treatment clinical effect is lacking or unsatisfactory, continued treatment is unlikely to be beneficial.

UPPER ENDOSCOPY

Endoscopy in a symptomatic patient is still considered the gold standard of diagnostics. The utility of upper endoscopy in the workup of dyspepsia depends on the pretest probability of clinically significant findings, specifically reflux esophagitis, peptic ulcer disease, and tumors. The prevalence of gastric cancer and *H. pylori* impacts this decision as does age and alarm symptoms. Most guidelines designate endoscopy in patients >50–55 or those with alarm symptoms. The role of *H. pylori* status to determine the role of endoscopy is more debatable (see below).

Endoscopy likely has a clinical impact in a significant proportion of patients. In addition to specific diagnosis and therapy, the procedure has been shown to decrease symptoms and PPI usage, and improve quality of life, independently of the findings [9].

One of the effects of endoscopy is the reassurance offered to the patient and the referring doctor. In many patients, the concern that a serious diagnosis is overlooked can severely worsen the impact of symptoms [10].

The arguments against widespread use of endoscopy are partly economic, questioning the cost-effectiveness compared to the noninvasive alternative. However, cost estimation studies suffer from variable and nonrepresentative calculations of item costs; hence, conflicting conclusions have been published in this respect. Moreover, the access to upper endoscopy is not universal, and extensive access to endoscopy may have to be balanced towards unduly long waiting lists, risking delayed diagnosis of significant pathology.

H. PYLORI TESTING

While the role of *H. pylori* in the pathogenesis of peptic ulcer disease is noncontroversial, the implications in functional dyspepsia are more debatable. Still, the latest European recommendations consider dyspepsia a valid indication for *H. pylori* eradication [11].

The utility of widespread testing relies on the accuracy of the test and the *H. pylori* prevalence in the population. The declining prevalence of *H. pylori* infection in several Western countries will impact the situation, reducing the role of *H. pylori* testing strategies [12]. Also, extended eradication activity will increase the number of antibiotics-associated side effects, which may in some cases present as prolonged diarrhea, bloating, or irritable bowel syndrome (IBS)-like symptoms. Finally, resistance to, e.g., clarithromycin is likely to increase with nondifferentiated use.

Test-and-treat implies testing dyspeptic patients by serology, breath, or fecal tests and treating accordingly. Low prevalence in the target population will lead to overtreatment from false-positive tests; however, the strategy has been shown to be effective in recent meta-analysis and would likely be a valid means of reducing the number of referrals to endoscopy in low-capacity areas [13].

Test and scope is another approach where a positive *H. pylori* test implies endoscopy, the rationale being an increased diagnostic output of the endoscopic activity, specifically by detecting ulcers. With this strategy, endoscopy-negative patients would not be offered eradication therapy. However, with the increasing adaptation of eradicating *H. pylori* even for nonulcer dyspepsia (NUD), the basis for test-and-scope is declining. Also, a number of the patients have already received PPI therapy while waiting for endoscopy, healing the ulcer that initially implicated the referral.

Finally, this strategy is likely to increase the rate of referrals to endoscopy, which will extend from age/alarm symptom-based patients to include all patients with a positive (true or false) *H. pylori* test [14].

PH AND MOTILITY TESTING

Intraesophageal pH monitoring has emerged as an objective measure of documenting pathological acid reflux, even in the context of negative upper endoscopy. With typical symptoms and a 24-h value of >3.4% (percentage of time with pH below 4), the diagnosis of nonerosive reflux disease (NERD) can formally be called. The test is among the most useful investigations in patients with noncardiac chest pain (after negative coronary workup). Its value in classical heartburn patients with a normal upper endoscopy is less well established. Nevertheless, if the symptoms are typical, the test is often recommended to objectively document the disease. Moreover, it is helpful to assess the effect of treatment (or in the workup of treatment failures) preoperatively before Nissen fundoplication.

However, it is becoming increasingly clear that a subset of patients do have acid reflux-related symptoms with normal pH-metry. If the symptom episodes correlate closely in time with the pH detected reflux episodes, the patient is likely to have reflux disease and a favorable response to PPI therapy. This entity may bear similarities to the IBS with augmented sensory signaling from the esophageal mucosa. Within research protocols, as much as 30% to 50% of patients with typical symptoms and normal endoscopy also exhibit normal pH measurements [15]. According to the Rome criteria, this does not fulfill criteria to call NERD, and the diagnosis should be functional heartburn [16]. Esophageal manometry is often performed in conjunction with pH monitoring, to determine the location of the sphincter and to document a physiological correlate to the reflux disease, e.g., low lower esophageal sphincter (LES) pressure or impaired tubular clearance motility. However, motility testing per se is rarely helpful in the workup of classical dyspepsia, being more valuable in the assessment of chest pain and dysphagia.

OTHER FUNCTIONAL DIAGNOSTICS

Functional tests for the stomach include gastric emptying tests, barostat tests to assess gastric distension sensitivity, and antroduodenal motility testing. While these tests offer interesting data for research purposes, they yet have not been found to yield much in the workup of dyspepsia [17]. This is partially due to difficulties in interpretation of the study results and also because the therapeutic consequences of the findings are limited. In clear cases of delayed emptying, therapeutic options are available prokinetics or even gastric pacemaker.

Breath tests are available for a number of gastrointestinal indications [18]. However, they are rarely helpful in the situation of unexplained dyspepsia. Most of them address issues related to general or specific malabsorption or bacterial overgrowth. One obvious exception is, however, the 13C urease breath test to determine *H. pylori* colonization in patients where endoscopy is not warranted. In summary, however, functional tests play a limited role in the clinical context of dyspepsia. Indeed, their lack of specificity may lead the diagnostic process astray.

DIAGNOSTIC ALGORITHM

Dyspepsia is a basket concept of a number of different diagnoses, and one diagnostic strategy is unlikely to be appropriate in all cases. Among the various available strategies, the challenge is to pick the right one according to the clinical setting. In the following, a few keywords are given to each of the diagnostic options (Fig. 6.1) [1].

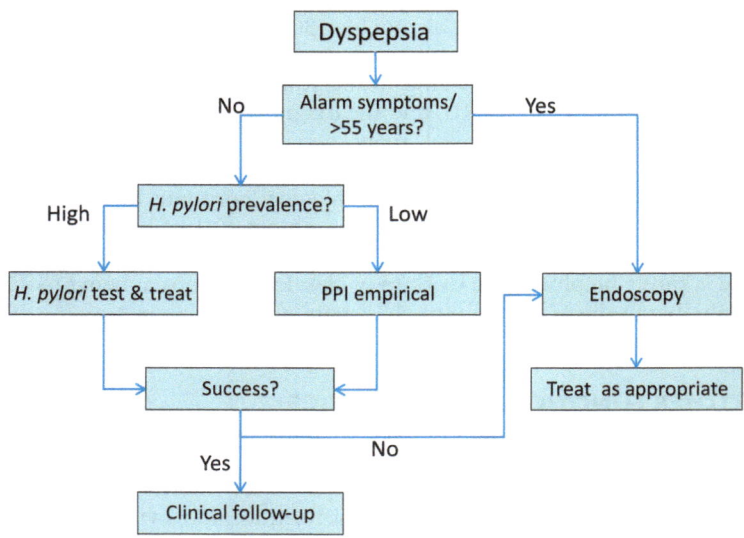

FIG. 6.1 Simplified diagnostic algorithm for simple dyspepsia.

Clinical Diagnosis

Unreliable, even in the context of minute symptom subgrouping or computer aided scoring systems

Empirical Acid Suppressant Therapy

Likely cost-effective in low-prevalence *H. pylori* areas, particularly in young patients without alarm symptoms

H. pylori Test-and-Treat

Offers cure for *H. pylori* positive subjects
Avoids endoscopy in a number of patients
May be superior to empirical PPI therapy

H. pylori Test and Scope

Unlikely to be useful due to increasing tendency to eradicate regardless of ulcer disease

Early Endoscopy

Costly, but directs further treatment accurately
Offers reassurance
Prefer in elderly population or with alarm symptoms

CONCLUSIONS

The diagnostic algorithm in dyspepsia must be adjusted according to the a priori probability of relevant diagnosis. Prevalence of *H. pylori* in the region as well as access to endoscopy will influence the priorities of the workup. However, presence of alarm symptoms and high age of the patient remain crucial factors dictating upper endoscopy. Endoscopy retains a vital role in the workup of these patients, and avoiding the procedure often just delays the diagnostic process, which in many cases will include endoscopy anyway.

References

1. Bytzer P. Diagnostic approach to dyspepsia. Best Pract Res Clin Gastroenterol. 2004;18:681–93.
2. Kapoor N, Bassi A, Sturgess R, Bodger K. Predictive value of alarm features in a rapid access upper gastrointestinal cancer service. Gut. 2005;54:40–5.
3. Wallace MB, Durkalski VL, Vaughan J, et al. Age and alarm symptoms do not predict endoscopic findings among patients with dyspepsia: a multicentre database study. Gut. 2001;49:29–34.
4. Graham DY, Rugge M. Clinical practice: diagnosis and evaluation of dyspepsia. J Clin Gastroenterol. 2010;44:167–72.

5. Talley NJ, Zinsmeister AR, Schleck CD, Melton 3rd LJ. Dyspepsia and dyspepsia subgroups: a population-based study. Gastroenterology. 1992;102:1259–68.

6. Talley NJ, Weaver AL, Tesmer DL, Zinsmeister AR. Lack of discriminant value of dyspepsia subgroups in patients referred for upper endoscopy. Gastroenterology. 1993;105:1378–86.

7. Spiegel BM, Vakil NB, Ofman JJ. Dyspepsia management in primary care: a decision analysis of competing strategies. Gastroenterology. 2002;122:1270–85.

8. Laheij RJ, Severens JL, Jansen JB, van de Lisdonk EH, Verbeek AL. Management in general practice of patients with persistent dyspepsia. A decision analysis. J Clin Gastroenterol. 1997;25:563–7.

9. Delaney BC, Wilson S, Roalfe A, et al. Cost effectiveness of initial endoscopy for dyspepsia in patients over age 50 years: a randomised controlled trial in primary care. Lancet. 2000;356:1965–9.

10. Rabeneck L, Wristers K, Souchek J, Ambriz E. Impact of upper endoscopy on satisfaction in patients with previously uninvestigated dyspepsia. Gastrointest Endosc. 2003;57:295–9.

11. Malfertheiner P, Megraud F, O'Morain C, et al. Current concepts in the management of *Helicobacter pylori* infection: the Maastricht III Consensus Report. Gut. 2007;56:772–81.

12. Kang JY, Tinto A, Higham J, Majeed A. Peptic ulceration in general practice in England and Wales 1994–98: period prevalence and drug management. Aliment Pharmacol Ther. 2002;16:1067–74.

13. Delaney BC, Moayyedi P, Forman D. Initial management strategies for dyspepsia. Cochrane Database Syst Rev. 2003:CD001961.

14. Delaney BC, Wilson S, Roalfe A, et al. Randomised controlled trial of *Helicobacter pylori* testing and endoscopy for dyspepsia in primary care. BMJ. 2001;322:898–901.

15. Martinez SD, Malagon IB, Garewal HS, Cui H, Fass R. Non-erosive reflux disease (NERD) – acid reflux and symptom patterns. Aliment Pharmacol Ther. 2003;17:537–45.

16. Winter JW, Heading RC. The nonerosive reflux disease-gastroesophageal reflux disease controversy. Curr Opin Gastroenterol. 2008;24:509–15.

17. Tack J. Mandatory and optional function tests in gastroduodenal disorders. Best Pract Res Clin Gastroenterol. 2009;23:387–93.

18. Braden B. Methods and functions: breath tests. Best Pract Res Clin Gastroenterol. 2009;23:337–52.

Chapter 7
Differential Diagnosis: Overlap Between Gastroesophageal Reflux Disease and Irritable Bowel Syndrome

Michael Häfner

Keywords: Gastroesophageal reflux, Irritable bowel syndrome, Barrett's esophagus, Functional dyspepsia

INTRODUCTION

Symptoms of dyspepsia, gastroesophageal reflux, and intestinal disorders like diarrhea or constipation are among the most common complaints in patients seeking the advice of a gastroenterologist. Although these symptom complexes are summarized in three distinct disease entities – functional dyspepsia, gastroesophageal reflux disease (GERD), and irritable bowel syndrome – several studies suggest considerable overlap between these conditions. This chapter covers the basics about the latter two diseases and the various aspects of overlap with functional dyspepsia.

GASTROESOPHAGEAL REFLUX DISEASE
Definition
Based on the Montreal consensus of 2005, GERD exists when there is reflux of contents of the stomach into the esophagus and

M. Häfner (✉)
Department of Medicine, St. Elisabeth Hospital, Vienna, Austria
e-mail: Michael.Haefner@elisabethinen-wien.at

M. Duvnjak (ed.), *Dyspepsia in Clinical Practice*,
DOI 10.1007/978-1-4419-1730-0_7,
© Springer Science+Business Media, LLC 2011

leads to symptoms with or without further complications [1]. The most common symptoms include acid reflux, heartburn, and regurgitation. Other symptoms – often referred to as extra-esophageal symptoms – include noncardiac chest pain, chronic cough of otherwise unexplained origin, asthma, or laryngitis. There is a second group of extra-esophageal manifestations referred to as proposed associations with GERD as the evidence for a direct link is weaker than for established associations like the reflux cough syndrome. Those proposed associations include pharyngitis, sinusitis, idiopathic pulmonary fibrosis, and recurrent otitis media among others (Tables 7.1 and 7.2).

Erosive lesions are not mandatory for the diagnosis of GERD but may result in complications like the formation of ulcers or strictures, hemorrhage, metaplastic change of the mucosa (Barrett's esophagus), and, ultimately, adenocarcinoma of the esophagus.

Although the term GERD is usually used in patients with erosive mucosal lesions at the gastroesophageal junctions, a majority of patients presenting with symptoms of reflux disease show no erosions on endoscopy. These patients are classified as suffering from nonerosive reflux disease (NERD). Although during white light endoscopy no lesions are found at the gastroesophageal junctions, NERD is not just a milder form of GERD as patients show life impairment similar to those suffering from erosive changes.

TABLE 7.1. Esophageal syndromes associated with gastro-esophageal reflux disease [1].

Symptomatic syndromes	Typical reflux syndrome
	Reflux chest pain syndrome
Syndromes with esophageal injury	Reflux esophagitis
	Reflux stricture
	Barrett's esophagus
	Esophageal adenocarcinoma

TABLE 7.2. Extra-esophageal syndromes associated with gastro-esophageal reflux disease [1].

Established associations	Reflux cough syndrome
	Reflux laryngitis syndrome
	Reflux asthma syndrome
	Reflux dental erosion syndrome
Proposed associations	Pharyngitis
	Sinusitis
	Idiopathic pulmonary fibrosis
	Recurrent otitis media

Additionally, patients with NERD seem to respond less well to acid suppression. Recent data suggest that 70% of reflux patients suffering from typical symptoms show no erosive changes at endoscopy making NERD the most common form of GERD [2, 3].

While symptoms related to gastroesophageal reflux, which are troublesome for a patient, are referred to as GERD, the mere presence of reflux symptoms, not troublesome to an individual, should not be classified as GERD. Usually, in population-based studies mild symptoms occurring 2 or more days a week or moderate-to-severe symptoms occurring more than 1 day a week are considered as troublesome. According to the Montreal consensus, in daily clinical practice, it is the patient who should determine if their reflux symptoms are troublesome.

Prevalence of Gastroesophageal Reflux Disease

GERD is a very common affection; however, its prevalence varies considerably over the world. The rates are highest in Europe and the USA, ranging from 10% to 20% in the adult population [4, 5]. In Asia, the prevalence is generally lower ranging from 2% to 6% [6, 7]. However, data from Singapore suggest that GERD is becoming more frequently in the Asian population over the years [8].

Diagnosis of Gastroesophageal Reflux Disease

The diagnosis of reflux disease can be challenging as the clinical presentation is extremely variable: there are asymptomatic patients presenting with Barrett's mucosa on endoscopy, while others suffer from troublesome symptoms like retrosternal burning or chest pain. The Montreal working group allows therefore basing the diagnosis of GERD on typical symptoms alone or on the basis of investigations that show the reflux of stomach contents including pH testing or impedance monitoring. Another way of diagnosing GERD is by showing the injurious effect of acid reflux, for example, by endoscopy and histology [1].

Overlap Between Gastroesophageal Reflux and Dyspepsia

The issue of overlap between functional dyspepsia (FD) on one side and gastroesophageal reflux and irritable bowel syndrome (IBS) on the other side is a controversial one and the discussion is still ongoing. While working groups in the late 1980s considered a group of reflux-like dyspepsia within FD, it was excluded later [9–11].

In a population-based study in Olmsted County, Minnesota, occurrence of heartburn and/or acid reflux was recorded at least once a week using a self-report questionnaire in 19.8% of all participants. Other frequently reported symptoms included noncardiac chest pain (23.1%), dysphagia (13.5%), and dyspepsia (10.6%). In a logistic regression model, all three symptoms were found to be associated with typical reflux. The odds ratio for dyspepsia in this study was 3.1 [12].

In a recent paper, Savarino et al. studied 200 patients with typical reflux symptoms and normal endoscopy by using 24-h impedance–pH monitoring [13]. Fifty-four patients (27%) had normal esophageal acid exposure time and a negative symptom association probability for reflux. These patients significantly suffered more frequently from postprandial fullness, bloating, early satiety, and nausea compared with patients with NERD or positive symptom association probability for acid/non-acid reflux, suggesting that functional gastrointestinal disorders occur regardless of anatomical boundaries and that there might be considerable overlap between reflux symptoms and dyspeptic complaints.

In another recent study from Korea, Lee et al. examined the prevalence for overlap between gastroesophageal reflux, dyspepsia, and IBS [14]. In a sample of 1,443 subjects (out of 1,688 randomly selected Koreans), enough data was available to calculate the risk factors and prevalence of above-mentioned affections. The prevalence of GERD, dyspepsia, and IBS was 8.5%, 9.5%, and 9.6%, respectively. An overlap between GERD and dyspepsia could be observed in 2.3% of all subjects studied. Approximately 27% of patients suffering from GERD also suffered from dyspepsia according to the Rome II criteria, while 24% of dyspeptic patients also had GERD. There was a higher risk for dyspepsia overlap compared with dyspepsia alone associated with the presence of anxiety (OR 3.1). The authors conclude that overlap between GERD, dyspepsia, and IBS is common and that mostly individuals with anxiety disorders are affected.

A Belgian study tried to assess the prevalence of dyspeptic symptoms, with and without overlapping reflux symptoms, and their impact on daily life and to compare the symptom groupings, in the general population, to patients with FD. A total of 2,025 subjects were studied using a validated questionnaire for dyspeptic and reflux symptoms [15]. A total of 417 individuals (20.6%) reported significant symptoms of dyspepsia which affected daily life in a high percentage (61.2%) and induced weight loss and absenteeism in 12.7% and 12.4%, respectively. Most interestingly, overlapping with reflux symptoms occurred in 417 of 2,025 subjects (33.8%). Furthermore, patients suffering from both dyspepsia and gastroesophageal reflux-like symptoms showed higher scores for symptom intensity and frequency. One limiting factor of the study is the fact that no specific diagnostic procedures for GERD were performed. Nonetheless, this chapter – apart from assessing the impact of dyspepsia on patient's life – shows a considerable overlap between dyspeptic and reflux-associated symptoms.

Neumann et al. evaluated the presence of functional dyspepsia and IBS in patients with erosive or NERD or Barrett's esophagus according to the Montreal classification [16]. A total of 71 patients were studied prospectively using the Rome III criteria for IBS and FD. Symptoms indicative for FD were found more frequently in patients with NERD compared with erosive reflux disease or Barrett's esophagus. However, the difference was only statistically significant when comparing the prevalence of gastric pain between patients with NERD and Barrett's esophagus. Symptoms typical for FD like bothersome fullness were extremely common, ranging from 38.5% (in patients with Barrett's esophagus) to 45.5% (patients with NERD). Prevalence was even higher for epigastric pain, being between 30.8% (Barrett's) and 69.7% (NERD). Again, this study shows a considerable overlap between various forms of GERD and symptoms of dyspepsia.

A different approach was chosen by De Vries et al. The group examined the prevalence of FD and IBS in patients with proven GERD [17]. Their study population consisted of 263 patients with GERD as diagnosed by means of 24-h pH-metry. They assessed the patient's symptoms by using a questionnaire and evaluated the prevalence of both FD and IBS, as well as health-related quality of life. Approximately 25% of patients suffering from GERD also showed symptoms of FD compared with 13% to 14% in the Dutch general population. An additional 5% had both FD and IBS. Especially in the subgroup of care-seeking patients with GERD, the percentage of patients with FD and IBS was significantly higher. While in the non-care-seeking group only 54% suffered from GERD, 30% of the care-seeking group had no concomitant functional disorder. Additionally, patients with GERD also suffering from FD/IBS had a significantly lower health-related quality of life. The authors therefore conclude that quality of life in patients with GERD is mainly affected by the existence or nonexistence of FD or IBS.

In a random sample of 730 Australian subjects, Talley et al. tried to identify distinct symptom groupings in an urban population [18]. Symptoms of gastroesophageal reflux were the most common, followed by dyspepsia (17.5% and 11.5%, respectively). In total, 92 subjects met the Rome criteria for dyspepsia. Again, there was considerable overlap of symptoms: 36.8% met both ulcer-like and reflux-like criteria and 32.9% met both dysmotility-like and reflux-like criteria. Apart from showing that gastrointestinal symptoms occur frequently in the population, this study also shows considerable overlap between IBS, FD, and GERD. The authors performed a factor analysis and found seven distinct groups of symptoms. One of the groups comprised symptomatic gastroesophageal reflux; in this group, subjects with IBS and dyspepsia according to the Rome classification had the highest scores, underlining the hypothesis of overlap between the various gastrointestinal affections.

This overlap might also explain the treatment failures seen in patients with reflux disease. A better definition and categorization of the various subgroups of patients suffering from dyspepsia, reflux symptoms, and IBS has implications for the patient's management as it allows for clearer strategies for each condition.

IRRITABLE BOWEL SYNDROME
Definition and Diagnosis

IBS consists of a group of intestinal disorders identified only by symptoms. The diagnostic criteria and management recommendation have been established by working groups and are referred to as the Rome criteria. The current version of these criteria has been published in 2006 and is known as Rome III [19]. In order to be diagnosed with IBS, patients have to complain with recurrent abdominal pain or discomfort at least 3 days per month in the last months and a symptom onset of at least 6 months prior to diagnosis. Additionally, two or more criteria consisting of improved symptoms after defecation, an initial change in stool frequency or form must be present (Table 7.3).

Supportive symptoms, according to the Rome III working group, include abnormal stool frequency, abnormal stool form, defecation straining, urgency, or feeling of incomplete bowel movement. In order to assess misleading descriptions by patients regarding constipation or diarrhea, a tool like the Bristol Stool Form Scale is frequently used to achieve reproducible results both in research and in general practice (Table 7.4) [20].

TABLE 7.3.   Diagnostic criteria for irritable bowel syndrome [19].

Recurrent abdominal pain or discomfort at least 3 days per month in the last 3 months associated with two or more of the following:
  Improvement with defecation
  Onset associated with a change in frequency of stool
  Onset associated with a change in form (appearance) of stool

TABLE 7.4. The Bristol Stool Form Scale [20].

Type	Description
1	Separate hard lumps like nuts (difficult to pass)
2	Sausage shaped but lumpy
3	Like a sausage but with cracks on its surface
4	Like a sausage or snake, smooth and soft
5	Soft blobs with clear-cut edges (passed easily)
6	Fluffy pieces with ragged edges, a mushy stool
7	Watery, no solid pieces, entirely liquid

Before diagnosing IBS, the patient's state has to be evaluated carefully. Especially, so called "alarm symptoms" like fever, anemia, obscure or overt gastrointestinal bleeding, weight loss, or the presence of an abdominal mass be taken seriously and an underlying pathology ruled out. Also, pain or discomfort associated with urination, menstruation, physical exercise, or movement is not likely to be caused by IBS. On the other hand, in women, pelvic pain, worsening of symptoms during menstruation may lead to a delayed diagnosis of IBS. Investigations, to rule out conditions other than IBS, usually include lab testing that includes the test for celiac disease. Stool examinations aim at ruling out bacterial or parasitic infections or occult blood. Breath tests for lactose and fructose intolerance should usually be performed to exclude frequent malabsorption syndromes. Finally, complete colonoscopy with intubation of the terminal ileum and multiple biopsies is usually necessary to exclude chronic inflammatory bowel diseases like Crohn's disease, ulcerative colitis, ischemic colitis or microscopic colitis, or the presence of a tumor.

Prevalence
Prevalence reported for symptoms consistent with IBS is about 10% and 20% worldwide and shows a female predominance. Symptoms may come and go, and overlap with other functional disorders that occur frequently as shown later. IBS leads to reduced quality of life and higher health care costs [19].

Overlap Between Irritable Bowel Syndrome and Dyspepsia
As already shown for the relationship between gastroesophageal reflux and dyspepsia, there seems to be considerable overlap between IBS and dyspepsia as well.

The already cited study by Lee et al. also shows an overlap of IBS and dyspepsia in 1.3% of 1,443 randomly selected Korean subjects.

While this reflects the presence of overlap in the general Korean population, overlap between dyspepsia, reflux, and IBS seems to be frequent in patients affected by gastrointestinal symptoms. In the group of patients suffering from dyspepsia, 14% had also IBS. Again, anxiety in patients with IBS leads to significantly more overlap with dyspepsia and reflux compared with IBS alone (OR 4.92) [14].

In a Spanish study on a sample of randomly chosen 264 subjects, the prevalence of dyspepsia was high, being 23.9% [21]. IBS was diagnosed based on the Rome criteria and found in 13.6%. Again, the subgroup affected by IBS also complained of dyspepsia in a high percentage (55.6%), while the prevalence of symptoms characteristic for IBS was equally high in patients with predominantly dyspepsia (31.7%) and significantly low in patients without dyspepsia (7.9%). The authors conclude that overlap between dyspepsia and IBS is very frequent suggesting various presentations of a general gastrointestinal disorder.

Choung et al. looked for dyspepsia subgroups in the Olmested county community by performing a cross-sectional study using a valid questionnaire mailed to more than 4,000 subjects (response rate 55%) [22]. They found three distinct subgroups of dyspepsia characterized by frequent upper abdominal pain, nausea and/or vomiting, and early satiety. More interestingly, overlapping with IBS was reported frequently. Among the patients with nausea and/ or vomiting, overlapping with IBS was highest, being 41%. In the group predominantly suffering from upper abdominal pain, overlapping IBS was found in 21%, and in the early satiety group in 32%. Again, the authors struggle in stating whether dyspepsia and IBS are two distinct processes or simply different manifestations of an irritable gut.

An interesting paper was recently published by Agréus et al. [23]. They tested the stability, consistency, and relevance of the current classifications for dyspepsia and IBS in an unselected population of subjects with gastrointestinal symptoms. In this Swedish cohort, the prevalence of dyspepsia was 14%. In the subgroup of subjects with IBS, 87.5% also fulfilled the criteria for dyspepsia. Even by excluding persons reporting reflux symptoms, the overlap diminished but did not fall below 50%. The authors conclude that, because of the lack of natural symptom clusters and the resulting high percentage of overlap, as well as flux between symptom classes over time, the current separation of various gastrointestinal symptoms into dyspepsia, its subgroups, and IBS might be inappropriate. They conclude that there might be a common underlying mechanism explaining all functional gastrointestinal symptoms or that the symptoms may represent unspecific responses to a variety of pathophysiological (and eventually psychological) disorders.

Agréus et al. also found that approximately 50% of subjects with IBS and dyspepsia changed their symptom profile over a 1-year period. They showed a considerable flux between the syndromes, as well as appearance or disappearance of symptoms over time. About 20.4% of persons who were symptom-free at the first survey showed symptoms of either dyspepsia or IBS a year later, and 17.9% of subjects who complained of symptoms at baseline were symptom-free after a year. Only 37.3% of the responders were free of symptoms at the time of both surveys.

A change of the predominant diagnosis over time was also found by Papatheodoridis and Karamanolis in a Greek urban population [24]. Out of 700 persons studied, 53% reported one or more gastrointestinal symptoms during the week prior to answering the questionnaire and 55% during the past 6 months. The most common affection reported was dyspepsia (48%), followed by GERD (38%) and IBS (21%). However, only one disorder was diagnosed in 25%, while 75% of symptomatic subjects were diagnosed of having two or all three disorders. The combination of dyspepsia and IBS was recorded to be present during the last week prior to the study in 6.1% of all individuals and during the last 6 months in 5.6%, respectively. Although the authors did not use the Rome criteria for the diagnosis of IBS and therefore its prevalence might be overestimated, the published data is in line with other studies. In accordance with the findings of Agréus et al., the predominant symptom changed over time in a number of patients. IBS was predominant in 28% according to the severity of the previous week's symptoms compared with 19% of the preceding 6 months. Dyspepsia was predominant in the previous week in 7% and in 16% in the preceding 6 months, respectively.

IBS can be arbitrarily divided into two groups, defined by primary bowel patterns of constipation (IBS-C) and diarrhea (IBS-D). Talley et al. studied 121 patients with IBS for the presence of FD and divided the cohort into two groups according to their bowel habits [25]. They found statistically significant more overall gastrointestinal symptoms in IBS patients with predominantly constipation when compared with those suffering from diarrhea (6.67 vs. 4.62, respectively). Upper abdominal pain was more frequent in patients with IBS-C (36.8%) than in those with IBS-D (24.4%), as well as bloating (75% vs. 40.9%, respectively). In general, overlap between IBS and dyspepsia (and GERD) was found frequently in both groups: 85.5% of patients with IBS-C were also diagnosed with FD, while 75% of subjects with IBS-D fulfilled the criteria for FD.

While this study potentially reflects pathophysiological differences between the two subgroups of patients with IBS, it also clearly shows the considerable overlap between IBS and other gastrointestinal affections like FD and GERD.

Finally, in a recent study by Wang and colleagues, the clinical overlap between FD and IBS based on the Rome III criteria was examined in a Chinese population [26]. Although the study suffers from some limitations like a potential selection bias, it adds to our knowledge regarding the relationship between dyspepsia and IBS. In total 3,014 patients, attending a gastroenterology outpatient clinic, returned a questionnaire based on the Rome III criteria (response rate 89.2%). Based on this self-report questionnaire, 15.2% of the subjects fulfilled the criteria for FD alone and 10.9% for IBS alone. An additional 5.0% presented with an overlap between FD and IBS. If the patient fulfilled the Rome III criteria for IBS, the risk for also suffering from FD was doubled compared with non-IBS subjects (OR 2.09). Additionally, patients with overlap between the two conditions had higher severity scores for postprandial fullness (2.35 vs. 1.49, respectively) and a higher overall FD score (6.65 vs. 5.82, respectively). Again, this study shows that overlap between FD and other gastrointestinal affections like IBS occurs frequently and that the disorders seem to be associated. This particular paper suggests that the presence of postprandial fullness may predict an overlap between the two conditions.

CONCLUSIONS

As we have shown, in recent years several studies have addressed the overlap between FD and IBS. Both affections are very common and are among the most frequent conditions that lead to the consultation of a gastroenterologist. As shown above, they are usually considered to be distinct entities, although overlapping seems to occur frequently. Published data suggest that at least 40% of patients presenting to gastroenterologists show overlapping between FD and IBS [27, 28]. In the study by Agréus et al., this overlap even reached 90%. Early satiety and postprandial fullness are more common in patients with constipation-predominant IBS and also seem to be predictive for an overlap between dyspepsia and IBS. Also, the presence of overlap seems to be associated with a significantly higher symptom severity than the presence of IBS alone [29].

Overlap is not only reported in studies from tertiary referral centers but also from primary care, suggesting a natural pattern of the condition more than a matter of selection bias. Although there are many studies showing overlap between dyspepsia and IBS, most authors conclude that the current evidence is insufficient to determine whether both affections are two separate processes or different manifestations of a single condition. Cremonini and Talley hypothesize that the distinction between FD and IBS is artificial and that we are most likely dealing with a single disease leading to various symptoms and disturbances [30].

In line with these assumptions, others too suggested the existence of an irritable gut leading to various symptoms like dyspepsia, IBS, or gastroesophageal reflux. This is further emphasized by the fact that there is considerable flux between the various symptom groups over time. Despite the ongoing discussion, the key consideration has to be whether distinguishing between the various forms of functional gastrointestinal disorders leads to improved treatment outcomes. Current evidence suggests that this is not the case and that treatment of functional disorders remains a complex issue leading to combination therapies in clinical practice [31].

References

1. Vakil N, van Zanten SV, Kahrilas P, Dent J, Jones R, Global Consensus Group. The Montreal definition and classification of gastroesophageal reflux disease: a global evidence-based consensus. Am J Gastroenterol. 2006;101:1900–20.
2. Smout AJPM. Endoscopy-negative acid reflux disease. Aliment Pharmacol Ther. 1997;11 Suppl 2:81–5.
3. Lind T, Havelund T, Carlsson R, et al. Heartburn without esophagitis: efficacy of omeprazole therapy and features determining therapeutic response. Scand J Gastroenterol. 1997;32:974–9.
4. Dent J, El-Serag HB, Wallander MA, Johansson S. Epidemiology of gastro-oesophageal reflux disease: a systematic review. Gut. 2005;54:710–7.
5. Stanghellini V. Relationship between upper gastrointestinal symptoms and lifestyle, psychosocial factors and co-morbidity in the general population: results from the domestic/international gastroenterology surveillance study (DIGEST). Scand J Gastroenterol Suppl. 1999;231:29–37.
6. Chen M, Xiong L, Chen H, Xu A, He L, Hu P. Prevalence, risk factors and impact of gatroesophageal reflux disease symptoms: a population based study in South China. Scand J Gastroenterol. 2005;40:750–67.
7. Wong WM, Lai KC, Lam KF, et al. Prevalence, clinical spectrum and health care utilization of gastro-esophageal reflux disease in a Chinese population: a population-based study. Aliment Pharmacol Ther. 2003;18:595–604.
8. Lim SL, Goh WT, Lee JM, Community Medicine GI Study Group, et al. Changing prevalence of gastro-esophageal reflux with changing time: longitudinal study in an Asian population. J Gastroenterol Hepatol. 2005;20:995–1001.

9. Colin-Jones DG, Bloom B, Bodemar G, et al. Management of dyspepsia: report of a working party. Lancet. 1988;1:576–9.

10. Barbara L, Camilleri M, Corinaldesi R, et al. Definition and investigation of dyspepsia. Consensus of an international ad hoc working party. Dig Dis Sci. 1989;34:1272–6.

11. Talley NJ, Stanghellini V, Heading RC, Koch KL, Malagelada JR, Tytgat GNJ. Functional gastroduodenal disorders. Gut. 1999;45 Suppl 2:37–42.

12. Locke GR, Talley NJ, Fett SL, et al. Prevalence and clinical spectrum of gastro-esophageal reflux: a population-based study in Olmstead County, Minnesota. Gastroenterology. 1997;112:1448–56.

13. Savarino E, Pohl D, Zentilin P, et al. Functional heartburn has more in common with functional dyspepsia than with non-erosive reflux disease. Gut. 2009;58:1185–91.

14. Lee SY, Lee KJ, Kim SJ, Cho SW. Prevalence and risk factors for overlaps between gastroesophageal reflux disease, dyspepsia, and IBS: a population-based study. Digestion. 2009;79:196–201.

15. Piessevaux H, De Winter B, Louis E, et al. Dyspeptic symptoms in the general population: a factor and cluster analysis of symptom groupings. Neurogastroenterol Motil. 2009;21:378–88.

16. Neumann H, Monkemuller K, Kandulski A, Malfertheiner P. Dyspepsia and IBS symptoms in patients with NERD, ERD and Barrett's esophagus. Dig Dis. 2008;26:243–7.

17. De Vries DR, Van Herwaarden MA, Baron A, Smout AJ, Samsom M. Concomitant functional dyspepsia and irritable bowel syndrome decrease health-related quality of life in gastroesophageal reflux disease. Scand J Gastroenterol. 2007;42:951–6.

18. Talley NJ, Boyce P, Jones M. Identification of distinct upper and lower gastrointestinal symptom groupings in an urban population. Gut. 1998;42:690–5.

19. Longstreth GF, Thompson WG, Chey WD, Houghton LA, Mearin F, Spiller RC. Functional bowel disorders. Gastroenterology. 2006; 130:1480–91.

20. O'Donnell LJD, Virjee J, Heaton KW. Detection of pseudodiarrhoea by simple clinical assessment of intestinal transit rate. Br Med J. 1990;300:439–40.

21. Caballero-Plasencia AM, Sofos-Kontoyannis S, Valenzuela-Barranco M, Martín-Ruiz JL, Casado-Caballero FJ, López-Mañas JG. Irritable bowel syndrome in patients with dyspepsia: a community-based study in southern Europe. Eur J Gastroenterol Hepatol. 1999;11:517–22.

22. Choung RS, Locke GR, Schleck CD, Zinsmeister AR, Talley NJ. Do distinct dyspepsia subgroups exist in the community? A population-based study. Am J Gastroenterol. 2007;102:1983–9.

23. Agréus L, Svärdsudd K, Nyrén O, Tibblin G. Irritable bowel syndrome and dyspepsia in the general population: overlap and lack of stability over time. Gastroenterology. 1995;109:671–80.

24. Papatheodoridis GV, Karamanolis DG. Prevalence and impact of upper and lower gastrointestinal symptoms in the Greek urban general population. Scand J Gastroenterol. 2005;40:412–21.

25. Talley NJ, Dennis EH, Schettler-Duncan VA, Lacy BE, Olden KW, Crowell MD. Overlapping upper and lower gastrointestinal symptoms in irritable bowel syndrome patients with constipation or diarrhea. Am J Gastroenterol. 2003;98:2454–9.
26. Wang A, Liao X, Xiong L, et al. The clinical overlap between functional dyspepsia and irritable bowel syndrome based on Rome III criteria. BMC Gastroenterol. 2008;8:43.
27. Stanghellini V, Tosetti C, Barbara G, et al. Dyspeptic symptoms and gastric emptying in the irritable bowel syndrome. Am J Gastroenterol. 2002;97:2738–43.
28. Holtmann G, Goebell H, Talley NJ. Functional dyspepsia and irritable bowel syndrome: is there a common pathophysiological basis? Am J Gastroenterol. 1997;92:954–9.
29. Corsetti M, Caenepeel P, Fischler B, Janssens J, Tack J. Impact of co-existing irritable bowel syndrome on symptoms and pathophysiological mechanisms in functional dyspepsia. Am J Gastroenterol. 2004;99:1152–9.
30. Cremonini F, Talley NJ. Review article: the overlap between functional dyspepsia and irritable bowel syndrome: a tale of one or two disorders? Aliment Pharmacol Ther. 2004;20 Suppl 7:40–9.
31. Gwee KA, Chua AS. Functional dyspepsia and irritable bowel syndrome, are they different entities and does it matter? World J Gastroenterol. 2006;12:2708–12.

Chapter 8
Management of Uninvestigated Dyspepsia

Marko Duvnjak, Marija Gomerčić, and Sanja Stojsavljević

Keywords: Uninvestigated dyspepsia, Diagnosis, Treatment, Management, Guidelines, Test-and-treat, Acid suppressive therapy, Endoscopy

INTRODUCTION

Patients with new-onset or recurrent dyspeptic symptoms, but without previous investigations (diagnostic procedures), primarily upper gastrointestinal (GI) endoscopy, are defined as having "uninvestigated dyspepsia." Based on the results of performed diagnostic workup, patients are redefined as having organic (structural) or functional dyspepsia that subsequently requires appropriate specific management. Test-and-treat, empiric acid suppressive therapy, test-and-scope, and prompt endoscopy are diagnostic and therapeutic tools commonly applied in the management of uninvestigated dyspepsia. The choice of management strategy is determined by degree of possibility of underlying disease and cost effectiveness. Due to numerous randomized controlled trials (RCTs) that have compared these different strategies, the evidence base for the management of uninvestigated dyspepsia is one of the largest and most extensive ones, although

M. Gomerčić (✉)
Division of Gastroenterology and Hepatology,
Department of Medicine, 'Sestre milosrdnice' University Hospital,
Zagreb, Croatia
e-mail: marijagomercic@yahoo.com

M. Duvnjak (ed.), *Dyspepsia in Clinical Practice*,
DOI 10.1007/978-1-4419-1730-0_8,
© Springer Science+Business Media, LLC 2011

RCTs have often been underpowered to observe plausible minor dissimilarities in symptom outcomes [1–8]. Majority of countries, in an attempt to diminish healthcare expenses and standardize clinical practice, embraced evidence-based guidelines for the management of dyspepsia. Since a detailed comparison of utility and cost effectiveness of each strategy is elaborated in other chapters, here we will provide an insight into differences and similarities of present guidelines. Variations in the definition of dyspepsia, structure of development group, efficacy of alarm symptoms in the detection of underlying serious disease, age threshold, initial management, and management of nonresponders will be described in detail. The guidelines evaluated in this chapter have been created by the American College of Gastroenterology (ACG), American Gastroenterological Association (AGA), Canadian Dyspepsia (CanDys) Working Group, England and Wales National Institute of Clinical Excellence (NICE), Scottish Intercollegiate Guidelines Network (SIGN), and the Asia-Pacific Working Party (Fig. 8.1) [9–15]. Management of the underlying diseases exceeds the content of this chapter and is elaborated in others.

DEFINITION AND GUIDELINE DEVELOPMENT GROUPS
Although majority of guidelines, ACG, AGA, SIGN, and Asia-Pacific Working Party, used the Rome criteria in classifying patients with dyspepsia [those with gastroesophageal reflux disease (GERD) were excluded], there was a difference in the composition of development groups [10, 11, 14, 15]. The ACG and AGA guidelines are most alike since they were both written by gastroenterologists together with the ACG Practice Parameters Committee and AGA Clinical Practice and Economics Committee, respectively [10, 11]. In contrast, SIGN guidelines were developed from general health practice perspective by diverse specialists such as gastroenterologists, primary care physicians, pharmacists, dieticians, general surgeons, nurses, radiologists with involvement of patient representatives, and methodology experts [14]. Asia-Pacific Working Party consisted of four invited speakers and audience of medical practitioners who with joined forces established algorithms for management of dyspepsia in this specific geographical region [15]. NICE guidelines and CanDys Working Group were both developed from a primary care perspective, with the involvement of gastroenterologists and pharmacists to a lesser extent in NICE group, but they differ in defining of dyspepsia symptoms. NICE group defined dyspepsia as presence of any symptom of the upper gastrointestinal tract including recurrent epigastric pain, heartburn,

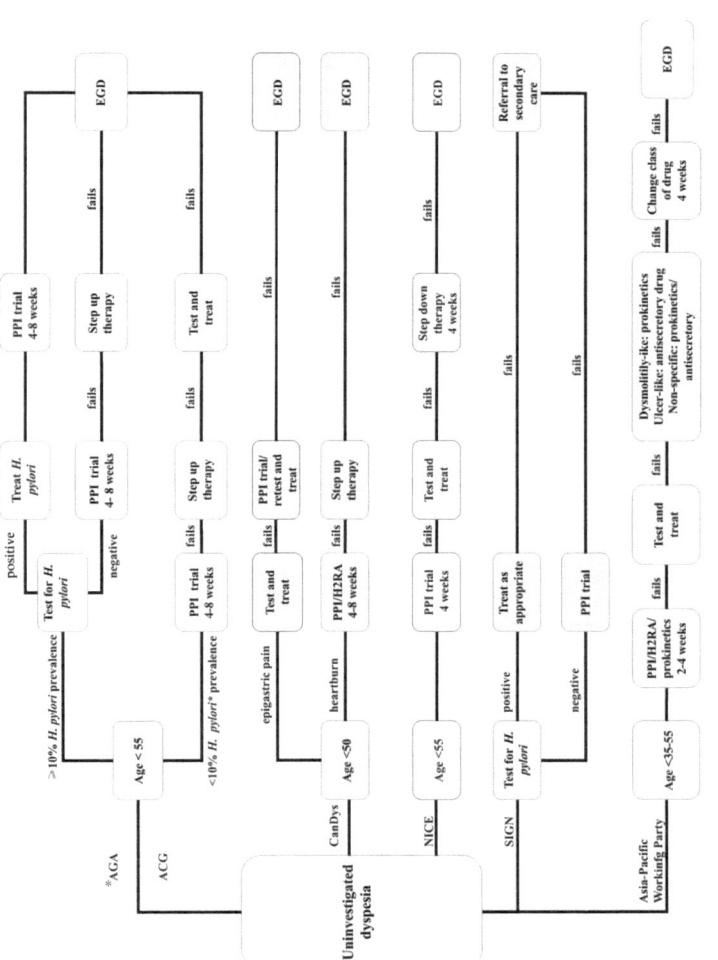

*AGA: ≥ 10% H. pylori prevalence-test and treat; 5-10%-therapy is uncertain; <5%-PPI trial.

FIG. 8.1   Summary of algorithm guidelines in young patients without alarm symptoms [10–15].

or acid regurgitation, with or without bloating, nausea, or vomiting [13]. CanDys Working Group defined dyspepsia as all upper GI symptoms, except isolated heartburn [12].

PROMPT ENDOSCOPY
Alarm Symptoms (Red Flags, Alert Features, Warning Signs)

Even though existing national guidelines and recommendations on managing dyspepsia differ in initial steps for patients without alarm symptoms, they all agree in necessity of performing upper GI endoscopy in dyspeptic patients with the alarm signs (Table 6.1). Since alarm signs warn clinicians of possibility of serious clinical illness (e.g., malignancy) or pathology (e.g., peptic ulcer), all national guidelines recommend referral to endoscopic investigation for dyspeptic patients of any age with alarm symptoms [10–15]. Even though present guidelines agree on the management of these patients, prospective studies provide little evidence that alarm symptoms anticipate upper GI malignancy.

Vakil et al. conducted a systematic review and meta-analysis of 15 studies, evaluating a total of 57,363 patients with 458 (0.8%) cases of cancer, to assess the diagnostic accuracy of alarm symptoms in predicting the presence of otherwise unsuspected underlying malignancy in dyspeptic patients [16]. Alarm signs were appraised by three modalities: direct assessment of presence or absence of alarm features, assessment by physician (general practitioner or specialist), and computer models derived from symptom questionnaires. Sensitivity of assessed alarm symptoms varied from 0% to 83% with pooled sensitivity 67%, specificity from 40% to 98%, and pooled specificity 66%. Accuracy of other tools used for assessment of alarm signs also varied widely. Furthermore, clinical opinion made by a physician was very specific (97% to 98%) but not very sensitive (11% to 53%), in contrast to computer models which were very sensitive (75% to 100%), but had a modest specificity (21% to 49%). The disappointing performance of alarm symptoms was reflected in the generally poor diagnostic odds ratios (DORs). The pooled DOR was 7.49 (95% CI: 4.37–12.8) and area under the curve was 0.80 (95% CI: 0.73–0.85), indicating that there was moderate accuracy in investigated methods for diagnosing upper GI malignancy. In conclusion, based on presented data, neither clinical opinion, nor computer models, nor alarm features by themselves are accurate predictors of underlying severe GI pathology. Under presumption that unsatisfactory accuracy of summarized alarm signs in predicting possible underlying malignancy is due to different predictive value of each sign, several alarm signs were assessed individually. Weight loss, anemia, and dysphagia were appraised, resulting in pooled sensitivities that varied between 13% and 49%, and specificity from 85% to 95%. Alarm features had low positive predictive value meaning that GI malignancy increases slightly when alarm features are present but absolute increase of GI malignancy in detected cases was small, and therefore inadequate for a meaningful conclusion. Even though all individual alarm signs presented with high negative predicative value, they are not a specific attribute, when absent, in ruling out malignancy. Therefore, results only reflected a low prevalence of malignancy (0.8%) in dyspeptic patients. It seems that the major problem lies in the varying prevalence of GI malignancy and varying thresholds for the determination of whether alarm features were present (e.g., severity or duration of the alarm feature that would lead to inclusion is not defined). Unfortunately, at this time there is no evidence for a particular threshold that would determine whether a symptom qualifies as an alarm feature and this should be a priority for further studies. Although it might seem that the most logical alternative strategy is to recommend endoscopy based on age when alarm symptoms arise, all studies that evaluated computer models in this meta-analysis included age and gender but there was no significant improvement in accuracy of alarm signs. Possibly, combinations of alarm symptoms (e.g., weight loss and dysphagia) and physical signs could improve diagnostic accuracy and have greater predictive value than alarm signs individually. However, it should be taken in consideration that study results obtained in Western countries, which have a lower prevalence of GI malignancy. In the end, clinicians have to be aware that more efficient ways of predicting underlying GI malignancy are emerging. Accurate prediction of upper GI malignancy and reduction in the number of dyspeptic patients undergoing unnecessary GI endoscopy is a final goal, but until better approaches emerge alarm symptoms should not be abandoned. We assume that identifying features with high specificity, quantifying thresholds of each alarm feature or their specific combinations will be more successful in revealing underlying malignancy.

Age Threshold

All national guidelines, except SIGN, have determined an age threshold that is considered as an alarm symptom and therefore implies urgent GI endoscopy. Present national guidelines tried to set an appropriate age threshold with acceptable level of risk for missing upper GI malignancy, based on the significantly increased risk of upper GI malignancy with age. The main rationale for accepted age thresholds of 50 or 55 years in Western countries for performing endoscopy in the investigation of dyspepsia is due to increased incidence of gastric and esophageal cancer above this age [10, 13, 17–19]. The age threshold recommended by ACG, AGA, and NICE guidelines is 55 years [11–13]. The CanDys Working Group, based on expert opinion, accepted an age cut-off of 50 years since there is no randomized controlled data to state differently [12]. SIGN, however, did not suggest an age cut-off due to the lack of evidence that GI cancer found during upper GI endoscopy in dyspeptic patients is more prevalent than in age matched [14]. The age threshold given by Asia-Pacific Party is lower when compared with other working groups due to the higher risk of gastric cancer or other GI pathology; therefore, age cut-off is set between 35 and 55 years depending on the country in this geographical region (e.g., Australia: 55 years old, Japan: 35 years old) [15]. Even though age thresholds have been determined by national guidelines, it is opinion of GI community that age threshold should be assessed locally, based on known regional correlation between age and incidence of upper GI malignancies.

Trials that determinate age thresholds for upper endoscopy in dyspeptic patients in European developing countries are surprisingly rare, where one should expect age cut-offs to be at a lower level because of relatively higher incidences of upper GI malignancies in younger age groups [20, 21]. For example, study conducted in Poland reported that 24% of patients with gastric cancer were younger than 45 [21]. Also, age in combination with gender seems to enhance the capability for predicting upper GI malignancy in patients with uninvestigated dyspepsia, resulting in different age thresholds depending on gender. This means that age threshold should be lower in males and higher in females [22]. In addition, Salkic et al. showed that thresholds of 45 years for males and 50 years for females in Bosnia and Herzegovina have a small level of risk of missing upper GI malignancy and are acceptable to use in areas with low availability of endoscopy [23]. Another important axiom is that in many of the Western nations, the number of immigrants originating from developing countries is increasing, where upper GI malignancy is not so rare at a younger age and they should be managed bearing in mind their native age thresholds.

INITIAL MANAGEMENT OF PATIENTS UNDER AGE THRESHOLD WITHOUT ALARM SYMPTOMS

ACG Guidelines Recommend as Initial Management Strategy

- In populations with moderate to high prevalence of *Helicobacter pylori* (*H. pylori*) infection (≥10%), patients should undergo test-and-treat strategy
- In low-prevalence populations (<10%, high socioeconomic standard areas), an empirical acid suppression with proton pump inhibitor (PPI) for 4–8 weeks is proposed

These recommendations are based on the RCT trials in which rationale for test-and-treat strategy, in populations with high *H. pylori* infection prevalence, was supported by the identification of an underlying peptic ulcer disease even though cure of *H. pylori* infection will lead only to a minority of patients with symptom improvement. RCT trials showed no difference in symptom outcome when comparing test-and-treat with prompt endoscopy and that empiric antisecretory therapy can lead to inappropriately treated peptic ulcer disease, misdiagnosis at subsequent endoscopy, and long-term inappropriate maintenance therapy, which the patient does not require. Therefore, prompt GI endoscopy and empiric PPI therapy are not the management options of choice in *H. pylori*-positive patients in areas with high *H. pylori* prevalence [10].

AGA Guidelines Recommend as Initial Management Strategy

- In populations with moderate-to-high prevalence of *H. pylori* infection (≥10%), patients should undergo test-and-treat strategy
- In 5% to 10% prevalence of *H. pylori* infection strategy is uncertain
- In low-prevalence populations (high socioeconomic standard areas), an empirical acid suppression with PPI for 4–8 weeks is proposed

Test-and-treat strategy in regions with >10% prevalence is a first-line strategy even though it offers a cure to a small number of patients, but benefits of symptom relief are increased by the potential prevention of distal gastric cancer and subsequently reduced mortality. It seems that benefit of test-and-treat over acid suppression therapy in infected patients is greater, but in *H. pylori*-negative patients or population with low prevalence of *H. pylori* infection it vanishes, and therefore in those groups of patients acid suppression trial is recommended. Although endoscopy compared with test-and-treat and empirical acid suppression strategies shows more benefit, its invasiveness and costs diminish it [11].

CanDys Working Group Recommend as Initial Management Strategy

- Empiric acid suppression (PPIs) for 4–8 weeks if heartburn is predominant symptom and in *H. pylori*-negative dyspeptic patients
- Test-and-treat strategy if epigastric pain is predominant symptom

PPI over H2RA, standard dose of PPI over lower dose, longer duration of the PPI treatment (4–8 weeks) over shorter showed in patients with heartburn as predominant symptom better effect on symptom resolution and healing in patient with erosive gastritis and nonerosive reflux disease (NERD), and thereby PPIs are recommended as a first-line therapy in this group.

The benefits of the test-and-treat strategy lie in identification of underlying ulcer disease and in improving symptoms in a small proportion of patients with functional dyspepsia [12].

NICE Guidelines Recommend as Initial Management Strategy

- Empirical treatment with a PPI for a month or test-and-treat strategy (there is no recommendation which should be offered first)

Recommendations for empirical treatment with PPIs are based on data which show that PPIs are more effective than H2RAs and antacids at reducing dyspeptic symptoms, and early endoscopy has not been presented to give better patient outcomes when compared with empirical treatment. In addition, test-and-treat strategy showed to be more effective than empirical acid suppression at reducing dyspeptic symptoms after 1 year in trials of *H. pylori*-positive patients and reduced number of endoscopies resulting in portentous cost savings [13].

SIGN Guidelines Recommend as Initial Management Strategy

- *H. pylori* Test-and-treat

H. pylori test-and-treat seems to be an appropriate strategy when compared with empirical antisecretory therapy, early endoscopy, and test-and-scope. Endoscopy is more costly, acid suppression therapy deprives those with underlying ulcer disease from being cured by eradication of *H. pylori,* and test-and-scope is no more effective than selective endoscopy. Since the prevalence of *H. pylori* in Scottish is high, test-and-treat seems to be noninvasive and cheaper strategy compared with GI endoscopy and so preferred strategy [14].

Asia-Pacific Party Recommend as Initial Management Strategy
- Antisecretory therapy (PPI or H2RA) at standard dose or prokinetics with a duration less than 2–4 weeks

This recommendation is based on the fact that significant percentage of patients will respond to this treatment, due to given drug or placebo, and subsequently have a long-term remission without implying further investigation (GI endoscopy). Therefore, the Asia-Pacific Working Party considers this approach to be a less expensive alternative and appropriate strategy in countries with limited health resources [15].

MANAGEMENT OF NONRESPONDERS TO FIRST-LINE STRATEGY (PATIENTS UNDER AGE THRESHOLD WITHOUT ALARM SYMPTOMS)
ACG Guidelines Recommend
- In populations with moderate to high prevalence of *H. pylori* infection (≥10%), *H. pylori*-positive patients in whom eradication is successful but symptoms do not resolve, a trial of acid suppression is indicated
- In populations with moderate to high prevalence of *H. pylori* infection (≥10%), in *H. pylori*-negative patients, if acid suppression fails after 2–4 weeks it is reasonable to step up therapy (changing dose or drug class). In patients who do respond to initial 4–8 weeks acid suppression in whom symptoms recur, same treatment is justified.
- In low-prevalence populations (<10%, high socioeconomic standard areas), if the patients fail to respond or relapse rapidly after ceasing empiric antisecretory therapy, test-and-treat strategy is indicated before referral for upper GI endoscopy

Their recommendations are based on an opinion that endoscopy adds little to young patients who are nonresponders to *H. pylori* test-and-treat or initial PPI therapy due to a very low probability of finding relevant organic disease in this group of patients, decision whether to endoscope is based on clinical judgment. Although they state that some patients, particularly those who are anxious, may require the reassurance gained by endoscopy, it should not be routinely offered [10].

AGA Guidelines Recommend
- In *H.* pylori-negative patients or *H. pylori*-positive patients who had successful eradication but symptoms continue, a short course of PPI is proposed

- If standard PPI doses fail, a trial of a double dose is proposed

These recommendations are based under assumption that some patients will respond and PPIs can be discontinued after 4 weeks without recurrence. In a case of relapse, long-term PPI therapy is recommended [11].

CanDys Working Group Recommends
- For patients with nonheartburn-dominant dyspepsia who tested positive for *H. pylori* and have symptoms despite successful treatment, possible options are retest and subsequent therapy, empiric PPI trial, or endoscopy if indicated
- For *H.pylori*-negative or heartburn-dominant nonresponders after initial empiric acid therapy, step-up approach is recommended, PPI if an H2RA was given, or double dose of a PPI, or treatment for a further 4–8 weeks with the same dose. PPI should be discontinued and endoscopy should be performed in a case patient fails to improve with the course of double-dose PPI for 4–8 weeks. Also recommendations for partial responders were given. They are defined by one or more of the following: partial symptom control, returning clinic visits, or hesitation to continue with given therapy. In these patients, most likely medication compliance has a big role; therefore, it is rationale to switch medications (H2RA to PPI) or increase the dose for another 4- to 8-week period

It should be pointed out that majority of the patients, who presented with heartburn as dominant symptom, with erosive gastritis or NERD will require maintenance therapy in a shape of continuous or intermittent acid suppression therapy, endoscopic antireflux procedures, or surgery [12].

NICE Guidelines Recommend
- If the patient relapses after first-line approach, step-down PPI therapy is proposed to the lowest dose required to control symptoms. Attempt with H2RA or prokinetic therapy is advised if there is an inadequate response to a PPI due to a possibility of poor individual response to a drug [13]

SIGN Guidelines Recommend
- There is no explicit statement for this topic [14].

Asia-Pacific Working Party Recommends
- If there is no response or patients relapse after initial empiric acid suppression and/or prokinetics therapy, test-and-treat is

option of choice. For patients who test negative for *H. pylori* and symptoms are still present the following is proposed:

- Patients with ulcer-like symptoms should be treated with antisecretory therapy at standard dose
- Patients with dysmotility-like symptoms should be treated with prokinetics
- Patients with nonspecific symptoms should be treated with either of these alternatives

After 4 weeks of empiric therapy and no response, another class of therapy should be prescribed, e.g., antisecretory therapy should be substituted with prokinetics [15].

CONCLUSIONS

Despite the fact that the guideline development groups are characterized by their varying structure and methodology used, their recommendations were outstandingly similar. Guidelines are based on regional H. pylori prevalence, prevalence of underlying diseases and healthcare standard. Although guidelines are based on a wide variety of clinical research and systematical reviews, there are questions that still cry out for their answers. Utility of each alarm symptom and their combination, age threshold based on known regional correlation between age and incidence in detecting underlying GI malignancy and prevalence of *H. pylori* at which test-and-treat is cost effective point out that new trials are still needed.

References

1. Arents NLA, Thijs JC, van Zwet AA, et al. Approach to treatment of dyspepsia in primary care: a randomized trial comparing 'test-and-treat' with prompt endoscopy. Arch Intern Med. 2003;163:1606–12.
2. Bytzer P, Hansen JM, Schaffalitzky de Muckadell OB. Empirical H2-blocker therapy or prompt endoscopy in management of dyspepsia. Lancet. 1994;343:811–6.
3. Delaney BC, Wilson S, Roalfe A, et al. Cost effectiveness of initial endoscopy for dyspepsia in patients over age 50 years: a randomised controlled trial in primary care. Lancet. 2000;356:1965–9.
4. Delaney BC, Wilson S, Roalfe A, et al. Randomised controlled trial of *Helicobacter pylori* testing and endoscopy for dyspepsia in primary care. Br Med J. 2001;322:898–901.
5. Duggan AE, Elliott CA, Miller P, et al. Clinical trial: a randomized trial of endoscopy, *Helicobacter pylori* testing and empirical therapy for the management of dyspepsia in primary care. Aliment Pharmacol Ther. 2009;29:55–68.

6. Jarbol DE, Kragstrup J, Stovring H, et al. Proton pump inhibitor or testing for *Helicobacter pylori* as the fi rst step for patients presenting with dyspepsia? A cluster-randomized trial. Am J Gastroenterol. 2006;101:1200–8.

7. Lassen AT, Pedersen FM, Bytzer P, et al. *Helicobacter pylori* test and eradicate versus prompt endoscopy for management of dyspeptic patients: a randomised trial. Lancet. 2000;356:455–60.

8. Lewin van den Broek NT, Numans ME, Buskens E, et al. A randomised controlled trial of four management strategies for dyspepsia: relationships between symptom subgroups and strategy outcome. Br J Gen Pract. 2001;51:619–24.

9. Ford AC, Moayyedi P. Current guidelines for dyspepsia management. Dig Dis. 2008;26(3):225–30. http://content.karger.com/produktedb/produkte.asp?typ=fulltext&file=000121351. Accessed 20 Apr 2010.

10. Talley NJ, Vakil N, the Practice Parameters Committee of the American College of Gastroenterology. Guidelines for the management of dyspepsia. Am J Gastroenterol. 2005;100:2324–37.

11. American Gastroenterological Association. American Gastroenterological Association technical review on the evaluation of dyspepsia. Gastroenterology. 2005;129:1756–80.

12. Veldhuyzen van Zanten S, Bradette M, Chiba N, Armstrong D, Barkun A, Flook N, et al. Evidence-based recommendations for short- and long-term management of uninvestigated dyspepsia in primary care: an update of the Canadian Dyspepsia Working Group (CanDys) clinical management tool. Can J Gastroenterol. 2005;19:285–303.

13. Dyspepsia: managing dyspepsia in adults in primary care, 2004. National Institute for Clinical Excellence Web Site. http://www.nice.org.uk/. Updated August 2004. Accessed 20 Apr 2010

14. Dyspepsia: a national clinical guideline, 2003. Scottish Intercollegiate Guidelines Network. www.sign.ac.uk/pdf/sign68.pdf. Updated March 2003. Accessed Apr 2010

15. Talley NJ, Lam SK, Goh KL, Fock KM. Management guidelines for uninvestigated and functional dyspepsia in the Asia-Pacific region: first Asian Pacific working party on functional dyspepsia. J Gastroenterol Hepatol. 1998;13:335–53.

16. Vakil N, Moayyedi P, Fennerty MB, Talley NJ. Limited value of alarm features in the diagnosis of upper gastrointestinal malignancy: systematic review and meta-analysis. Gastroenterology. 2006;131:390–401. quiz 659–60.

17. Christie J, Shepherd NA, Codling BW, Valori RM. Gastric cancer below the age of 55: implications for screening patients with uncomplicated dyspepsia. Gut. 1997;41:513–7.

18. Gillen D, McColl KE. Does concern about missing malignancy justify endoscopy in uncomplicated dyspepsia in patients aged less than 55? Am J Gastroenterol. 1999;94:75–9.

19. Eisen GM, Dominitz JA, Faigel DO, et al. The role of endoscopy in dyspepsia. Gastrointest Endosc. 2001;54:815–7.

20. Ferlay J BF, Pisani P, Parkin DM. GLOBOCAN 2002: Cancer Incidence, Mortality and Prevalence Worldwide. IARC CancerBase No. 5, version 2.0, 2004

21. Boldys H, Marek TA, Wanczura P, Matusik P, Nowak A. Even young patients with no alarm symptoms should undergo endoscopy for earlier diagnosis of gastric cancer. Endoscopy. 2003;35:61–7.

22. Marmo R, Rotondano G, Piscopo R, et al. Combination of age and sex improves the ability to predict upper gastrointestinal malignancy in patients with uncomplicated dyspepsia: a prospective multicentre database study. Am J Gastroenterol. 2005;100:784–91.

23. Salkic NN, Zildzic M, Zerem E, et al. Simple uninvestigated dyspepsia: age threshold for early endoscopy in Bosnia and Herzegovina. Eur J Gastroenterol Hepatol. 2009;21:39–44.

Chapter 9
Management of *Helicobacter pylori* Infection

Marko Duvnjak and Ivan Lerotić

Keywords: *Helicobacter pylori*, Noninvasive tests, Invasive tests, Treatment, Indications for treatment, Eradication control

INTRODUCTION

The discovery of *Helicobacter pylori* (*H. pylori*) in 1982 by Barry Marshall and Robin Warren was the starting point of a new era in understanding and management of gastroduodenal diseases. *H. pylori* is a spiral-shaped, gram-negative, microaerophilic, urease-producing bacterium. It is one of the most common human infections worldwide, and it is estimated that about one half of the world's population is infected [1]. The risk of acquiring *H. pylori* infection is related to socioeconomic status, living conditions, and habits that we acquire from early childhood. Person-to-person transmission through either fecal-to-oral or oral-to-oral exposure seems to be the most probable way of acquiring the infection. In developing nations, where the majority of children are infected before the age of 10, the prevalence in adults exceeds 80% [1]. In developed countries, detection of the infection in children is unusual but becomes more common during adulthood, and the prevalence increases up to 50% in the elderly population [1].

I. Lerotić (✉)
Division of Gastroenterology and Hepatology, Department
of Medicine, 'Sestre milosrdnice' University Hospital, Zagreb, Croatia
e-mail: ilerotic@kbsm.hr

M. Duvnjak (ed.), *Dyspepsia in Clinical Practice*,
DOI 10.1007/978-1-4419-1730-0_9,
© Springer Science+Business Media, LLC 2011

Approximately 30% to 40% of the United States (US) population is infected with *H. pylori* [2]. In North America, the prevalence of *H. pylori* among Asian Americans, African Americans, and Hispanics is similar to the one found in developing countries [3]. Once acquired, infection persists in the stomach for years and may or may not produce a gastroduodenal disease. Over 80% of individuals infected with the bacterium are asymptomatic. However, *H. pylori* infection is the main risk factor for a broad variety of chronic gastrointestinal diseases such as chronic gastritis, peptic ulcer disease, gastric adenocarcinoma, and gastric mucosa-associated lymphoid tissue (MALT) lymphoma.

H. PYLORI TESTING

It is important to emphasize that *H. pylori* testing should be performed only if the clinician plans to offer treatment in the case of a positive result [2].

Diagnostic tests for *H. pylori* can be divided into two groups: noninvasive tests, which do not require endoscopy, and invasive methods, which require upper endoscopy and are based on the analysis of gastric biopsy specimens. The choice of the test depends on availability, clinical setting, pretest probability of infection, and expenditure. Upper gastrointestinal bleeding, use of antisecretory drugs, bismuth, or antibiotics can influence the results of certain tests and therefore also influence the choice of test. Table 9.1 summarizes the characteristics of different diagnostic tests used for the detection of *H. pylori* infection.

Noninvasive methods should be preferred in all situations where the extra information yielded by an endoscopy is not necessary. They can also be used along with the invasive tests to improve diagnostic accuracy. A great number of patients infected with

TABLE 9.1.   Diagnostic tests for *Helicobacter pylori* infection.

	Sensitivity (%)	Specificity (%)	Comments
Noninvasive tests			
$^{13/14}$C-urea breath test[a]	95–100	98–100	Excellent PPV and NPV The most accurate non-invasive test Useful before and after treatment
^{13}C-bicarbonate assay[a]	92–100	96–97	Rarely used in clinical practice Reliable before and after treatment

(continued)

TABLE 9.1. (continued)

	Sensitivity (%)	Specificity (%)	Comments
Stool antigen test[a]	96	97	Inexpensive Useful before treatment (polyclonal and monoclonal) and after treatment (monoclonal more reliable) Excellent PPV and NPV irrespective of *H. pylori* prevalence False positive in bleeding peptic ulcer
Serology	85–96	73–93	Inexpensive and convenient Requires local validation Very good NPV, but variable PPV (depends on *H. pylori* prevalence) Alternative to urea breath test and stool antigen test before treatment Not useful in the control of eradication
Invasive tests			
Biopsy urease test[a]	90–95	95–100	The cheapest biopsy-based test Sensitivity higher when biopsies from both antrum and corpus are taken Some commercial tests not fully sensitive before 24 h Less sensitive than histology in the control of eradication
Histology[a]	>95	100	Multiple biopsies of antrum and corpus required Gives additional histologic information
Culture[a]	78–80	100	Expensive, difficult to perform Poor sensitivity, excellent specificity Allows antibiotic susceptibility testing

PPV positive predictive value
NPV negative predictive value
[a]Sensitivity reduced by antisecretory therapy, antibiotics, and bismuth-containing compounds. Patient should be off antibiotics and bismuth for at least 4 weeks and off proton pump inhibitors for at least 2 weeks

H. pylori who present with dyspeptic symptoms initially consult their primary care physician. The underlying pathology of dyspepsia is often unknown; nevertheless, many of these cases can be managed in primary care by using "test-and-treat" strategy. It is strongly recommended that noninvasive tests should be used in this setting [4].

NONINVASIVE TESTS

A variety of noninvasive tests for the diagnosis of *H. pylori* infection is available. These include urea breath tests (UBTs), ^{13}C-bicarbonate assay, stool antigen tests, and antibody tests (serology). UBT and stool antigen test identify the presence of active *H. pylori* infection, while antibody tests identify an immunological reaction to the infection.

$^{13/14}$C-Urea Breath Tests

The $^{13/14}$C-UBTs identify active *H. pylori* infection by the detection of urease enzyme in the stomach of an infected person. Since human stomach does not produce urease normally and *H. pylori* is the most common urease-producing gastric pathogen, detection of urease enzyme generally denotes the presence of *H. pylori* infection.

In this simple test, the patient drinks a solution of urea, labeled with either the non-radioactive isotope ^{13}C or the radioactive isotope ^{14}C. If *H. pylori* urease is present in the stomach, the urea is hydrolyzed into ammonia and carbon dioxide, and labeled carbon dioxide is quantified in expired breath samples (Fig. 9.1) [5]. Both ^{13}C- and ^{14}C-UBT can be performed in about 20 min, and they have similar accuracy. However, UBT using ^{13}C-labeled urea is preferred by most physicians and has become the most widely used since it is completely innocuous. Although the dose of radiation in the tests using radioactive ^{14}C isotope is minimal (less than daily background radiation exposure), it should not be used in children and pregnant women, and it is also not approved in many countries [6, 7]. The main problem of the ^{13}C-UBT is its high cost due to high initial economical investment in the necessary equipment. At the moment, it is more costly than the antibody test or stool antigen test. However, it is becoming increasingly more available.

UBT is the most accurate noninvasive test for the diagnosis of *H. pylori* infection with very high sensitivity and specificity, both over 95% [5]. It provides excellent accuracy both for the initial diagnosis of *H. pylori* infection and for the confirmation of its eradication after the treatment [8–11].

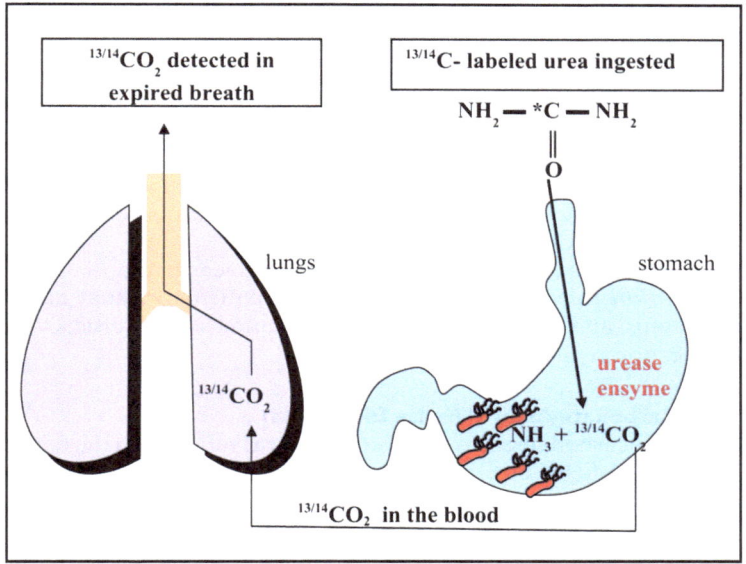

Fig. 9.1   The principle of the urea breath test.

Use of proton pump inhibitors (PPIs), bismuth-containing compounds, or antibiotics can induce false negative results by reducing intragastric bacterial load (density) or inhibiting urease activity [5, 12, 13]. Therefore, in order to reduce false negative results, the patient should discontinue antibiotic and bismuth therapy for at least 4 weeks and PPI therapy for at least 2 weeks prior to the UBT [2, 14, 15]. Although it is still controversial whether the H2-receptor antagonists can decrease the sensitivity, most studies suggest that this actually does occur and it is reasonable that the H2-receptor antagonist treatment is withheld for 1–2 weeks prior to the UBT [16–18]. Antacids on the other hand do not reduce the sensitivity of UBT and therefore need not be stopped prior to testing [12]. False positive results of UBT are uncommon.

A clinical situation where *H. pylori* diagnosis is indispensable and challenging is the one where the patient is hospitalized due to the bleeding peptic ulcer. In such cases, early diagnosis of *H. pylori* is essential because it is of great importance that the patient is conclusively discharged with prescribed eradication therapy, which will guarantee the treatment of the underlying infection. In this clinical setting, UBT is more accurate than biopsy-based testing. To preclude false negative results due to PPI therapy, testing should be performed as soon as possible. However, most *H. pylori*-positive patients with bleeding ulcers, despite previous treatment with high-dose PPIs, have a positive UBT when performed after resuming oral feeding [19]. In some cases, the infection cannot be detected with this first UBT; therefore, *H. pylori* needs to be definitively excluded with a second UBT performed after stopping PPIs or with another invasive or noninvasive (serology) test.

In summary, UBT is the method of choice in the diagnosis of *H. pylori* infection in young dyspeptic patients without alarm symptoms and in the noninvasive evaluation of the efficacy of eradication regimens [2, 4].

[13]C-Bicarbonate Assay (Urease Blood Test)

The ^{13}C-bicarbonate assay (urease blood test) relies upon the detection of ^{13}C-labeled bicarbonate in a blood sample taken before and 60 min after ingestion of a ^{13}C-urea rich meal. It reliably identifies active *H. pylori* infection before and after treatment. Available data, although limited, suggest high-level sensitivity, specificity, and accuracy of up to 100, 97, and 97%, respectively [20, 21]. However, this test is rarely used in clinical practice, and it is not approved in most countries. Further clinical trials are needed to evaluate its accuracy.

Stool Antigen Test

The stool antigen test is based on the finding that *H. pylori* is present in the stool of infected patients [22]. Testing identifies *H. pylori* antigen in the stool by enzyme immunoassay with the use of polyclonal or monoclonal (developed more recently) anti-*H. pylori* antibodies. It utilizes anti-*H. pylori* capture antibody adsorbed to microwells. A diluted stool sample and a peroxidase-conjugated antibody are added to the wells and incubated for 1 h at room temperature. Unbound material is removed by washing. After addition of a substrate solution, color changes in the presence of a bound enzyme. The results are interpreted visually or spectrophotometrically, and the color change indicates the presence of *H. pylori* antigen. This can be performed in less than 90 min by any laboratory, since no special equipment is needed.

A systematic review of 89 studies, evaluating the stool antigen tests before and after eradication therapy, demonstrated very good sensitivity, specificity, and positive and negative predictive values for the polyclonal test before treatment (91, 93, 92, and 87%, respectively), but sensitivity and positive predictive value were not satisfactory after therapy (86 and 76%, respectively), leading to significant proportion of false positive results. On the other hand, the monoclonal test had excellent sensitivity, specificity, positive and negative predictive values before (96, 97, 96, and 97%, respectively) as well as after therapy (95, 97, 91, and 98%, respectively) [23]. A meta-analysis of 22 studies, evaluating the performance of monoclonal stool antigen test in diagnosing *H. pylori* infection, confirmed that it is an accurate noninvasive method both for the initial diagnosis of *H. pylori* infection and for the confirmation of its eradication after treatment and that the monoclonal technique has higher sensitivity than the polyclonal one, especially in the posttreatment setting [24]. Most of the available data suggest that the stool antigen test should be performed not earlier than 4–8 weeks after *H. pylori* treatment in evaluation of eradication success [23]. Although some data indicate that the test may be effective as early as 7–14 days after eradication, studies evaluating the stool antigen test performance within 4 weeks after treatment have reached contradictory conclusions [25, 26].

Sensitivity of the stool antigen tests is reduced, equally common as in UBT, by the use of PPIs, antibiotics, and bismuth-containing compounds [12, 27, 28]. Therefore, recommendations regarding the use of these medications related to UBT can also be applied to the stool antigen testing. On the other hand, specificity is significantly reduced in the setting of upper gastrointestinal bleeding, resulting in a great number of false positive results [29–31]. This is probably due to the presence of blood constituents that cross-react in the enzyme immunoassay [30]. Therefore, the stool antigen test is not reliable for diagnosing *H. pylori* infection in patients with bleeding peptic ulcers.

At the moment, the stool antigen test is considered acceptable on the same grounds as UBT for *H. pylori* diagnosis, especially in the case of implementation of test-and-treat strategy [4]. Both polyclonal and monoclonal stool antigen tests can be used as an alternative to UBT in the diagnosis of *H. pylori* infection prior to therapy, but monoclonal antibody-based test is more reliable in confirming eradication [2].

A novel rapid *H. pylori* stool antigen test (in-office stool test) that can be performed during outpatient visits (provides results in 5 min) has recently become available [32]. However, additional clinical trials are needed for better evaluation of its accuracy.

Serology

Serologic testing relies upon the detection of *H.pylori*-specific IgG antibodies in serum, mostly by enzyme-linked immunosorbent assay.

Laboratory-based serology is the simplest, cheapest, and the most widely available noninvasive diagnostic test for the evaluation of *H. pylori* status.

However, there are certain concerns regarding its accuracy. A systematic review of studies evaluating the performance characteristics of different serological assays reported that their overall sensitivity was 92% (range 85% to 96%), specificity 83% (range 73% to 92%), and the diagnostic accuracy was low (<90%) [33]. Diagnostic performances of various serology kits differed substantially because commercially available serology kits were based on various antibody preparations and were used with different study populations. However, recent study showed that some kits may have high diagnostic accuracy (>90%), with sensitivity and specificity of 95 and 92.6%, respectively [34]. It is important to note that serology assays using bacterial antigens from one part of the world may not perform well when applied to another population, since the antigenic properties of local bacterial strains may differ [35]. Every serologic test should therefore be validated locally before routine use [4].

It is also important to emphasize that the positive predictive value of serology is greatly influenced by the prevalence of *H. pylori* infection in the population. Low positive predictive value in populations with low prevalence of infection limits its usefulness in clinical practice because of great number of false positive results [36]. If the pretest probability of infection is low in a specific patient (e.g., patient with dyspeptic symptoms without evidence of peptic ulcer disease, with low prevalence of infection in the population), negative serologic test helps to exclude infection. In this setting, positive test is more likely to be false positive and should be confirmed with another noninvasive test (UBT or stool antigen test) before starting treatment. This approach would reduce the number of unnecessarily treated patients [37, 38].

Serologic tests are not appropriate for monitoring the treatment success, since the IgG anti-*H. pylori* antibodies remain detectable even 18 months after successful eradication [39].

Considering all available data, serology may be used as an alternative to UBT and stool antigen test for diagnosis prior to treatment, but it is less efficient and requires local validation for appropriate accuracy. On the other hand, it is not useful in the control of eradication [4].

There are some conditions in which intragastric bacterial density is low, which reduces the accuracy of all noninvasive and invasive diagnostic tests, except serology. These conditions include bleeding ulcers, extensive gastric atrophy, MALT lymphoma, and the current use of PPIs, bismuth, or antibiotics. In these cases, serology testing should be considered, especially if negative result is obtained with another test [4, 27, 40, 41].

Whole blood tests and office-based serology tests, although very convenient, have not reached acceptable accuracy for the diagnosis of *H. pylori* infection and currently have no role in the management of *H. pylori* infection [4, 42, 43]. The detection of *H. pylori* antibodies in urine and saliva is possible but has also no role in patient management [4].

INVASIVE TESTS

Endoscopy is not indicated if the establishment of *H. pylori* status is the only goal. However, if endoscopy is indicated based upon the patient's clinical presentation, biopsy-based tests are the most appropriate tool for the diagnosis of *H. pylori* infection. Invasive or biopsy-based diagnostic techniques include biopsy urease test, histology, culture, and polymerase chain reaction.

Diagnostic accuracy (sensitivity in particular) of all invasive tests is diminished in patients taking antisecretory therapy, antibiotics, or bismuth-containing compounds. If the patient has not recently been taking these medications, rapid urease test offers the optimal combination of reliability and availability. Unfortunately, many patients referred to endoscopy are taking some of these medications, most often a PPI. In this situation, histological testing of samples taken from both antrum and corpus with or without additional biopsy urease test may be performed, but false negative results are still possible and a negative result should be reevaluated. In this setting, it is even more reasonable not to perform invasive diagnostics, but to plan noninvasive testing after withholding the previously mentioned medications for a certain period of time. Therefore, it would be the best if the patient could discontinue PPI, antibiotic, and bismuth therapy as previously mentioned in the section on UBT [2].

During an acute phase of ulcer bleeding, the sensitivity and negative predictive value of the biopsy urease test and, although less significantly, histology, are also reduced [44–47]. Therefore, a positive result of these tests is reliable, but negative result should be confirmed with another test to prevent false negative findings. Noninvasive tests seem to be more sensitive than invasive tests in detecting *H. pylori* infection in the clinical setting of bleeding peptic ulcer [45]. Serologic tests represent a reasonable choice due to their high positive predictive value in the setting of high pretest probability of *H. pylori* infection, and the prevalence of the infection in these patients with bleeding ulcer is expected to be high. UBT can be used as soon as possible, but the negative result has to be reassessed due to the aforementioned reasons.

Biopsy Urease Test or Rapid Urease Test

Biopsy urease test or rapid urease test identifies active *H. pylori* infection by the detection of urease enzyme in the gastric biopsy specimen. It is the most convenient and the cheapest biopsy-based test, and it should be the first choice among invasive diagnostic tests for *H. pylori* infection.

When endoscopy is performed, one antral biopsy specimen is placed into a medium containing urea and a pH-indicator. Obtaining tissue samples from two sites, antrum and corpus, may increase the sensitivity of the test, especially in the setting of recent or ongoing antisecretory therapy [48–50]. In the presence of *H. pylori's* urease, urea is metabolized to bicarbonate and ammonia, leading to a pH increase. pH-indicator changes color (e.g., pH-indicator phenol red changes color from yellow to red or violet), which often occurs within minutes but can require up to 24 h (depending on bacterial density in the biopsy spacemen and the type of the test used). A change of color signifies active infection [50].

The first-generation commercial kits were agar based (e.g., CLO-test, Hp-fast, HUT-test). These tests may become positive as early as 1 h after collection, but if negative, a final reading after 24 h is strongly recommended. The second-generation kits are strip-based tests with two areas separated by a microporous membrane, one where the urease hydrolyzes urea and the other where NH_3 is trapped and causes a change in the pH (e.g., PyloriTek, ProntoDry). The strip-based tests provide results within 1 h [50].

The sensitivity of both biopsy urease tests is approximately 90% to 95%, and specificity is 95% to 100% [51–53]. Therefore, considering the strip-based tests, the sensitivity of the final reading is not significantly different from that of the CLO-test, but the last reading can be done after 1 h instead of 24 h for the CLO-test [50]. A significant proportion of endoscopists read the CLO-test earlier than recommended, which leads to a marked decrease in sensitivity (about 20% reduction) [50].

False positive results of the biopsy urease tests are uncommon, and a positive result is considered to be sufficient to initiate treatment [4]. As mentioned above, false negative results can occur in patients taking antisecretory drugs, antibiotics, or bismuth-containing compounds, and in the setting of recent upper gastrointestinal bleeding (sensitivity reduced by up to 25%) [44, 51, 54, 55].

Histology

Histology was the first diagnostic method applied for the detection of *H. pylori*. It relies upon the microscopic examination of biopsy specimens of gastric mucosa. In addition to *H. pylori* detection, histological study yields information regarding the presence, degree, and pattern of inflammation (gastritis). It also provides the detection of mucosal atrophy, intestinal metaplasia, dysplasia, MALT lymphoma, and carcinoma. This ability to evaluate pathologic changes associated with *H. pylori* infection is a great advantage of this diagnostic method.

Since the distribution and density of *H. pylori* varies within the stomach, particularly with the ongoing antisecretory therapy, multiple biopsies of both the corpus and antrum are required for accurate diagnosis. Biopsy site preferences and number vary in clinical practice, but sensitivity increases with the number of biopsies taken [56]. The usual recommendation derived from the Sydney system is to obtain two biopsy specimens from the antrum and two specimens from the corpus for the diagnosis of *H. pylori* infection and classification of gastritis, as it was confirmed by a recent study [57, 58]. An additional specimen taken from the gastric angle improves the determination of gastritis [57]. According to the American College of Gastroenterology recommendations, a minimum of three biopsies should be obtained to optimize the diagnostic accuracy of histology in the diagnosis of *H. pylori:* one from the greater curvature of the antrum, one from the angulus, and one from the greater curvature of the corpus [2, 59].

Biopsy specimens are immediately introduced into a fixative of 10% formaldehyde, which maintains the morphology of the bacteria. The sample can be sent to the laboratory at room temperature. Storage in formaldehyde is limited because, after a week, the diagnosis becomes difficult [50]. The routine hematoxylin-eosin stain is not well suited for *H. pylori* detection. There are several special stains that allow for better visualization, and Giemsa stain is the most commonly used (Fig. 9.2) [50].

Histology is an accurate test for the detection of *H. pylori* infection, achieving sensitivity and specificity of over 95% [2]. Sensitivity is decreased in patients taking antisecretory therapy, antibiotics, and bismuth, but it is still higher than biopsy urease test in this setting. High cost of histology and its limited availability are the problems recognized worldwide.

Brush Cytology of Gastric Mucosa

Brush cytology of gastric mucosa to detect *H. pylori* infection is not routinely used in clinical practice, but the available data are

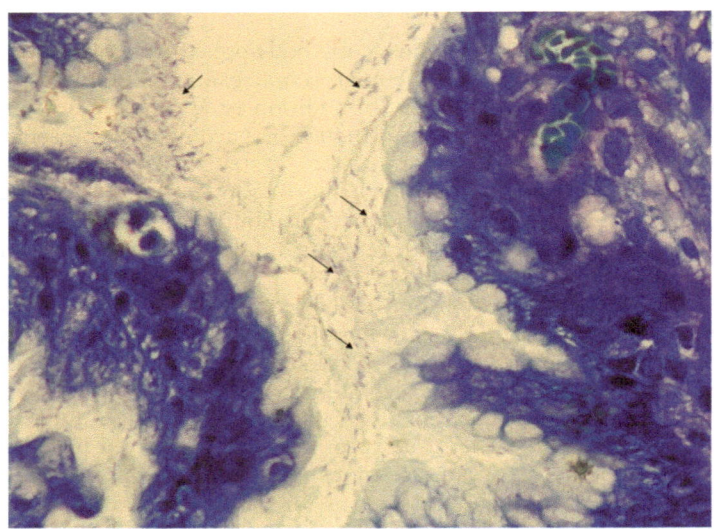

FIG. 9.2 The Giemsa stained gastric biopsy spacemen showing large colonies of *H. pylori* (*arrows*) on the cell epithelial surface (Courtesy of Drinko Baličević, MD, PhD, "Sestre milosrdnice" University Hospital, Zagreb, Croatia).

encouraging. Published studies report sensitivity and specificity to be over 95% [60, 61].

Bacterial Culture and Antibiotic Susceptibility Testing

Bacterial culture and antibiotic susceptibility testing is a demanding and expensive method that is not widely available. Therefore, it is not routinely used for the diagnosis of *H. pylori* infection but only when antibiotic susceptibility testing is necessary. However, culturing *H. pylori* after repeated therapy failure and testing the strains for antimicrobial susceptibility is becoming increasingly important with higher prevalence of drug resistance. Furthermore, in areas with a high primary resistance to a certain antibiotic (e.g., clarithromycin), it may be performed even before the initial eradication protocol to optimize the therapy.

The best samples used to culture *H. pylori* are gastric biopsy specimens obtained during endoscopy. It is of paramount importance that the patient is not taking antisecretory drugs (at least 2 weeks) and antibiotics (at least 4 weeks) prior to the procedure. The number of biopsies needed to maximize the accuracy of the test remains a subject of controversy. *H. pylori* may have a patchy distribution, and the more biopsy specimens analyzed, the higher is the chance of organism detection. It is recommended to take two biopsy specimens from the antrum and two specimens from the corpus [50]. After antisecretory therapy, the corpus may be the only site that remains positive. If we plan to take a biopsy for both culture and histology during the same endoscopy, biopsy specimens for culture must be taken first (before specimens for histological examination), in order to eliminate the risk of contamination of this sample with formaldehyde (fixative for histology sample), which kills the bacteria [50].

Another key point is the transport of the biopsy specimens from the endoscopy department to the laboratory. It is important not to expose the biopsy specimens to air. They should be placed either in a saline solution for short-term transport (4 h maximum) or in a transport medium (usually semisolid agar) maintained at 4°C for long-term transport (up to 24 h). If these transport conditions cannot be provided, biopsy specimens should be frozen at –70°C or in liquid nitrogen in a dry tube and transported to the laboratory in a frozen condition [50, 62].

Once the organism is cultured, its identity can be confirmed by its typical appearance on Gram's stain and its positive reactions in oxidase, catalase, and urease tests. Moreover, the organism's susceptibility to antibiotics can be determined. Culture requires from 3 to 10 days depending on the growth, and further susceptibility testing will take 3–4 additional days [50].

Microbiologic culture has extremely high specificity in diagnosing *H. pylori* (up to 100%), but it is very insensitive (sensitivity 70% to 80%) because of the difficulties with *H. pylori* isolation [63].

Polymerase Chain Reaction
Polymerase chain reaction is a very sensitive technique that can be used to detect *H. pylori* in various samples, including gastric biopsies. This method can also identify some mutations associated with antibiotic resistance, which is of great importance. However, it is not routinely used in clinical practice [64–67].

INDICATIONS FOR *H. PYLORI* ERADICATION THERAPY

As *H. pylori* has consistently been associated with a wide range of upper gastrointestinal disorders, use of the treatment aimed at clearance of the infection has an important role in the management of these entities and has been extensively investigated in numerous studies.

TABLE 9.2.   Indications for the treatment of *Helicobacter pylori* infection.

Gastric mucosa-associated lymphoid tissue (MALT) lymphoma
Peptic ulcer disease (active or not)
Following gastric surgery for peptic ulcer
Gastritis with severe abnormalities
Post-gastric cancer resection
Patients who are first degree relatives of gastric cancer patients
Uninvestigated dyspepsia
Functional dyspepsia (after full investigation)
Chronic NSAID therapy
Patients with otherwise unexplained iron deficiency anemia
Patients with chronic idiopathic thrombocytopenic purpura
In response to patients' wishes after appropriate consultation with physician

Indications for *H. pylori* eradication therapy are summarized in Table 9.2, and the rationale for each of these indications is given in the following text.

H. pylori and Gastric Mucosa-Associated Lymphoid Tissue Lymphoma

An increasing amount of evidence suggests that *H. pylori* infection plays a key role in the pathogenesis and natural history of gastric MALT lymphoma [68, 69]. Because of the fact that localized disease often responds to the eradication of *H. pylori*, accurate staging is of paramount importance for appropriate management of these patients [70, 71]. A series of studies have shown that *H. pylori* eradication alone leads to a complete remission in 62% to 85% of patients with localized low-grade gastric MALT lymphoma [72, 73]. Therefore, eradication therapy is strongly recommended in *H. pylori* positive patients with low-grade gastric MALT lymphoma and, moreover, it is the treatment of choice in stage 1 disease [4]. Recurrence rate of such cases of MALT lymphoma is 3% to 13% over 5 years of follow up, and subsequent life-long follow up with histological surveillance and testing for *H. pylori* is necessary [73–75].

A recent study suggests that individual patients with an early stage gastric high-grade MALT lymphoma (diffuse large B cell lymphoma) who are *H. pylori* positive may also benefit from *H. pylori* eradication therapy [76].

H. pylori and Peptic Ulcer Disease

Globally, more than 80% of duodenal ulcers and more than 60% of gastric ulcers are related to *H. pylori* infection [77, 78]. Infected individuals have a four- to tenfold higher risk of peptic ulcer development than those who are not infected [79, 80]. All this points out that there is an apparent link between *H. pylori* infection and pathogenesis of peptic ulcer disease [81]. A meta-analysis revealed that 12-month remission rate was 97% for gastric ulcer and 98% for duodenal ulcer in patients successfully treated for *H. pylori* infection. In contrast, remission rate was only 61% for gastric ulcer and 65% for duodenal ulcer in those patients with persistent infection [82]. Several other meta-analyses confirmed that *H. pylori* eradication, compared to other treatment options, significantly reduces the risk of peptic ulcer recurrence, development of complications, rebleeding rate, and is cost-effective [83–85].

Therefore, *H. pylori* eradication is strongly recommended in all infected patients with documented duodenal or gastric ulcer disease (both active ulcer disease and past history) and patients following gastric surgery for peptic ulcer [2, 4].

H. pylori and Gastric Cancer

H. pylori has been identified as a group 1 carcinogen (definitely carcinogenic) by the World Health Organization. The risk of developing gastric cancer is increased by three to six times in infected persons [86, 87]. *H. pylori* is the most important cause of chronic gastritis, a condition that initiates the pathophysiological sequence of adverse events leading to atrophic gastritis, metaplasia, dysplasia, and subsequently, cancer [88]. A number of studies have demonstrated a clear association between *H. pylori* infection and both histological types of gastric cancer, intestinal and diffuse [89–91]. It was also observed that eradication of *H. pylori* prevents development of preneoplastic lesions (atrophic gastritis and intestinal metaplasia) and appears to reduce the risk of gastric cancer in high-risk populations [92–95]. Therefore, *H. pylori* eradication is strongly recommended in patients with severe forms of chronic gastritis and those who have already undergone early gastric cancer resection [4]. *H. pylori* eradication is also strongly recommended in patients who are first-degree relatives of gastric cancer patients because they are at a significantly higher risk of developing gastric cancer than the general population [4, 96, 97]. At present, there is still insufficient data to recommend screening asymptomatic patients for *H. pylori* to prevent gastric cancer on a widespread basis.

H. pylori and Uninvestigated Dyspepsia

The test and treat strategy for *H. pylori* infection is a proven management strategy for patients with symptoms of dyspepsia who are under the age of 45–55 and have no "alarm symptoms" (bleeding, anemia, early satiety, anorexia, unexplained weight loss, dysphagia, odynophagia, recurrent vomiting, abdominal mass, family history of gastrointestinal malignancy) [2, 4, 98]. The age cutoff value may vary locally, considering the differences in the incidence of gastric malignancy and the mean age of gastric cancer onset. This group of patients under the cutoff limit should be tested for *H. pylori* using one of the noninvasive methods and, if positive, treated with *H. pylori* eradication therapy. Test-and-treat strategy is safe, improves symptoms, reduces the number of endoscopies performed, reduces administration of antisecretory drugs, and is cost-effective [99–103]. Patients over the recommended age and those with alarm symptoms regardless of their age should be referred to a specialist for endoscopy and are candidates for invasive diagnostics.

H. pylori and Functional (Nonulcer) Dyspepsia

Eradication of *H. pylori* in patients with functional dyspepsia (after careful exclusion of other pathologies that can cause symptoms of dyspepsia) remains controversial. A recent meta-analysis has reported that *H. pylori* eradication provides modest but statistically significant benefit in patients with functional dyspepsia and may be cost-effective. Therapeutic gain of eradication over placebo is 8%, and 15 infected patients need to be treated to cure one case of functional dyspepsia [104, 105]. However, when effective, this therapy leads to long-term symptom improvement. Therefore, *H. pylori* eradication is considered appropriate for patients infected with *H. pylori* and functional dyspepsia [4, 106, 107].

H. pylori and Gastroesophageal Reflux Disease

The relationship between *H. pylori* infection and gastroesophageal reflux disease (GERD) still has not been defined completely. There is no clear evidence to support the suggestion that *H. pylori* eradication can provoke the development of GERD, exacerbate pre-existing GERD, or affect the outcome of PPI therapy [108–112]. Therefore, planned eradication should not be abandoned due to concerns of causing or worsening GERD.

On the other hand, most *H. pylori* positive patients with GERD have a corpus-predominant gastritis, and there are conflicting data whether the long-term profound acid suppression can accelerate the progression of *H. pylori*-induced corpus-predominant atrophic gastritis. Some studies suggested that patients who are infected with *H. pylori* and maintained on PPI therapy are at risk for developing atrophic gastritis, but this finding has not been confirmed in other reports [113–115]. Based upon these observations, routine testing for *H. pylori* cannot be recommended in GERD [2]. However, some authorities suggest that *H. pylori* testing and eradication should be considered in patients receiving long term PPI therapy for GERD [4]. In conclusion, due to the inconsistency of published data, further prospective studies are necessary to give a final verdict on this topic.

H. pylori and the Use of Nonsteroidal Anti-Inflammatory Drugs

The use of nonsteroidal anti-inflammatory drugs (NSAIDs) and *H. pylori* infection are independent risk factors for peptic ulcer disease and ulcer bleeding. Furthermore, *H. pylori* infection increases the risk of peptic ulcer disease and ulcer bleeding in NSAID users. A meta-analysis of 16 studies reported that *H. pylori* infection increases the risk of peptic ulcer disease in NSAID users by 3.53-fold in addition to the risk associated with NSAID use [116]. *H. pylori* infection and NSAIDs also increase the risk of ulcer bleeding by 1.79- and 4.85-fold, respectively, compared to the general population. The risk of ulcer bleeding is increased by 6.13-fold when both factors are present together [116].

Results of *H. pylori* eradication studies in NSAID users are complicated. Due to the complexity of pathogenesis of ulcer disease in *H. pylori*-infected NSAID users, we can expect eradication therapy to reduce the risk of ulcer disease but not to eliminate it. Identification and treatment of *H. pylori* infection in NSAID-naive individuals who are to be treated with NSAIDs has been shown to reduce the risk of peptic ulcer disease and ulcer bleeding and can therefore be recommended [117–120]. On the other hand, in patients who need to be treated with NSAIDs or aspirin and have a history of ulcer complications, *H. pylori* eradication should be followed by continuous PPI therapy [121]. In patients already taking NSAIDs who develop ulcer disease and/or ulcer bleeding, *H. pylori* eradication alone appears to be less effective in reducing recurring peptic ulcers or ulcer bleeding than PPI maintenance therapy only [117, 122, 123]. In conclusion, it seems reasonable to test all NSAIDs users who develop peptic ulcer disease for *H. pylori* and treat, if positive, with eradication and subsequent PPI maintenance therapy [121].

H. pylori and Extra-Alimentary Diseases

An increasing number of studies suggest an association between *H. pylori* infection and iron deficiency anemia, although the pathogenetic mechanism remains unknown [124, 125]. Possible explanations include reduced intestinal iron absorption due to pangastritis with subsequent achlorhydria, occult blood loss from erosive gastritis, and utilization of iron by *H. pylori* itself [126]. There is also a growing amount of evidence that eradication of

H. pylori may improve anemia [127–129]. Therefore, patients with otherwise unexplained iron deficiency anemia should be tested for *H. pylori* and treated if positive.

Idiopathic thrombocytopenic purpura (ITP) also seems to be associated with *H. pylori* infection, and up to 60% of patients with chronic ITP have been shown to be infected with *H. pylori* [130–132]. Eradication therapy was demonstrated to induce a significant increase in the platelet count in approximately one half of patients [131]. However, these results have not been consistent, and more studies are needed to reach firmer conclusions [133, 134].

Other Indications

Eradication therapy should also be considered in asymptomatic *H. pylori* positive patients in response to their preferences, after full consultation with their physician [4].

TREATMENT OF *H. PYLORI* INFECTION

Despite many years of experience in *H. pylori* treatment and many therapeutic algorithms evaluated, the optimal therapy regimen still has to be defined. The therapy should be effective (achieve eradication rate of at least 80%), well tolerated, simple, easy to comply, and cost-effective [135]. However, *H. pylori* infection is not easily cured, probably because of inadequate antibiotic activity in the colonization niche. Although the bacterium is very sensitive to a wide range of antibiotics in vitro, monotherapy has been disappointing in vivo, with cure rates ranging from 0 to 35% and rapid development of resistance [136]. This is the reason why various multidrug therapeutic protocols have been extensively studied.

Based on the published literature, it is strongly recommended that the treatment regimen should include PPI-based triple or quadruple therapy, consisting of a PPI and two or three antimicrobial agents given for 7–14 days [2, 4].

Most commonly used antimicrobial agents are clarithromycin, amoxicillin, metronidazole, tetracycline, bismuth subsalicylate/subcitrate, and recently, levofloxacin. PPIs improve the efficacy of antibiotics by reducing the acidity of gastric content, but they also have a direct inhibitory effect on the bacterial growth. Therefore, PPIs are an extremely important component of most protocols. Available PPIs and their doses in the eradication protocols are: omeprazole 20 mg twice daily, esomeprazole 20 mg twice daily (or 40 mg once daily), lansoprazole 30 mg twice daily, pantoprazole 40 mg twice daily, and rabeprazole 20 mg twice daily. These PPIs perform comparably when used in eradication protocols [137]. H2-receptor antagonists are less effective in the treatment protocols, but ranitidine bismuth citrate (400 mg twice daily) can be used as an alternative to PPIs [138]. However, H2-receptor antagonists may still be used if the patient cannot tolerate PPIs and ranitidine bismuth citrate [139].

A detailed description of different therapy regimes, including doses, is summarized in the Table 9.3.

PPI-based triple or quadruple therapies result in *H. pylori* eradication rates of >90% in many trials and >75% in clinical practice [140, 141]. Although currently the best available option for *H. pylori* eradication, standard PPI-based therapy is still not successful in a significant proportion of patients. The two most important factors that have a great influence on efficacy of *H. pylori* treatment are the patient's compliance with the therapeutic regimen and the use of drugs to which *H. pylori* has not acquired resistance [142]. These two factors intertwine with each other, meaning that patient compliance to the eradication protocol is of great importance not only for the eradication success in a particular patient but also in the prevention of the development of antibiotic resistance. Furthermore, careful provision of information to the patient is necessary to achieve optimal compliance and avoid any interruption of the therapy. Side effects are reported in up to one half of patients taking one of the triple agent regimens, but they are usually mild and patients should be nevertheless encouraged to continue with the therapy. Still we have to bear in mind that 5% to 20% of patients experience significant side effects; so in the end, almost one fifth of the patients do not complete therapy [143]. The most commonly reported adverse effects are nausea, vomiting, diarrhea, headache, alternated taste, metallic taste in the mouth, and darkening of the tongue and the stool (bismuth compounds).

Antibiotic Resistance

The efficacy of PPI-based regimens seems to be decreasing in the last few years, probably due to increasing antibiotic resistance, which is a growing concern. Primary resistance to antibiotics exists even before commencing with the treatment, while secondary resistance develops during therapy with a certain antibiotic. Attempts of eradication that fail can elicit secondary antibiotic resistance. Prior use of macrolides or metronidazole for other indications also appears to increase the risk of *H. pylori* resistance against these antibiotics [144]. Therefore, a history of the patient's antibiotic use should be obtained, and, even if only distant exposure is identified, use of certain agents should be avoided if possible.

TABLE 9.3.   Eradication protocols for *H. pylori* infection [2, 4, 156].

Regimen	Drug 1	Drug 2	Drug 3	Drug 4
First-line treatment				
Clarithromycin-based triple therapy (7–14 days)	Standard dose of PPI[a] twice daily	Clarithromycin 500 mg twice daily	Metronidazole 500 twice daily or Amoxicillin 1 g twice daily	–
Bismuth-based quadruple therapy (10–14 days)	Standard dose of PPI[a] twice daily	Bismuth subsalicylate 525 mg four times daily	Metronidazole 250 mg four times daily	Tetracycline 500 mg four times daily
		Bismuth subcitrate potassium 420 mg four times daily	Metronidazole 375 mg four times daily	Tetracycline 375 mg four times daily
Sequential therapy (10 days)	Standard dose of PPI[a] twice daily and amoxicillin 1 g twice daily for the first 5 days	Standard dose of PPI[a] twice daily, clarithromycin 500 mg twice daily, and tinidazole 500 twice daily for the remaining 5 days		
Second-line treatment				
Bismuth-based quadruple therapy (10–14 days)	Standard dose of PPI[a] twice daily	Bismuth subsalicylate 525 mg four times daily	Metronidazole 250 mg four times daily	Tetracycline 500 mg four times daily
		Bismuth subcitrate potassium 420 mg four times daily	Metronidazole 375 mg four times daily	Tetracycline 375 mg four times daily
PPI-metronidazole-amoxicillin/tetracycline (10–14 days)	Standard dose of PPI[a] twice daily	Metronidazole 500 twice daily	Amoxicillin 1 g twice daily or Tetracycline 500 mg twice daily	–
Levofloxacin-based triple therapy (10 days)	Standard dose of PPI[a] twice daily	Levofloxacin 500 mg once daily or 250 mg twice daily	Amoxicillin 1 g twice daily	–

PPI proton pump inhibitor

In the eradication protocol, esomeprazole can be used 20 mg twice daily or 40 mg ones daily

[a]Standard doses of PPIs are: omeprazole 20 mg, esomeprazole 20 mg, lansoprazole 30 mg, pantoprazole 40 mg, rabeprazole 20 mg

The European study conducted in 1997–1998 estimated the overall resistance to clarithromycin, metronidazole, and amoxicillin to be 9.9, 33.1, and 0.8%, respectively. Concerning clarithromycin resistance, there were important differences between northern and southern Europe (resistance rate of 4 and 18.5%, respectively) [145]. A recent large US study has estimated the overall resistance to clarithromycin, metronidazole, and amoxicillin to be 13, 25, and 0.9%, respectively [146].

Resistance to clarithromycin has been identified as one of the major factors affecting the efficacy of eradication therapy and is associated with a very high rate of treatment failure when clarithromycin-based protocols are used [147, 148]. Unfortunately, the rate of resistance to this antibiotic seems to be increasing in many geographical areas [142, 144, 149]. The situation is somewhat different with metronidazole, whose in vitro resistance does not completely correlate with in vivo resistance. Therefore, metronidazole susceptibility testing is not routinely necessary [4].

In conclusion, although clarithromycin resistance is less prevalent than metronidazole resistance, it usually results in treatment failure if present. Metronidazole-resistant strains of *H. pylori* are much more common, but these strains still may be treated by metronidazole-containing regimens.

Duration of Treatment

The recommended duration of therapy for *H. pylori* eradication is 7–14 days [2, 4]. Some studies have shown that a 14-day course of therapy is more effective than a 7-day course by about 12% [150–152]. However, a recent meta-analysis suggested that extension of PPI-based triple therapy from 7 to 14 days was associated with only a 5% increase in eradication rates [153]. Therefore, a 7-day treatment may be acceptable in areas where local studies show that it is effective. European guidelines suggest 7- to 14-day regimens, while the US guidelines recommend 10- to 14-day protocols [2, 4].

First-Line Therapy

According to the current European and US guidelines, the recommended first-line therapy is clarithromycin-based triple therapy, which consists of a PPI, clarithromycin, and amoxicillin or metronidazole [2, 4]. There are some advantages when using metronidazole instead of amoxicillin, and this combination was therefore found to be preferable in areas where the prevalence of metronidazole resistance was lower than 40% [4, 154]. Metronidazole should also be used in individuals allergic to penicillin, and amoxicillin should be preferred when alcohol abuse is suspected (metronidazole can cause a disulfuram-like reaction when taken together with alcohol). Tinidazole, another nitroimidazole, can be used instead of metronidazole (equal dosage). In order to optimize first-line therapies, it is important to monitor the primary antibiotic resistance of *H. pylori* in different populations. If clarithromycin resistance is greater than 15% to 20% in the respective population, according to the European guidelines, clarithromycin should not be used or clarithromycin susceptibility testing should be performed prior to clarithromycin-based triple therapy [4]. US guidelines do not emphasize this requirement because susceptibility testing is not widely available [2].

Bismuth-based quadruple therapy, where available, is an alternative first-line therapy [2, 4]. It should always be considered in individuals who have previously been treated with clarithromycin or metranidazole for any indication because they could be resistant to these antibiotics. This therapy protocol consists of a PPI, bismuth subsalicylate or bismuth subcitrate, metronidazole, and tetracycline [155, 156]. Recently published systematic review and meta-analysis comparing efficacy and tolerability of clarithromycin-based triple therapy and bismuth-based quadruple therapy concluded that both the therapies yielded similar eradication rates as primary therapy for *H. pylori* infection (77.0 and 78.3%, respectively) [157]. Patient compliance and side effects were also similar. The main disadvantage of this quadruple protocol is the complexity of the protocol (four times daily dosing, great number of pills – up to 18). A solution to this problem is found in a combination capsule containing bismuth subcitrate, metronidazole, and tetracycline, which has been approved by the FDA [156].

Sequential therapy consisting of a PPI and amoxicillin for 5 days followed by a PPI, clarithromycin, and tinidazole for an additional 5 days, offers promising results. Several studies confirmed the superiority of sequential therapy over the standard clarithromycin-based triple therapy, especially in those infected with clarithromycin-resistant strains [158–163]. In contrast, recent randomized trial of 232 *H. pylori*-infected patients showed that both the therapy protocols were equally effective [164]. Therefore, sequential therapy may provide an alternative to clarithromycin-based triple or bismuth-based quadruple therapy but requires further validation before it can be recommended as a first-line therapy.

Second-Line Therapy
If the patient has already been treated and *H. pylori* was not eradicated, he can be retreated using a regimen avoiding antibiotics used

previously to which the bacterium may be resistant. Alternatively, culture and sensitivity testing can be used to ensure the choice of the appropriate antimicrobial therapy, but the sensitivity testing is usually performed after the second-line therapy failure.

Bismuth-based quadruple therapy with a PPI, bismuth, metronidazole, and tetracycline is the best option for the second-line therapy [4]. An average eradication rate in this setting is 76% [140].

If bismuth-based therapy is not available or has already been used as the first-line therapy, protocol including a PPI, metronidazole, and amoxicillin or tetracycline can be used [4]. If a patient has not previously been treated with clarithromycin, although it is rare, clarithromycin-based triple therapy may also be an option for the second-line therapy [2].

Levofloxacin-based triple therapy is another option in patients with persistent infection, which seems to be effective, but requires further validation before it can be recommended [165, 166].

Rescue Therapy

The rescue therapy, after failure of two different therapy protocols, should be based on antibiotic susceptibility testing [4].

Vaccination Against *H. pylori*

Despite a large source of evidence in animals that vaccination against *H. pylori* (both preventive and therapeutic) is feasible, not many clinical studies have been carried out to evaluate whether the positive results obtained in animals can be reproduced in humans [167–171].

CONFIRMATION OF ERADICATION

Post-treatment testing for *H. pylori* infection used to be recommended only for patients with peptic ulcer disease, malignancy, or those with persistent/recurrent symptoms after therapy. Since the costs of noninvasive tests have fallen and they are getting increasingly available, it is now recommended to confirm eradication of *H. pylori* in all treated patients, at least 4 weeks after the completion of treatment [4]. The tests used are dependent on *H. pylori* load, and control of eradication within 4 weeks from completion of therapy may therefore lead to a false negative result. Furthermore, recent treatment with antisecretory drugs, antibiotics taken for some other reason, or bismuth can affect the results of diagnostic testing. For that reason, antibiotics and bismuth should be discontinued for at least 4 weeks and PPIs at least 2 weeks prior to testing of eradication to reduce the probability of a false negative result.

The UBT, the stool antigen test, and the biopsy-based tests can all be used to assess the success of treatment. Noninvasive tests should always be preferred, except in cases where endoscopy is clinically indicated for other reasons.

The UBT is the best option, with a sensitivity of 94% and a specificity of 95% in this setting [2, 4, 5]. If urea breath testing is not available, a laboratory based stool antigen test, preferably the one using monoclonal antibodies, is the alternative [4, 10, 23, 172]. Serologic tests are not an appropriate means of determining the eradication of the infection, as the gradual drop in titer of *H. pylori*-specific antibodies is too slow for the purpose.

Biopsy-based invasive testing is acceptable in any situation when, in addition to confirming eradication, there is a need for histological (re)assessment of any mucosal abnormalities (e.g., in the case of gastric ulcer, gastric MALT lymphoma, and after resection of early gastric carcinoma). In this setting, histological testing or histological testing in combination with biopsy urease test, which is even more sensitive (96%), is most commonly used [2, 173]. Biopsy urease test has lower sensitivity than histology when used alone in the control of eradication [173]. Endoscopy with biopsy for culture should be performed only when antibiotic resistance is suspected.

CONCLUSIONS

H. pylori infection is one of the most common chronic infections worldwide, and it is estimated that about one half of the world's population is infected. It is the main risk factor for a broad variety of chronic gastrointestinal diseases such as chronic gastritis, peptic ulcer disease, gastric adenocarcinoma, and MALT lymphoma.

In the current practice, noninvasive testing is generally used to establish the diagnosis of *H. pylori* infection before therapy and in the control of eradication. Invasive biopsy-based testing should be reserved for those patients who require endoscopy based upon their clinical presentation because of the need for extra information provided by endoscopy.

H. pylori treatment should consist of a PPI-based triple or quadruple therapy, including a PPI and two or three antimicrobial agents given for 7–14 days. Clarithromycin-based triple therapy and bismuth-based quadruple therapy represent the first-line treatment options. A 14-day course of therapy is slightly more effective than a 7-day course. *H. pylori* eradication should be confirmed in all treated patients at least 4 weeks after the completion of treatment.

Acknowledgments   The unselfish help of our esteemed colleagues Lucija Virović-Jukić, MD, PhD, and Neven Baršić, MD, is highly appreciated.

References

1. Pounder RE, Ng D. The prevalence of *Helicobacter pylori* infection in different countries. Aliment Pharmacol Ther. 1995;9 Suppl 2:33–9.
2. Chey WD, Wong BC, Practice Parameters Committee of the American College of Gastroenterology. American College of Gastroenterologoy guideline on the management of *Helicobacter pylori* infection. Am J Gastroenterol. 2007;102:1808–25.
3. Staat MA, Kruszon-Moran D, McQuillan GM, Kaslow RA. A population-based serologic survey of *Helicobacter pylori* infection in children and adolescents in the United States. J Infect Dis. 1996;174:1120–3.
4. Malfertheiner P, Megraud F, O'Morain C, et al. Current concepts in the management of *Helicobacter pylori* infection: the Maastricht III Consensus Report. Gut. 2007;56:772–81.
5. Gisbert JP, Pajares JM. Review article: 13C-urea breath test in the diagnosis of *Helicobacter pylori* infection: a critical review. Aliment Pharmacol Ther. 2004;20:1001–17.
6. Leide-Svegborn S, Stenström K, Olofsson M, et al. Biokinetics and radiation doses for carbon-14 urea in adults and children undergoing the *Helicobacter pylori* breath test. Eur J Nucl Med. 1999;26:573–80.
7. Chey WD. Accurate diagnosis of *Helicobacter pylori*. 14C-urea breath test. Gastroenterol Clin N Am. 2000;29:895–902.
8. Leodolter A, Domínguez-Muñoz JE, von Arnim U, Kahl S, Peitz U, Malfertheiner P. Validity of a modified 13C-urea breath test for pre- and posttreatment diagnosis of *Helicobacter pylori* infection in the routine clinical setting. Am J Gastroenterol. 1999;94:2100–4.
9. Chey WD, Metz DC, Shaw S, Kearney D, Montague J, Murthy U. Appropriate timing of the 14 C-urea breath test to establish eradication of *Helicobacter pylori* infection. Am J Gastroenterol. 2000;95:1171–4.
10. Perri F, Manes G, Neri M, Vaira D, Nardone G. *Helicobacter pylori* antigen stool test and 13C-urea breath test in patients after eradication treatments. Am J Gastroenterol. 2002;97:2756–62.
11. Gatta L, Ricci C, Tampieri A, et al. Accuracy of breath tests using low doses of 13C-urea to diagnose *Helicobacter pylori* infection: a randomised controlled trial. Gut. 2006;55:457–562.
12. Gatta L, Vakil N, Ricci C, et al. Effect of proton pump inhibitors and antacid therapy on 13C urea breath tests and stool test for *Helicobacter pylori* infection. Am J Gastroenterol. 2004;99:823–9.
13. Mana F, Van Laer W, Bossuyt A, Urbain D. The early effect of proton pump inhibitor therapy on the accuracy of the 13C-urea breath test. Dig Liver Dis. 2005;37:28–32.
14. Graham DY, Opekun AR, Hammoud F, et al. Studies regarding the mechanism of false negative urea breath tests with proton pump inhibitors. Am J Gastroenterol. 2003;98:1005–9.
15. Laine L, Estrada R, Trujillo M, Knigge K, Fennerty MB. Effect of proton-pump inhibitor therapy on diagnostic testing for *Helicobacter pylori*. Ann Intern Med. 1998;129:547–50.

16. Savarino V, Tracci D, Dulbecco P, et al. Negative effect of ranitidine on the results of urea breath test for the diagnosisity of *Helicobacter pylori*. Am J Gastroenterol. 2001;96:348–52.

17. Adachi K, Fujishiro H, Mihara T, Komazawa Y, Kinoshita Y. Influence of lansoprazole, famotidine, roxatidine and rebamipide administration on the urea breath test for the diagnosis of *Helicobacter pylori* infection. J Gastroenterol Hepatol. 2003;18:168–71.

18. Graham DY, Opekun AR, Jogi M, et al. False negative urea breath tests with H2-receptor antagonists: interactions between *Helicobacter pylori* density and pH. Helicobacter. 2004;9:17–27.

19. Gisbert JP, Esteban C, Jiminez I, Moreno-Ortero R. 13C-urea breath test during hospitalization for the diagnosis of *Helicobacter pylori* infection in peptic ulcer bleeding. Helicobacter. 2007;12:231–7.

20. Chey WD, Murthy U, Toskes P, Carpenter S, Laine L. The 13C-urea blood test accurately detects active *Helicobacter pylori* infection: a United States, multicenter trial. Am J Gastroenterol. 1999;94:1522–4.

21. Ahmed F, Murthy UK, Chey WD, Toskes PP, Wagner DA. Evaluation of the Ez-HBT Helicobacter blood test to establish *Helicobacter pylori* eradication. Aliment Pharmacol Ther. 2005;22:875–80.

22. Kelly SM, Pitcher MC, Farmery SM, Gibson GR. Isolation of *Helicobacter pylori* from feces of patients with dyspepsia in the United Kingdom. Gastroenterology. 1994;107:1671–4.

23. Gisbert JP, Pajares JM. Stool antigen test for the diagnosis of *Helicobacter pylori* infection: a systematic review. Helicobacter. 2004;9:347–68.

24. Gisbert JP, de la Morena F, Abraira V. Accuracy of monoclonal stool antigen test for the diagnosis of *H. pylori* infection: a systematic review and meta-analysis. Am J Gastroenterol. 2006;101:1921–30.

25. Viara D, Vakil N, Menegatti M, et al. The stool antigen test for detection of *Helicobacter pylori* after eradication therapy. Ann Intern Med. 2002;136:280–7.

26. Odaka T, Yamaguchi T, Koyama H, Saisho H, Nomura F. Evaluation of the *Helicobacter pylori* stool antigen test for monitoring eradication therapy. Am J Gastroenterol. 2002;97:594–9.

27. Bravo LE, Realpe JL, Campo C, Mera R, Correa P. Effects of acid suppression and bismuth medications on the performance of diagnostic tests for *Helicobacter pylori* infection. Am J Gastroenterol. 1999;94:2380–3.

28. Manes G, Balzano A, Iaquinto G, et al. Accuracy of the stool antigen test in the diagnosis of *Helicobacter pylori* infection before treatment and in patients on omeprazole therapy. Aliment Pharmacol Ther. 2001;15:73–9.

29. Griñó P, Pascual S, Such J, et al. Comparison of stool immunoassay with standard methods for detection of *Helicobacter pylori* infection in patients with upper-gastrointestinal bleeding of peptic origin. Eur J Gastroenterol Hepatol. 2003;15:525–9.

30. van Leerdam ME, van der Ende A, ten Kate FJ, Rauws EA, Tytgat GN. Lack of accuracy of the noninvasive *Helicobacter pylori* stool antigen test in patients with gastroduodenal ulcer bleeding. Am J Gastroenterol. 2003;98:798–801.

31. Lin HJ, Lo WC, Perng CL, et al. *Helicobacter pylori* stool antigen test in patients with bleeding peptic ulcers. Helicobacter. 2004;9:663–8.

32. Leodolter A, Wolle K, Peitz U, Schaffranke A, Wex T, Malfertheiner P. Evaluation of a near-patient fecal antigen test for the assessment of *Helicobacter pylori* status. Diagn Microbiol Infect Dis. 2004;48:145–7.

33. Laheij RJ, Straatman H, Jansen JB, Verbeek AL. Evaluation of commercially available *Helicobacter pylori* serology kits: a review. J Clin Microbiol. 1998;36:2803–9.

34. Monteiro L, de Mascarel A, Sarrasqueta AM, et al. Diagnosis of *Helicobacter pylori* infection: non-invasive methods compared to invasive methods and evaluation of two new tests. Am J Gastroenterol. 2001;96:353–8.

35. Hoang TT, Wheeldon TU, Bengtsson C, Phung DC, Sörberg M, Granström M. Enzyme-liked immunosorbent assay for *Helicobacter pylori* needs adjustment for the population investigated. J Clin Microbiol. 2004;42:627–30.

36. Nurgalieva ZZ, Graham DY. Pearls and pitfalls of assessing *Helicobacter pylori* status. Dig Liver Dis. 2003;35:375–7.

37. Chey WD, Fendrick AM. Noninvasive *Helicobacter pylori* testing for the "test-and-treat" strategy: a decision analysis to assess the effect of past infection on test choice. Arch Intern Med. 2001;161:2129–32.

38. Vakil N, Rhew D, Soll A, Ofman JJ. The cost-effectiveness of diagnostic testing strategies for *Helicobacter pylori*. Am J Gastroenterol. 2000;95:1691–8.

39. Ho B, Marshall BJ. Accurate diagnosis of *Helicobacter pylori*. Serologic testing. Gastroenterol Clin North Am. 2000;29:853–62.

40. Kokkola A, Rautelin H, Puolakkainen P, et al. Diagnosis of *Helicobacter pylori* infection in patients with atrophic gastritis: comparison of histology, 13C-urea breath test, and serology. Scand J Gastroenterol. 2000;35:138–41.

41. Lehours P, Ruskone-Fourmestraux A, Lavergne A, et al. Which test to use to detect *Helicobacter pylori* infection in patients with low-grade gastric mucosa-associated lymphoid tissue lymphoma? Am J Gastroenterol. 2003;98:291–5.

42. Duggan A, Elliott C, Logan R. Testing for *Helicobacter pylori* infection: validation and diagnostic yield of a near patient test in primary care. BMJ. 1999;319:1236–9.

43. Wong BC, Wong W, Tang VS, et al. An evaluation of whole blood testing for *Helicobacter pylori* infection in the Chinese population. Aliment Pharmacol Ther. 2000;14:331–5.

44. Lee JM, Breslin NP, Fallon C, O'Morain CA. Rapid urease tests lack sensitivity in *Helicobacter pylori* diagnosis when peptic ulcer disease presents with bleeding. Am J Gastroenterol. 2000;95:1166–70.

45. Tu TC, Lee CL, Wu CH, et al. Comparison of invasive and noninvasive tests for detecting *Helicobacter pylori* infection in bleeding peptic ulcers. Gastrointest Endosc. 1999;49:302–6.

46. Griñó P, Pascual S, Such J, et al. Comparison of diagnostic methods for *Helicobacter pylori* infection in patients with upper gastrointestinal bleeding. Scand J Gastroenterol. 2001;36:1254–8.

47. Schilling D, Demel A, Adamek HE, Nüsse T, Weidmann E, Riemann JF. A negative rapid urease test is unreliable for exclusion of *Helicobacter pylori* infection during acute phase of ulcer bleeding. A prospective case control study. Dig Liver Dis. 2003;35:217–21.

48. Woo JS, el-Zimaity HM, Genta RM, Yousfi MM, Graham DY. The best gastric site for obtaining a positive rapid urease test. Helicobacter. 1996;1:256–9.

49. Weston AP, Campbell DR, Hassanein RS, Cherian R, Dixon A, McGregor DH. Prospective multivariate evaluation of CLOtest performance. Am J Gastroenterol. 1997;92:1310–5.

50. Mégraud F, Lehours P. *Helicobacter pylori* detection and antimicrobial susceptibility testing. Clin Microbiol Rev. 2007;20:280–322.

51. Midolo P, Marshall BJ. Accurate diagnosis of *Helicobacter pylori*. Urease tests. Gastroenterol Clin North Am. 2000;29:871–8.

52. Perna F, Ricci C, Gatta L, et al. Diagnostic accuracy of a new rapid urease test (Pronto Dry), before and after treatment of *Helicobacter pylori* infection. Minerva Gastroenterol Dietol. 2005;51:247–54.

53. Rogge JD, Wagner DR, Carrico RJ, et al. Evaluation of a new urease reagent strip for detection of *Helicobacter pylori* in gastric biopsy specimens. Am J Gastroenterol. 1995;90:1965–8.

54. Laine LA, Nathwani RA, Naritoku W. The effect of GI bleeding on *Helicobacter pylori* diagnostic testing: a prospective study at the time of bleeding and 1 month later. Gastrointest Endosc. 2005;62: 853–9.

55. Gisbert JP, Abraira V. Accuracy of *Helicobacter pylori* diagnostic tests in patients with bleeding peptic ulcer: a systematic review and meta-analysis. Am J Gastroenterol. 2006;101:848–63.

56. Bayerdörffer E, Oertel H, Lehn N, et al. Topographic association between active gastritis and *Campylobacter pylori* colonisation. J Clin Pathol. 1989;42:834–9.

57. Dixon MF, Genta R, Yardley JH, Correa P. Classification and grading of gastritis: the updated Sydney System. International Workshop on the Histopathology of Gastritis, Houston 1994. Am J Surg Pathol. 1996;20:1161–81.

58. van IJzendoorn MC, Laheij RJ, de Boer WA, Jansen JB. The importance of corpus biopsies in the determination of *Helicobacter pylori* infection. Neth J Med. 2005;63:141–5.

59. el-Zimaity HM. Accurate diagnosis of *Helicobacter pylori* with biopsy. Gastroenterol Clin North Am. 2000;29:863–9.

60. Huang MS, Wang WM, Wu DC, et al. Utility of brushing cytology in the diagnosis of *Helicobacter pylori* infection. Acta Cytol. 1996;40: 714–8.

61. Mostaghni AA, Afarid M, Eghbali S, Kumar P. Evaluation of brushing cytology in the diagnosis of *Helicobacter pylori* gastritis. Acta Cytol. 2008;52:597–601.

62. Meunier O, Walter P, Chamouard P, Piemont Y, Monteil H. Isolation of *Helicobacter pylori*: necessity of control of transport conditions. Pathol Biol (Paris). 1997;45:82–5.

63. Makristathis A, Hirschl AM, Lehourst P, Mégraud F. Diagnosis of *Helicobacter pylori* infection. Helicobacter. 2004;9 Suppl 1:7–14.

64. Liu H, Rahman A, Semino-Mora C, Doi SQ, Dubois A. Specific and sensitive detection of *H. pylori* in biological specimens by real-time RT-PCR and in situ hybridization. PLoS ONE. 2008;3:e2689.

65. Zsikla V, Hailemariam S, Baumann M, et al. Increased rate of *Helicobacter pylori* infection detected by PCR in biopsies with chronic gastritis. Am J Surg Pathol. 2006;30:242–8.

66. Rimbara E, Noguchi N, Yamaguchi T, Narui K, Kawai T, Sasatsu M. Development of a highly sensitive method for detection of clarithromycin-resistant *Helicobacter pylori* from human feces. Curr Microbiol. 2005;51:1–5.

67. de Francesco V, Margiotta M, Zullo A, et al. Primary clarithromycin resistance in Italy assessed on *Helicobacter pylori* DNA sequences by TaqMan real-time polymerase chain reaction. Aliment Pharmacol Ther. 2006;23:429–35.

68. Farinha P, Gascoyne RD. *Helicobacter pylori* and MALT lymphoma. Gastroenterology. 2005;128:1579–605.

69. Montalban C, Norman F. Treatment of gastric mucosa-associated lymphoid tissue lymphoma: *Helicobacter pylori* eradication and beyond. Expert Rev Anticancer Ther. 2006;6:361–71.

70. Muller AF, Maloney A, Jenkins D, et al. Primary gastric lymphoma in clinical practice 1973–1992. Gut. 1995;36:679–83.

71. Ruskoné-Fourmestraux A, Lavergne A, Aegerter PH, et al. Predictive factors for regression of gastric MALT lymphoma after anti-*Helicobacter pylori* treatment. Gut. 2001;48:297–303.

72. Fischbach W, Goebeler-Kolve ME, Dragosics B, Greiner A, Stolte M. Long term outcome of patients with gastric marginal zone B cell lymphoma of mucosa associated lymphoid tissue (MALT) following exclusive *Helicobacter pylori* eradication therapy: experience from a large prospective series. Gut. 2004;53:34–7.

73. Kim JS, Chung SJ, Choi YS, et al. *Helicobacter pylori* eradication for low-grade gastric mucosa-associated lymphoid tissue lymphoma is more successful in inducing remission in distal compared to proximal disease. Br J Cancer. 2007;96:1324–8.

74. Wündisch T, Thiede C, Morgner A, et al. Long-term follow-up gastric MALT lymphoma after *Helicobacter pylori* eradication. J Clin Oncol. 2005;23:8018–24.

75. Nakamura S, Matsumoto T, Suekane H, et al. Long-term clinical outcome of *Helicobacter pylori* eradication for gastric mucosa-associated lymphoid tissue lymphoma with a reference to second-line treatment. Cancer. 2005;104:532–40.

76. Chen LT, Lin JT, Tai JJ, et al. Long-term results of anti-*Helicobacter pylori* therapy in early-stage gastric high-grade transformed MALT lymphoma. J Natl Cancer Inst. 2005;97:1345–53.

77. Marshall BJ, McGechie DB, Rogers PA, Glancy RJ. Pyloric Campylobacter infection and gastroduodenal disease. Med J Aust. 1985;142:439–44.

78. Arroyo MT, Forne M, de Argila CM, et al. The prevalence of peptic ulcer not related to *Helicobacter pylori* or non-steroidal anti-inflammatory drug use is negligible in southern Europe. Helicobacter. 2004;9:249–54.

79. Sipponen P, Varis K, Fräki O, Korri UM, Seppälä K, Siurala M. Cumulative 10-year risk of symptomatic duodenal and gastric ulcer in patients with or without chronic gastritis: a clinical follow-up study of 454 outpatients. Scand J Gastroenterol. 1990;25:966–73.

80. Aro P, Storskrubb T, Ronkainen J, et al. Peptic ulcer disease in a general adult population: the Kalixanda study: a random population-based study. Am J Epidemiol. 2006;163:1025–34.

81. Paptheodoridis GV, Sougioultzis S, Archimandritis AJ. Effects of *Helicobacter pylori* and nonsteroidal anti-inflammatory drugs on peptic ulcer disease: a systematic review. Clin Gastroenterol Hepatol. 2006;4:130–42.

82. Leodolter A, Kulig M, Brasch H, Meyer-Sabellek W, Willich SN, Malfertheiner P. A meta-analysis comparing eradication, healing and relapse rates in patients with *Helicobacter pylori*-associated gastric or duodenal ulcer. Aliment Pharmacol Ther. 2001;15:1949–58.

83. Ford AC, Delaney BC, Forman D, Moayyedi P. Eradication therapy in *Helicobacter pylori* positive peptic ulcer disease: systematic review and economic analysis. Am J Gastroenterol. 2004;99:1833–55.

84. Sharma VK, Sahai AV, Corder FA, Howden CW. *Helicobacter pylori* eradication is superior to ulcer healing with or without maintenance therapy to prevent further ulcer haemorrhage. Aliment Pharmacol Ther. 2001;15:1939–47.

85. Gisbert JP, Khorrami S, Carballo F, Calvet X, Gené E, Dominguez-Muñoz JE. *H. pylori* eradication therapy vs. antisecretory non-eradication therapy (with or without long-term maintenance antisecretory therapy) for the prevention of recurrent bleeding from peptic ulcer. Cochrane Database Syst Rev. 2004; (2):CD004062

86. Sepulveda AR, Graham DY. Role of *Helicobacter pylori* in gastric carcinogenesis. Gastroenterol Clin North Am. 2002;31:517–35.

87. Hunt RH. Will eradication of *Helicobacter pylori* infection influence the risk of gastric cancer? Am J Med. 2004;117(Suppl 5A):86S–91.

88. Valle J, Kekki M, Sipponen P, Ihamäki T, Siurala M. Long-term course and consequences of *Helicobacter pylori* gastritis. Results of a 32-year follow-up study. Scand J Gastroenterol. 1996;31:546–50.

89. Eslick GD, Lim LL, Byles JE, Xia HH, Talley NJ. Association of *Helicobacter pylori* infection with gastric carcinoma: a meta-analysis. Am J Gastroenterol. 1999;94:2373–9.

90. Helicobacter and Cancer Collaborative Group. Gastric cancer and *Helicobacter pylori*: a combined analysis of 12 case control studies nested within prospective cohorts. Gut. 2001;49:347–53.

91. Uemura N, Okamoto S, Yamamoto S, et al. *Helicobacter pylori* infection and the development of gastric cancer. N Engl J Med. 2001;345:784–9.

92. Ohkuma K, Okada M, Murayama H, et al. Association of *Helicobacter pylori* infection with atrophic gastritis and intestinal metaplasia. J Gastroenterol Hepatol. 2000;15:1105–12.

93. Fuccio L, Zagari RM, Eusebi LH, et al. Meta-analysis: can *Helicobacter pylori* eradication treatment reduce the risk for gastric cancer? Ann Intern Med. 2009;151:121–8.

94. Leung WK, Lin SR, Ching JY, et al. Factors predicting progression of gastric intestinal metaplasia: results of a randomised trial on *Helicobacter pylori* eradication. Gut. 2004;53:1244–9.

95. Mera R, Fontham ET, Bravo LE, et al. Long term follow up of patients treated for *Helicobacter pylori* infection. Gut. 2005;54:1536–40.

96. El-Omar E, Oien K, Murray LS, et al. Increased prevalence of precancerous changes in relatives of gastric cancer patients: critical role of *H. pylori*. Gastroenterology. 2000;118:22–30.

97. Brenner H, Bode G, Boeing H. *Helicobacter pylori* infection among offspring of patients with stomach cancer. Gastroenterology. 2000;118:31–5.

98. Veldhuyzen van Zanten SJ, Bradette M, Chiba N, et al. Evidence-based recommendations for short- and long-term management of uninvestigated dyspepsia in primary care: an update of the Canadian Dyspepsia Working Group (CanDys) clinical management tool. Can J Gastroenterol. 2005;19:285–303.

99. Lassen AM, Pedersen FM, Bytzer P, Schaffalitzky de Muckadell OB. *Helicobacter pylori* test- and-eradicate versus prompt endoscopy for management of dyspeptic patients: a randomized trial. Lancet. 2000;356:455–60.

100. Moayyedi P, Feltbower R, Brown J, et al. Effect of population screening and treatment for *Helicobacter pylori* on dyspepsia and quality of life in the community: a randomised controlled trial. Leeds HELP Study Group. Lancet. 2000;355:1665–9.

101. Ladabaum U, Chey WD, Scheiman JM, Fendrick AM. Reappraisal of non-invasive management strategies for uninvestigated dyspepsia: a cost-minimization analysis. Aliment Pharmacol Ther. 2002;16:1491–501.

102. Chiba N, Veldhuyzen Van Zanten SJ, Escobedo S, et al. Economic evaluation of *Helicobacter pylori* eradication in the CADET-Hp randomized controlled trial of *H. pylori*-positive primary care patients with uninvestigated dyspepsia. Aliment Pharmacol Ther. 2004;19:349–58.

103. Lassen AT, Hallas J, Schaffalitzky de Muckadell OB. *Helicobacter pylori* test and eradicate versus prompt endoscopy for management of dyspeptic patients: 6.7 year follow up of a randomised trial. Gut. 2004;53:1758–63.

104. Moayyedi P, Soo S, Deeks J, et al. Systematic review and economic evaluation of *Helicobacter pylori* eradication treatment for non-ulcer dyspepsia. Dyspepsia Review Group. BMJ. 2000;321:659–64.

105. Moayyedi P, Deeks J, Talley NJ, Delaney B, Forman D. An update of the Cochrane systematic review of *Helicobacter pylori* eradication therapy in nonulcer dyspepsia: resolving the discrepancy between systematic reviews. Am J Gastroenterol. 2003;98:2621–6.

106. Talley NJ, Vakil N, Practice Parameters Committee of the American College of Gastroenterology. Guidelines for the management of dyspepsia. Am J Gastroenterol. 2005;100:2324–37.

107. Spiegel BM, Vakil NB, Ofman JJ. Dyspepsia management in primary care: a decision analysis of competing strategies. Gastroenterology. 2002;122:1270–85.

108. Yaghoobi M, Farrokhyar F, Yuan Y, Hunt RH. Is there an increased risk of GERD after *Helicobacter pylori* eradication? A meta-analysis. Am J Gastroenterol. 2010;105:1007–13.

109. Raghunath AS, Hungin APS, Wooff D, Childs S. Systematic review: the effect of *Helicobacter pylori* and its eradication on gastro-oesophageal reflux disease in patients with duodenal ulcers or reflux oesophagitis. Aliment Pharmacol Ther. 2004;20:733–44.

110. Laine L, Sugg J. Effect of *Helicobacter pylori* eradication on development of erosive esophagitis and gastroesophageal reflux disease symptoms: a post hoc analysis of eight double blind prospective studies. Am J Gastroenterol. 2002;97:2992–7.

111. Fallone CA, Barkun AN, Mayrand S, et al. There is no difference in the disease severity of gastro-oesophageal reflux disease between patients infected and not infected with *Helicobacter pylori*. Aliment Pharmacol Ther. 2004;20:761–8.

112. Vakil N, Traxler BM, Levine D. Symptom response and healing of erosive esophagitis with proton-pump inhibitors in patients with *Helicobacter pylori* infection. Am J Gastroenterol. 2004;99:1437–41.

113. Kuipers EJ, Lundell L, Klinkenberg-Knol EC, et al. Atrophic gastritis and *Helicobacter pylori* infection in patients with reflux esophagitis treated with omeprazole or fundoplication. N Engl J Med. 1996;334:1018–22.

114. McColl KE, Murray LS, Gillen D. Omeprazole and accelerated onset of atrophic gastritis. Gastroenterology. 2000;118:239.

115. Lundell L, Miettinen P, Myrvold HE, et al. Lack of effect of acid suppression therapy on gastric atrophy. Nordic Gerd Study Group. Gastroenterology. 1999;117:319–26.

116. Huang JQ, Sridhar S, Hunt RH. Role of *Helicobacter pylori* infection and non-steroidal anti-inflammatory drugs in peptic-ulcer disease: a meta-analysis. Lancet. 2002;359:14–22.

117. Vergara M, Catalán M, Gisbert JP, Calvet X. Meta-analysis: role of *Helicobacter pylori* eradication in the prevention of peptic ulcer in NSAID users. Aliment Pharmacol Ther. 2005;21:1411–8.

118. Labenz J, Blum AL, Bolten WW, et al. Primary prevention of diclofenac associated ulcers and dyspepsia by omeprazole or triple therapy in *Helicobacter pylori* positive patients: a randomised, double blind, placebo controlled, clinical trial. Gut. 2002;51:329–35.

119. Chan FK, Sung JJ, Chan SC, et al. Randomised trial of eradication of *Helicobacter pylori* before non-steroidal anti-inflammatory drug therapy to prevent peptic ulcers. Lancet. 1997;350:975–9.

120. Chey WD, Eswaren S, Howden CW, Inadomi JM, Fendrick AM, Scheiman JM. Primary care physician perceptions of non-steroidal anti-inflammatory drug and aspirin-associated toxicity: results of a national survey. Aliment Pharmacol Ther. 2006;23:655–68.

121. Papatheodoridis GV, Archimandritis AJ. Role of *Helicobacter pylori* eradication in aspirin or non-steroidal anti-inflammatory drug users. World J Gastroenterol. 2005;11:3811–6.

122. Hawkey CJ, Tulassay Z, Szczepanski L, et al. Randomised controlled trial of *Helicobacter pylori* eradication in patients on non-steroidal anti-inflammatory drugs: HELP NSAIDs study. Helicobacter Eradication for Lesion Prevention. Lancet. 1998;352:1016–21.

123. Chan FK, Chung SC, Suen BY, et al. Preventing recurrent upper gastrointestinal bleeding in patients with *Helicobacter pylori* infection who are taking low-dose aspirin or naproxen. N Engl J Med. 2001;344:967–73.

124. Baggett HC, Parkinson AJ, Muth PT, Gold BD, Gessner BD. Endemic iron deficiency associated with *Helicobacter pylori* infection among school-aged children in Alaska. Pediatrics. 2006;117:e396–404.

125. Cardenas VM, Mulla ZD, Ortiz M, Graham DY. Iron deficiency and *Helicobacter pylori* infection in the United States. Am J Epidemiol. 2006;163:127–34.

126. DuBois S, Kearney D. Iron-deficiency anemia and *Helicobacter pylori* infection: a review of evidence. Am J Gastroenterol. 2005;100:453–9.

127. Choe YH, Soon KK, Son BK, Lee DH, Hong YC, Pai SH. Randomized placebo-controlled trial of *Helicobacter pylori* eradication for iron-deficiency anemia in preadolescent children and adolescents. Helicobacter. 1999;4:135–9.

128. Hacihanefioglu A, Edebali F, Celebi A, Karakaya T, Senturk O, Hulagu S. Improvement of complete blood count in patients with iron deficiency anemia and *Helicobacter pylori* infection after the eradication of *Helicobacter pylori*. Hepatogastroenterology. 2004;51:313–5.

129. Annibale B, Marignani M, Monarca B, et al. Reversal of iron deficiency anemia after *Helicobacter pylori* eradication in patients with asymptomatic gastritis. Ann Intern Med. 1999;131:668–72.

130. Franchini M, Veneri D. *Helicobacter pylori* infection and immune thrombocytopenic purpura: an update. Helicobacter. 2004;9:342–6.

131. Fujimura K, Kuwana M, Kurata Y, et al. Is eradication therapy useful as the first line of treatment in *H. pylori*-positive idiopathic thrombocytopenic purpura? Analysis of 207 eradicated chronic ITP cases in Japan. Int J Hematol. 2005;81:162–8.

132. Franchini M, Veneri D. *Helicobacter pylori*-associated immune thrombocytopenia. Platelets. 2006;17:712–7.

133. Arnold DM, Bernotas A, Nazi I, et al. Platelet count response to *H. pylori* treatment in patients with immune thrombocytopenic purpura with and without *H. pylori* infection: a systematic review. Haematologica. 2009;94:850–6.

134. Stasi R, Sarpatwari A, Segal JB, et al. Effects of eradication of *Helicobacter pylori* infection in patients with immune thrombocytopenic purpura: a systematic review. Blood. 2009;113:1231–40.

135. Malfertheiner P, Mégraud F, O'Morain C, et al. Current European concepts in the management of *Helicobacter pylori* infection-the Maastricht Consensus Report. The European *Helicobacter Pylori* Study Group (EHPSG). Eur J Gastroenterol Hepatol. 1997;9:1–2.

136. Gisbert JP, Pajares R, Pajares JM. Evolution of *Helicobacter pylori* therapy from a meta-analytical perspective. Helicobacter. 2007;12 Suppl 2:50–8.

137. Vergara M, Vallve M, Gisbert JP, Calvet X. Meta-analysis: comparative efficacy of different proton-pump inhibitors in triple therapy for *Helicobacter pylori* eradication. Aliment Pharmacol Ther. 2003;18: 647–54.
138. Gisbert JP, Pajares JM, Valle J. Ranitidine bismuth citrate therapy regimens for treatment of *Helicobacter pylori* infection: a review. Helicobacter. 1999;4:58–66.
139. Graham DY, Hammoud F, El-Zimaity HM, Kim JG, Osato MS, El-Serag HB. Meta-analysis: proton pump inhibitor or H2-receptor antagonist for *Helicobacter pylori* eradication. Aliment Pharmacol Ther. 2003;17:1229–36.
140. Hojo M, Miwa H, Nagahara A, Sato N. Pooled analysis on the efficacy of the second-line treatment regimens for *Helicobacter pylori* infection. Scand J Gastroenterol. 2001;36:690–700.
141. Vakil N. Primary and secondary treatment for *Helicobacter pylori* in the United States. Rev Gastroenterol Disord. 2005;5:67–72.
142. Mégraud F, Lamouliatte H. Review article: the treatment of refractory *Helicobacter pylori* infection. Aliment Pharmacol Ther. 2003;17:1333–43.
143. Mégraud F, Marshall BJ. How to treat *Helicobacter pylori*. First-line, second-line, and future therapies. Gastroenterol Clin North Am. 2000;29:759–73.
144. McMahon BJ, Hennessy TW, Bensler JM, et al. The relationship among previous antimicrobial use, antimicrobial resistance, and treatment outcomes for *Helicobacter pylori* infections. Ann Intern Med. 2003;139:463–9.
145. Glupczynski Y, Mégraud F, Lopez-Brea M, Andersen LP. European multicentre survey of in vitro antimicrobial resistance in *Helicobacter pylori*. Eur J Clin Microbiol Infect Dis. 2001;20:820–3.
146. Duck WM, Sobel J, Pruckler JM, et al. Antimicrobial resistance incidence and risk factors among *Helicobacter pylori*-infected persons, United States. Emerg Infect Dis. 2004;10:1088–94.
147. Tankovic J, Lamarque D, Lascols C, Soussy CJ, Delchier JC. Impact of *Helicobacter pylori* resistance to clarithromycin on the efficacy of the omeprazole–amoxicillin–clarithromycin therapy. Aliment Pharmacol Ther. 2001;15:707–13.
148. Ducóns JA, Santolaria S, Guirao R, Ferrero M, Montoro M, Gomollón F. Impact of clarithromycin resistance on the effectiveness of a regimen for *Helicobacter pylori*: a prospective study of 1-week lansoprazole, amoxicillin and clarithromycin in active peptic ulcer. Aliment Pharmacol Ther. 1999;13:775–80.
149. Horiki N, Omata F, Uemura M, et al. Annual change of primary resistance to clarithromycin among *Helicobacter pylori* isolates from 1996 through 2008 in Japan. Helicobacter. 2009;14(5):86–90.
150. Fischbach LA, Goodman KJ, Feldman M, Aragaki C. Sources of variation of *Helicobacter pylori* treatment success in adults worldwide: a meta-analysis. Int J Epidemiol. 2002;31:128–39.
151. Vakil N, Connor J. *Helicobacter pylori* eradication: equivalence trials and the optimal duration of therapy. Am J Gastroenterol. 2005; 100:1702–3.

152. Paoluzi P, Iacopini F, Crispino P, et al. 2-week triple therapy for *Helicobacter pylori* infection is better than 1-week in clinical practice: a large prospective single-center randomized study. Helicobacter. 2006;11:562–8.

153. Fuccio L, Minardi ME, Zagari RM, Grilli D, Magrini N, Bazzoli F. Meta-analysis: duration of first-line proton-pump inhibitor based triple therapy for *Helicobacter pylori* eradication. Ann Intern Med. 2007;147:553–62.

154. Mégraud F. Update on therapeutic options for *Helicobacter pylori*-related diseases. Curr Infect Dis Rep. 2005;7:115–20.

155. Katelaris PH, Forbes GM, Talley NJ, Crotty B. A randomized comparison of quadruple and triple therapies for *Helicobacter pylori* eradication: The QUADRATE Study. Gastroenterology. 2002;123:1763–9.

156. Laine L, Hunt R, El-Zimaity H, Nguyen B, Osato M, Spénard J. Bismuth-based quadruple therapy using a single capsule of bismuth biskalcitrate, metronidazole, and tetracycline given with omeprazole versus omeprazole, amoxicillin, and clarithromycin for eradication of *Helicobacter pylori* in duodenal ulcer patients: a prospective, randomized, multicenter, North American trial. Am J Gastroenterol. 2003;98:562–7.

157. Luther J, Higgins PD, Schoenfeld PS, Moayyedi P, Vakil N, Chey WD. Empiric quadruple vs. triple therapy for primary treatment of *Helicobacter pylori* infection: systematic review and meta-analysis of efficacy and tolerability. Am J Gastroenterol. 2010;105:65–73.

158. De Francesco V, Zullo A, Margiotta M, et al. Sequential treatment for *Helicobacter pylori* does not share the risk factors of triple therapy failure. Aliment Pharmacol Ther. 2004;19:407–14.

159. De Francesco V, Margiotta M, Zullo A, et al. Clarithromycin-resistant genotypes and eradication of *Helicobacter pylori*. Ann Intern Med. 2006;144:94–100.

160. Scaccianoce G, Hassan C, Panarese A, Piglionica D, Morini S, Zullo A. *Helicobacter pylori* eradication with either 7-day or 10-day triple therapies, and with a 10-day sequential regimen. Can J Gastroenterol. 2006;20:113–7.

161. Vaira D, Zullo A, Vakil N, et al. Sequential therapy versus standard triple-drug therapy for *Helicobacter pylori* eradication: a randomized trial. Ann Intern Med. 2007;146:556–63.

162. Zullo A, De Francesco V, Hassan C, Morini S, Vaira D. The sequential therapy regimen for *Helicobacter pylori* eradication: a pooled-data analysis. Gut. 2007;56:1353–7.

163. Jafri NS, Hornung CA, Howden CW. Meta-analysis: sequential therapy appears superior to standard therapy for *Helicobacter pylori* infection in patients naive to treatment. Ann Intern Med. 2008;148:923–31.

164. Wu DC, Hsu PI, Wu JY, et al. Sequential and concomitant therapy with four drugs is equally effective for eradication of *H. pylori* infection. Clin Gastroenterol Hepatol. 2010;8:36–41.

165. Bilardi C, Dulbecco P, Zentilin P, et al. A 10-day levofloxacin-based therapy in patients with resistant *Helicobacter pylori* infection: a controlled trial. Clin Gastroenterol Hepatol. 2004;2:997–1002.

166. Saad RJ, Schoenfeld P, Kim HM, Chey WD. Levofloxacin-based triple therapy versus bismuth-based quadruple therapy for persistent *Helicobacter pylori* infection: a meta-analysis. Am J Gastroenterol. 2006;101:488–96.
167. Crabtree JE. Eradication of chronic *Helicobacter pylori* infection by therapeutic vaccination. Gut. 1998;43:7–8.
168. Corthésy-Theulaz I, Parta N, Glauser M, et al. Oral immunization with *Helicobacter pylori* urease B-subunit as a treatment against *Helicobacter* infection in mice. Gastroenterology. 1995;109:115–21.
169. DeLyria ES, Redline RW, Blanchard TG. Vaccination of mice against *H. pylori* induces a strong Th-17 response and immunity that is neutrophil dependent. Gastroenterology. 2009;136:247–56.
170. Michetti P, Kreiss C, Kotloff KL, et al. Oral immunization with urease and *Escherichia coli* heat-labile enterotoxin is safe and immunogenic in *Helicobacter pylori*-infected adults. Gastroenterology. 1999; 116:804–12.
171. Malfertheiner P, Schultze V, Rosenkranz B, et al. Safety and immunogenicity of an intramuscular *Helicobacter pylori* vaccine in noninfected volunteers: a phase I study. Gastroenterology. 2008;135:787–95.
172. Bilardi C, Biagini R, Dulbecco P, et al. Stool antigen assay (HpSA) is less reliable than urea breath test for post-treatment diagnosis of *Helicobacter pylori* infection. Aliment Pharmacol Ther. 2002;16:1733–8.
173. Laine L, Sugg J, Suchower L, Neil G. Endoscopic biopsy requirements for post-treatment diagnosis of *Helicobacter pylori*. Gastrointest Endosc. 2000;51:664–9.

Chapter 10
Management of Peptic Ulcer Disease

Marko Duvnjak and Vedran Tomašić

Keywords: Peptic ulcer disease, *Helicobacter pylori*, NSaids, Treatment, Proton pump inhibitors

INTRODUCTION

Peptic ulcer disease (PUD) is an important cause of the complex of symptoms known as dyspepsia. Although it can only be found in up to 5% of all upper GI endoscopies performed for investigation of dyspepsia, it can be associated with different complications with the potential for significant morbidity and mortality, such as recurrence, bleeding, perforation, and GI obstruction [1, 2]. The annual incidence rate of peptic ulcer ranges from 0.1% to 0.3% worldwide, but the prevalence of PUD, hospitalization, and surgery rates for uncomplicated ulcers have been in decline in the past few decades [3–6]. These facts are attributed to the better understanding of PUD multifactorial etiology [*Helicobacter pylori* (*H. pylori*) infection, nonsteroidal anti-inflammatory drugs (NSAIDs) use and smoking], change in environmental factors (improved food transportation and refrigeration, improved hygiene, socioeconomic conditions, and overall health), and powerful treatment options

V. Tomašić (✉)
Division of Gastroenterology and Hepatology, Department of Medicine,
University Hospital "Sestre milosrdnice", Zagreb, Croatia
e-mail: vtomasic@globalnet.hr

M. Duvnjak (ed.), *Dyspepsia in Clinical Practice*,
DOI 10.1007/978-1-4419-1730-0_10,
© Springer Science+Business Media, LLC 2011

(antisecretory and antimicrobial drugs) [2, 7]. Peptic ulcers have a variable natural history; they can heal spontaneously but can also have a high recurrence rate ranging between 50% and 80% annually. On the other hand, some can cause complications or remain refractory, despite the antisecretory therapy [8–11].

CAUSES OF PEPTIC ULCER DISEASE

In general, there are two major causes of PUD – *H. pylori* infection and the consumption of NSAIDs. Other factors associated with the risk of developing PUD are smoking, excessive alcohol consumption, drugs such as bisphosphonates, potassium chloride, mycofenolate mofetil, and sirolimus, Zollinger–Ellison syndrome, herpes simplex virus type I infections or cytomegalovirus (especially in immunocompromised patients), recent use of cocaine and/or amphetamines, radiotherapy, chemotherapy, sarcoidosis, and Crohn's disease.

TREATMENT OPTIONS

From the beginning of the twentieth century, it has been common understanding that abnormal gastric acid secretion and duodenal bicarbonate production cause the change in acid homeostasis, which in combination with abnormal gastroduodenal motility lead to development of gastric and duodenal peptic ulcers [12–17]. Therefore, a variety of acid-neutralizing agents, mucosa protective agents, and antisecretory drugs were, and practically still are, the mainstay of PUD treatment.

Antacids

Antacids such as aluminum hydroxide, magnesium hydroxide, calcium carbonate, or sodium bicarbonate are still commonly prescribed by practitioners as co-therapy for PUD. They also continue to be widely used as over-the-counter self-medications, which patients use for dyspepsia relief. They work as a weak base that reacts with gastric acid to form salt and water. Because of the proven superiority of antisecretory drugs in treating PUD, antacids are no longer recommended for this indication. Different potential adverse effects, such as diarrhea (magnesium), constipation (aluminum, calcium), gastric distension and belching (sodium/calcium carbonate), hypomagnesaemia, hypercalcemia, aluminum toxicity, and "the milk-alkali syndrome," as well as the ability to reduce intestinal absorption of other drugs (by binding mechanism), limit their further use, especially on a long-term basis.

Sucralfate

Sucralfate is a polysaccharide (sulfated sucrose) combined with aluminum hydroxide. It is considered a mucosa protective agent with little (if any) acid-neutralizing capacity. It has different potential beneficial effects (formation of protective mucous barrier over the damaged tissue, stimulation of angiogenesis, and prostaglandin and bicarbonate secretion) which promote ulcer healing. The drug has been proven to be as efficient as H_2 receptor antagonists in treating duodenal ulcers, though there are not enough studies which confirm these results [18, 19]. Encouraging results have been reported in unlabeled treatment of gastric ulcers, although it is not registered for this indication. There are no significant systemic adverse effects other than the potential aluminum toxicity.

Bismuth

Bismuth does not have any effect on the production of gastric acid or the change of its pH. Its mechanism in the healing of peptic ulcers is not clear. The proposed action is the formation of a protective barrier over the ulcer craters, the inhibition of pepsin activity, and the stimulation of mucus, bicarbonate, and prostaglandin secretion. Its main effect is a direct antimicrobial activity against *H. pylori*. It can therefore be used in combination with other antimicrobials and proton pump inhibitors for the "quadruple therapy" treatment of *H. pylori*-associated duodenal ulcer [20]. Bismuth formulations cause blackening of the stool, and prolonged usage can lead to bismuth toxicity.

Prostaglandin Analogs

Prostaglandins enhance gastric mucosal defense mechanisms and also inhibit gastric acid secretion. Only prostaglandin E analog misoprostol is used and registered for prevention of NSAID-induced gastric ulcers [21]. The main side effect of misoprostol is diarrhea, which occurs in up to 30% of patients and leads to loss of compliance with the treatment regimen. It is contraindicated during pregnancy because it can stimulate uterine smooth muscle contraction and can cause uterine bleeding.

Histamine H_2 Receptor Antagonists (H2RAs)

H2RAs exhibit their antisecretory action through the blockade of histamine H_2 receptors on the parietal cell. They continue to be widely used as over-the-counter agents and prescription agents for treatment and maintenance therapy of a variety of acid-peptic disorders. They have a marked effect on nocturnal acid secretion but only a modest effect on meal-stimulated acid secretion in comparison with proton pump inhibitors (PPIs) [22]. Four agents are available: ranitidine, cimetidine, nizatidine, and famotidine; all four share comparable efficacy in inhibiting acid secretion and in healing peptic ulcers. They need to be taken twice daily to maintain a satisfactory 24-h acid suppression. Ulcer healing rates ranging between 80% and 90% were reported after these agents had been administered for 6–8 weeks in treating uncomplicated gastric and duodenal ulcers [11, 23]. If the ulcers were caused by aspirin or NSAID, H2RAs provide rapid ulcer healing so long as NSAID is discontinued. In the group of patients with *H. pylori*-associated peptic ulcers, these agents do not play a significant therapeutic role any more. They are a safe group of drugs; adverse effects occur in up to 4% of patients (generally similar to placebo) [24]. Dose reduction is advised in patients with moderate to severe renal insufficiency. The problem is that tolerance to the antisecretory effect of H2RAs develops commonly; the mechanism of this effect is not clear.

Proton Pump Inhibitors

PPIs are the mainstay in treating different acid-peptic disorders, including PUD. They are the most effective acid blocking agents that decrease gastric acid secretion through the inhibition of H^+/K^+-ATPase, the proton pump of the parietal cell. Five agents are available: omeprazole, esomperazole, lansoprazole, rabeprazole, and pantoprazole. All share similar efficacy on acid secretion inhibition and consequent PUD healing rates. Because of their superior efficacy, quicker effect, absence of tolerance development, and long-lasting inhibition of acid secretion, they have virtually replaced all other agents in the treatment of PUD. In comparison with H2RAs, PPIs afford a more rapid symptom relief and have faster and better healing rates on both duodenal and gastric ulcers, although these differences tend to disappear after a longer duration of therapy [11, 23, 25, 26]. Food decreases the bioavailability of all PPIs to up to 50%; therefore, all of these agents should be administered on an empty stomach, 30 min to 1 h before a meal (usually breakfast) – PPIs inhibit only actively secreting pumps that are activated by food (only 5% to 10% are actively secreting during fasting states!). Usually 3–4 days of daily medication is needed to achieve full acid inhibition. Four weeks of treatment with these agents leads to over 90% healing rates for uncomplicated duodenal ulcers, and similar results were obtained after 6–8 weeks for gastric ulcers [27]. PPIs are an extremely safe group with reported adverse effects such as diarrhea, headaches, and abdominal pain occurring in up to 5% of patients (similar to placebo). There is a risk of developing enteric infection during treatment with PPIs because of the loss of gastric acid barrier – this risk is slightly increased when traveling to underdeveloped areas or in hospitalized patients (*Clostridium difficile*). Rebound acid hypersecretion can develop after the cessation of PPI treatment. The clinical relevance of PPI-induced hypergastrinemia remains unknown. Long-term maintenance therapy with PPIs is a somewhat controversial issue due to potential adverse effects of prolonged PPI usage, such as decreased calcium absorption and the increased risk of bone fractures [28].

The combination of different "antiulcer" medicaments has no added benefit on ulcer healing. Therefore, it is not recommended.

H. PYLORI-ASSOCIATED ULCERS

H. pylori is the predominant cause of PUD worldwide. Since its discovery by Warren and Marshall in 1983, the treatment has changed fundamentally [29]. The annual recurrence rate for peptic ulcers used to be as high as 80%, in spite of maintenance antisecretory therapy. Since the establishment of an adequate *H. pylori* eradication therapy, peptic ulcer can now not only be healed, but its recurrence can also be prevented.

Therefore, today's standard approach is that all patients with a detected peptic ulcer must be tested for *H. pylori* using noninvasive (carbon-13 urea breath test, stool antigen test, and laboratory-based serology) or invasive endoscopic tests (biopsy urease testing, rapid urease test, histology, bacterial culture, and sensitivity testing). If a *H. pylori*-associated ulcer is diagnosed, there are two therapeutic goals: ulcer healing and the eradication of the causing organism.

Duodenal Ulcer

H. pylori infection can be found in up to 90% of patients with uncomplicated duodenal ulcers [30–32]. As previously emphasized, the confirmation of infection must be obtained. Most duodenal ulcers are diagnosed endoscopically (Fig. 10.1). Therefore, invasive tests such as biopsy urease test or histology are commonly used. Gastric biopsy specimens should be taken from the antrum; if a patient is receiving antisecretory therapy 1 week prior to the endoscopic biopsy, specimens should be obtained from the antrum and the corpus. If *H. pylori* infection is diagnosed, eradication therapy with one of the regimen protocols should be offered to the patient and carried out accordingly. Successful *H. pylori*

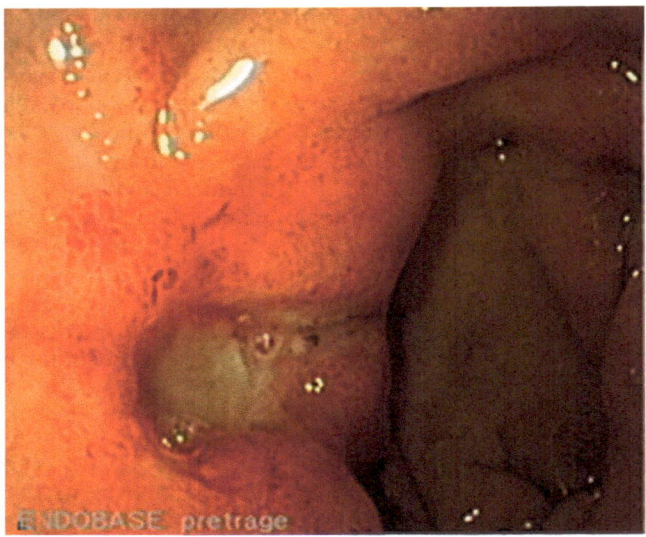

Fɪɢ. 10.1   Duodenal ulcer.

eradication therapy increases duodenal healing rate and reduces duodenal ulcer recurrence when compared with acid suppression therapy alone [33]. If the patient with uncomplicated duodenal ulcer has no symptoms after an adequate treatment regimen, no evidence supports further continuation of antisecretory agents [34]. A follow-up endoscopy to ensure ulcer healing and invasively confirm successful *H. pylori* infection is not recommended for uncomplicated duodenal ulcers. The eradication of infection should be confirmed by using the urea breath test 4 weeks after treatment discontinuation; the stool antigen test can be also performed, although it is less accurate. Serology testing is not useful for follow-ups. With patients suffering from complicated duodenal ulcers (especially if NSAIDs are a possible cause or there is a need to restart them), maintenance antisecretory therapy should be continued until successful ulcer healing is endoscopically confirmed and *H. pylori* eradication is achieved; follow-up endoscopy at least 4–12 weeks after the completion of *H. pylori* therapy should be performed [35, 36]. Special attention should be focused on a reliable interpretation of *H. pylori* test results. Concurrent use of PPIs can cause false-negative results. When we consider the group of patients with complicated duodenal ulcers, if the first control test after eradication therapy is negative (while still taking maintenance PPI therapy), the second control test (usually a noninvasive test, such as the urea breath test) should be obtained after PPI discontinuation (or switch to H2RAs 2 weeks prior to testing).

Gastric Ulcer

H. pylori infection can be found in 60% to 80% of patients with gastric ulcers (Fig. 10.2) [31, 37]. Multiple gastric biopsy specimens should be taken at the ulcer margin to exclude malignancy and separately from the antrum to search for a *H. pylori* infection. If gastric ulcer is diagnosed by radiography, a noninvasive test for *H. pylori* can be performed – when the appropriate eradication therapy is finished, endoscopic control is mandatory. If a *H. pylori* infection is diagnosed, eradication therapy with one of the regimen protocols should be offered to the patient and carried out accordingly. Results of some studies have shown that 1 week of *H. pylori* eradication therapy without additional acid suppression effectively heals uncomplicated gastric ulcers [38]. On the other hand, when compared with acid suppression therapy alone, *H. pylori* eradication combined with acid suppression does not increase gastric ulcer healing in trials of 4–8 weeks duration.

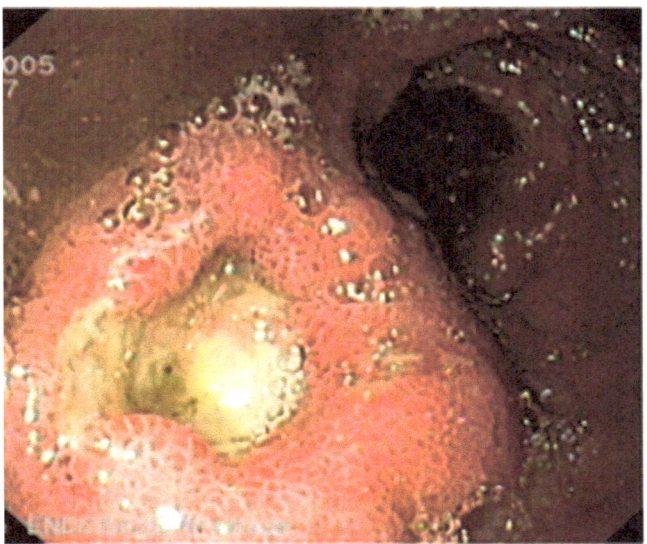

Fig. 10.2 Gastric ulcer.

Common clinical approach is to continue additional antisecretory therapy for 6–8 weeks after the eradication protocol in patients with *H. pylori*-associated gastric ulcer [39, 40]. In patients with giant gastric ulcers (>2–3 cm), 12 weeks of therapy is an effective and commonly used approach. Follow-up endoscopy is performed to confirm complete ulcer healing, to reconfirm that the ulcer was not gastric cancer, and to histologically confirm successful eradication of *H. pylori*. Successful *H. pylori* eradication therapy reduces gastric ulcer recurrence.

Treatment outcome in both types of peptic ulcers can be strongly influenced by several factors, most importantly the patient's adherence to therapy, concurrent aspirin or NSAID use, and smoking. Repeated counseling is advised.

In patients with complicated duodenal and gastric ulcers, long-term maintenance antisecretory therapy with H2RAs or PPIs is advised to prevent recurrence. It should be continued at least until the cure for the *H. pylori* infection has been confirmed. In patients who fail to eradicate *H. pylori* after repeated eradication regimens have been undertaken, the duration of treatment is guided by the clinical response.

NONSTEROIDAL ANTI-INFLAMMATORY DRUG-ASSOCIATED ULCERS

NSAIDs are one of the most commonly used drugs in the world. This is quite understandable when we appreciate different clinical uses of these agents. They are used for a variety of conditions due to their anti-inflammatory, analgesic, and antipyretic effects. Furthermore, their antiplatelet effect (especially one of aspirin) which leads to a significant reduction in the number of varieties of cardiovascular incidents has additionally "boostered up" their everyday usage. All of their effects are mainly mediated through the inhibition of cyclooxygenase (COX) pathway of biosynthesis of prostaglandins. There are distinct cyclooxygenase isoforms (COX-1 and COX-2); COX-2 is only induced at the site of inflammation as the COX-1 is commonly active in various tissues including the gastrointestinal (GI) tract where it is involved in gastric and duodenal cytoprotection. Nonselective COX inhibitors' (including aspirin) main adverse effects are upper GI intolerance and development of gastric and duodenal ulcers (mainly mediated through inhibition of COX-1). The risk of developing serious GI adverse effects ranges between 1% and 4% annually for nonselective NSAIDs and is probably dose dependant [4]. Therefore, COX-2 selective inhibitors were developed to reduce GI adverse effects, without limiting their anti-inflammatory, analgesic, or antipyretic effect. Also, COX-2 inhibitors do not have any impact on platelet aggregation (mediated by COX-1 isoenzyme), which further reduces potential bleeding complications in patients with peptic ulcers. For a while COX-2 inhibitors were widely considered to be an adequate substitution for conventional nonselective NSAIDs in patients with risk of GI adverse effects – unfortunately there are no data which support this approach. This was further "put on hold," especially after some of these agents had been withdrawn from the market because of the reported data suggestive of higher incidence of serious cardiovascular thrombotic events associated with COX-2 inhibitors [41–43].

Several risk factors have been associated as an additional influence on the development of PUD in patients taking NSAIDs. They include a prior history of PUD, patient age (>60 years) and comorbidities, *H. pylori* infection, higher dose and longer duration of NSAID therapy, co-therapy of NSAIDs with steroids, anticoagulants, other NSAIDs (including aspirin), and selective serotonin reuptake inhibitors or bisphosphonates [44–46].

Management of Active Ulcers Associated with NSAIDs

If possible, NSAIDs should be withdrawn in patients with NSAID-associated peptic ulcers [47]. Antisecretory therapy with PPIs should be the initial choice of therapy for ulcer healing; H2RAs are the alternative. *H. pylori* status should be assessed and eradication therapy should be offered to all *H. pylori*-infected patients. Antisecretory drugs can be discontinued after 8 weeks in patients with uncomplicated duodenal and gastric ulcers which are asymptomatic. Antacids, sucralfate and misoprostol, have no advantage over antisecretory agents for NSAID ulcer treatment and are not recommended for this purpose. If continuous NSAID (including aspirin) treatment is required, PPIs are the most effective agents for healing NSAID-associated peptic ulcers. Substitution of conventional NSAIDs with COX-2 inhibitors in patients with active ulcers is not recommended. Follow-up endoscopy is only recommended for gastric ulcers to confirm complete ulcer healing, to retest for *H. pylori* infection, and to exclude gastric cancer.

Prevention of NSAID-Induced Ulcers

Primary prevention focuses on the identification of patients who on the one hand must take NSAIDs and on the other hand have a high risk of developing symptomatic and complicated ulcers. As previously mentioned, several risk factors for NSAID-induced ulcers have been identified. These are prior history of PUD/ gastrointestinal hemorrhage, patient age (>60 years), higher dose and longer duration of NSAID therapy, co-therapy of NSAIDs with steroids, anticoagulants, other NSAIDs (including aspirin) or selective serotonin reuptake inhibitors, and presence of dyspepsia/GERD symptoms [46, 48, 49]. The choice of NSAIDs can also play an important role – NSAIDs such as meloxicam and ibuprofen have the lowest risk to induce PUD; aspirin, diclofenac, and naproxen have the relatively moderate risk to induce PUD; and indomethacin and ketoprofen have the highest relative risk to induce PUD [50]. Therefore, the choice of a particular agent should be individual with the emphasis on using the lowest possible dose and the shortest duration of NSAID therapy possible. Enteric-coated and buffered aspirins are nowadays commonly used under the presumption that they offer "protection" against the potential aspirin-induced GI toxicity. Although they do cause less dyspeptic symptoms and endoscopic signs of GI toxicity, they do not offer additional protection against ulcer bleeding when compared with "standard" aspirin [51]. Selective COX-2 inhibitors have been developed to offer significant gastroduodenal sparing effect while keeping the same anti-inflammatory effect when compared with nonselective NSAIDs. However, their wide usage is nowadays rather limited due to their potential cardiovascular toxicity. In addition, when COX-2 inhibitors are concomitantly used with low-dose aspirin or anticoagulants, their gastrointestinal sparing effect is lost [52, 53]. *H. pylori* testing should be offered to all patients with symptoms of dyspepsia or with a history of uncomplicated or complicated PUD prior to starting NSAID therapy. If positive, eradication therapy should be offered to patients. If patients are at high risk of developing NSAID-induced PUD (defined by previously described risk factors, especially if two or more are present), PPI should be co-administered as a primary prevention strategy [54]. Misoprostol offers a potential alternative to PPIs in these settings but is less frequently used because of its inconvenient dosing regimen and GI intolerance. H2RAs have no proven effect upon reducing the incidence of NSAID-induced GI injury. According to the guidelines issued by the American College of Gastroenterology [55]:

– Patients with high risk for development of GI complications (history of complicated ulcer or >2 risk factors present), as well with a high cardiovascular (CV) risk for which they are concomitantly using low-dose aspirin, should avoid NSAID or COX-2 inhibitor treatment
– Patients with high GI and low CV risk should be treated with COX-2 inhibitor in combination with PPI or misoprostol

- Patients with moderate GI risk (1–2 risk factors present) and low CV risk should be treated with COX-s inhibitor alone or with NSAID in combination with PPI or misoprostol
- Patients with low (no risk factors) to moderate GI risk and high CV risk should be treated with NSAID (preferably naproxen) in combination with either PPI or misoprostol
- Patients with low GI risk and low CV risk can be treated with NSAID alone, if possible with less ulcerogenic NSAID (e.g., ibuprofen and diclofenac)

Secondary prevention takes into account those patients who must continue NSAID therapy despite prior history of NSAID-induced uncomplicated or complicated PUD (including low-dose aspirin). All of those patients should be treated with concomitant PPI therapy for as long as NSAID (including low-dose aspirin) treatment is needed [56–58]. If patients are also infected with *H. pylori*, eradication therapy is co-administered to PPIs. Substitution of conventional NSAIDs with COX-2 inhibitors in patients with history of NSAID-induced PUD is not recommended over PPI maintenance therapy [59]. On the other hand, combination of COX-2 inhibitor and PPI may be effective in preventing recurrent ulcers but more data are needed before a clear recommendation can be made.

Regular review of a patient's need for continuous NSAID treatment is advised. Trial use of NSAID on "as needed" basis, NSAID dose reduction, substitution of one NSAID with another, less ulcerogenic NSAID, or use of alternative analgesic is recommended, if possible.

H. pylori and NSAIDs

The true relationship between *H. pylori* and NSAIDs is still widely debated but the current approach is to test-and-treat all, especially high-risk patients for development of PUD if they need to take NSAIDs or low-dose aspirin on long-term basis [60, 61]. If NSAID-induced peptic ulcer is diagnosed, *H. pylori* should also be looked for and treated appropriately. Still, the emphasis is on a continuous PPI maintenance therapy for prevention of ulcer recurrence if patients need to continue NSAID or low-dose aspirin.

PEPTIC ULCERS NOT ASSOCIATED WITH *H. PYLORI* OR NSAIDS

If an adequate evaluation has been performed and has excluded the presence of a *H. pylori* infection and NSAID use (including measuring serum salicylate levels or platelet aggregation), other rare causes of PUD should be considered. Medications such as potassium chloride, mycophenolate mofetil, or bisphosphonates, as well as corticosteroids and clopidogrel can be a potential cause of PUD, especially when combined with NSAIDs. Biopsies should be repeatedly obtained to search for signs of infection (HSV, CMV, and tuberculosis) or inflammation (sarcoidosis or Crohn's disease). Cocaine or amphetamine use can also be a cause of PUD. If clinical manifestations raise suspicion, patients should be evaluated for Zollinger–Ellison syndrome (serum gastrin levels). Full-dose PPI therapy lasting for 4–8 weeks heals peptic ulcers in majority of cases, although this group of patients appears to be predisposed to recurrent disease that is often associated with complications [62, 63].

REFRACTORY AND RECURRENT PEPTIC ULCER DISEASE

Refractory peptic ulcers should be suspected in all patients who present with persistent dyspeptic symptoms after the course of 8 weeks of adequate ulcer therapy. Endoscopy is used to differentiate between a group of patients who have refractory symptoms without ulceration and another group of patients who indeed have refractory ulcer. Gastric biopsy samples must be obtained during endoscopy from the ulcer margin and base, as well as from antrum and the body of the stomach. The following factors should be considered in patients with refractory ulcers:

(a) Patients' compliance with the treatment protocol
(b) Type and dose of antisecretory medications used – H2RA or PPI? A double dose of antisecretory agents is sometimes needed for induction and maintenance of ulcer healing
(c) Presence of persistent or previously undetected *H. pylori* infection – the question of adherence to eradication therapy, antibiotic resistance, false-negative tests, and concomitant use of NSAID
(d) Continuing NSAID use – if a patient denies taking those agents and clinical suspicion is high, measuring of serum salicylate levels or platelet aggregation is the recommended approach for further evaluation (in some reports up to 40% of patients denying the use of NSAIDs still abuse them)
(e) Ulcer size, depth, and scarring of surrounding tissue – average ulcer healing rate is approximately 3 mm per week; therefore, larger ulcers take longer time to heal (12 weeks of antisecretory therapy is advised for bigger ulcers, especially those greater than 20 mm)
(f) Smoking and cocaine and alcohol consumption can slow ulcer healing – patients should be advised to discontinue those habits

(g) Presence of other comorbidities that can impair ulcer healing such as uremia or liver cirrhosis

(h) Signs and symptoms of Zollinger–Ellison syndrome

(i) Repeat biopsy at the ulcer margin and base is advised to exclude malignancy and to search for or exclude gastric infection (HSV-1, CMV, tuberculosis) or some other inflammatory conditions (sarcoidosis, Crohn's disease)

Treatment approach is directed to the eradication of *H. pylori* (if present), withdrawal of NSAID, and adequate antisecretory therapy. PPIs in "full dose" and sometimes in "double dose" are recommended for additional 8 weeks [64, 65]. Control endoscopy is mandatory to search for signs of ulcer healing. The question of maintenance therapy after ulcer healing is individual. If potentially reversible causes are excluded (successful eradication of *H. pylori* accomplished, NSAID abuse stopped), maintenance therapy may not be necessary. If reversible causes are not excluded, maintenance antisecretory therapy is advised, especially for large and recurrent ulcers, sometimes for an indefinite period of time.

If ulcers stay refractory after a repeated adequate course of ulcer therapy, and if reversible causes and malignancy are carefully excluded, elective surgery can be recommended.

Recurrent PUD should be considered in those patients with a history of PUD who present with recurrent dyspeptic symptoms. Endoscopy is used to differentiate between a group of patients who have recurrent symptoms without ulceration and another group of patients who have recurrent ulcer. Gastric biopsy samples must be obtained from ulcer margin and base, as well as from antrum and body of stomach to exclude malignancy and to search for the cause of ulcer (*H. pylori*, other infectious and inflammatory conditions). The appropriate approach for the evaluation of NSAID abuse is previously depicted. Factors such as a history of complicated and/or recurrent peptic ulcers, smoking, and alcohol or cocaine use influence the development of recurrent disease. If present, *H. pylori* should be eradicated and potentially offending or contributing agents to the recurrence of PUD, such as NSAIDs, cigarettes, or alcohol, should be withdrawn. Full-dose antisecretory therapy is advised. If potentially reversible causes can be eliminated (successful eradication of *H. pylori*, discontinuation of NSAID use), the treatment can be stopped after an endoscopical confirmation of successful ulcer healing – repeated endoscopy after 8 weeks of treatment is a common approach. Long-term maintenance therapy is recommended for patients who fail to eradicate *H. pylori* or who have to continue NSAID treatment, especially if they have a positive history of a complicated and/or recurrent ulcer disease.

TREATMENT OF COMPLICATIONS OF PUD

Treatment of potential complications of PUD, such as bleeding, perforation, or obstruction, is often multidisciplinary and is almost always carried out in hospital settings. Combinations of different medical, endoscopical, radiological, and surgical methods are commonly used for treatment of those conditions. The depiction of different treatment approaches and modalities far surpasses the limits of this book. Therefore, readers are advised to look for those answers in other specialized gastroenterological books.

DIETARY RECOMMENDATIONS

No firm dietary recommendations are necessary for patients with PUD; patients should avoid foods that precipitate dyspepsia.

CONCLUSIONS

PUD is not a common cause of dyspepsia, but it can be associated with several life-threatening complications. Therefore, every practitioner should be aware of risk factors and alarm symptoms associated with PUD, which should help in directing potential patients to early endoscopic evaluation. Early recognition, testing and eradication of *H. pylori* (if present), discontinuation of potential offending causes (such as NSAIDs, smoking, and alcohol consumption), and adequate treatment with antisecretory agents (PPIs are preferred) are the fundamental modalities of PUD management. Patient's adherence to therapy regiments, patient's other comorbidities, unrecognized gastric malignancy, and unwillingness to stop NSAIDs can further influence treatment success. Refractory, recurrent, and complicated PUD should be in the domain of specialist care. There are no firm dietary recommendations for patients with PUD, although logical approach is to avoid foods that cause dyspeptic symptoms.

References

1. Ford AC, Marwaha A, Lim A, et al. Prevalence of clinically significant endoscopic findings in individuals with and without dyspepsia: systematic review and meta-analysis [abstract]. Gastroenterology. 2009;136 Suppl 1:A488.
2. el-Serag H, Sonnenberg A. Opposing time trends of peptic ulcer and reflux disease. Gut. 1998;43:327–33.
3. Garcia Rodriguez LA, Hernandez-Diaz S. Risk of uncomplicated peptic ulcer among users of aspirin and nonaspirin nonsteroidal antiinflammatory drugs. Am J Epidemiol. 2004;159:23–31.

4. Kurata JH. Epidemiology: peptic ulcer risk factors. Semin Gastrointest Dis. 1993;4:2.

5. Rosenstock SJ, Jorgensen T, Bonnevie O, Andersen LP. Does *Helicobacter pylori* infection explain all socio-economic differences in peptic ulcer incidence? Genetic and psychosocial markers for incident peptic ulcer disease in a large cohort of Danish adults. Scand J Gastroenterol. 2004;39:823–9.

6. Sung JJ, Kuipers EJ, El-Serag HB. Systematic review: the global incidence and prevalence of peptic ulcer disease. Aliment Pharmacol Ther. 2009;29:938–46.

7. Sonnenberg A. Time trends of ulcer mortality in Europe. Gastroenterology. 2007;132:2320–7.

8. Gudmand-Hoyer F, Jensen KB, Krag E, et al. Prophylactic effect of cimetidine in duodenal ulcer disease. Br Med J. 1978;1:1095.

9. Current status of maintenance therapy in peptic ulcer disease. The ACG Committee on FDA-Related Matters. Am J Gastroenterol. 1988;83:607–17.

10. Jorde R, Bostad L, Burhol PG. Asymptomatic gastric ulcer: a follow-up study in patients with previous gastric ulcer disease. Lancet. 1986; 1:119–21.

11. Howden CW, Hunt RH. The relationship between suppression of acidity and gastric ulcer healing rates. Aliment Pharmacol Ther. 1990;4:25–33.

12. Lam SK. Pathogenesis and pathophysiology of duodenal ulcer. Clin Gastroenterol. 1984;13:447–72.

13. Malagelada JR, Longstreth GF, Deering TB, et al. Gastric secretion and emptying after ordinary meals in duodenal ulcer. Gastroenterology. 1979;73:989–94.

14. Merki HS, Fimmel CJ, Walt RP, et al. Pattern of 24 hour intragastric acidity in active duodenal ulcer disease and in healthy controls. Gut. 1988;29:1583–7.

15. Samloff IM. Peptic ulcer: the many proteinases of aggression. Gastroenterology. 1989;96:586–95.

16. Isenberg JI, Selling JA, Hogan DL, Koss MA. Impaired proximal duodenal mucosal bicarbonate secretion in patients with duodenal ulcer. N Engl J Med. 1987;316:374–9.

17. Miller LJ, Malagelada JR, Longstreth GF, Go VL. Dysfunctions of the stomach with gastric ulceration. Dig Dis Sci. 1980;25:857–64.

18. McCarthy DM. Sucralfate[Rx]. N Engl J Med. 1991;325:1017–25.

19. Yeomans ND, Svedberg LE, Naesdal J. Is ranitidine therapy sufficient for healing peptic ulcers associated with non-steroidal anti-inflammatory drug use? Int J Clin Pract. 2006;60:1401–7.

20. Laine L, Hunt R, El-Zimaity H, et al. Bismuth-based quadruple therapy using a single capsule of bismuth biskalcitrate, metronidazole, and tetracycline given with omeprazole versus omeprazole, amoxicillin, and clarithromycin for eradication of *Helicobacter pylori* in duodenal ulcer patients: a prospective, randomized, multicenter, North American trial. Am J Gastroenterol. 2003;98:562–7.

21. Raskin JB, White RH, Jackson JE, et al. Misoprostol dosage in the prevention of nonsteroidal anti-inflammatory drug-induced gastric and duodenal ulcers: a comparison of three regimens. Ann Intern Med. 1995;123:344–50.

22. Lanzon-Miller S, Pounder RE, Hamilton MR, et al. Twenty-four-hour intragastric acidity and plasma gastrin concentration before and during treatment with either ranitidine or omeprazole. Aliment Pharmacol Ther. 1987;1:239–51.

23. Burget DW, Chiverton SG, Hunt RH. Is there an optimal degree of acid suppression for healing of duodenal ulcers? A model of the relationship between ulcer healing and acid suppression. Gastroenterology. 1990;99:345–51.

24. Reynolds JC. The clinical importance of drug interactions with antiulcer therapy. J Clin Gastroenterol. 1990;12:S54–63.

25. Holt S, Howden CW. Omeprazole. Overview and opinion. Dig Dis Sci. 1991;36:385–93.

26. Poynard T, Lemaire M, Agostini H. Meta-analysis of randomized clinical trials comparing lansoprazole with ranitidine or famotidine in the treatment of acute duodenal ulcer. Eur J Gastroenterol Hepatol. 1995;7:661–5.

27. Bader JP, Delchier JC. Clinical efficacy of pantoprazole compared with ranitidine. Aliment Pharmacol Ther. 1994;8 Suppl 1:47–52.

28. Yang YX, Lewis JD, Epstein S, et al. Long-term proton pump inhibitor therapy and risk of hip fracture. JAMA. 2006;296:2947–53.

29. Marshall BJ, Warren JR. Unidentified curved bacilli in the stomach of patients with gastritis and peptic ulceration. Lancet. 1984;1:1311–5.

30. Tytgat G, Langenberg W, Rauws E, et al. Campylobacter-like organism (CLO) in the human stomach. Gastroenterology. 1985;88:1620.

31. Marshall BJ, McGechie DB, Rogers PA, et al. Pyloric Campylobacter infection and gastroduodenal disease. Med J Aust. 1985;142:439–44.

32. Borody TJ, George LL, Brandl S, et al. *Helicobacter pylori*-negative duodenal ulcer. Am J Gastroenterol. 1991;86:1154–7.

33. Chiorean MV, Locke 3rd GR, Zinsmeister AR, et al. Changing rates of *Helicobacter pylori* testing and treatment in patients with peptic ulcer disease. Am J Gastroenterol. 2002;97:3015–22.

34. Ford AC, Delaney BC, Forman D, et al. Eradication therapy in *Helicobacter pylori* positive peptic ulcer disease: systematic review and economic analysis. Am J Gastroenterol. 2004;99:1833–55.

35. Buckley M, Culhane A, Drumm B, et al. Guidelines for the management of *Helicobacter pylori*-related upper gastrointestinal diseases. Irish *Helicobacter pylori* Study Group. Ir J Med Sci. 1996;165 Suppl 5:1–11.

36. Professional Advisory Panel (CRAG) and Scottish Intercollegiate Guidelines Network (SIGN). *Helicobacter pylori* eradication therapy in dyspeptic disease: a clinical guideline. 1996.

37. Lee J, O'Morain C. Who should be treated for *Helicobacter pylori* infection? A review of consensus conferences and guidelines. Gastroenterology. 1997;113(Suppl):S99–106.

38. Sung JJ, Chung SC, Ling TK, et al. Antibacterial treatment of gastric ulcers associated with *Helicobacter pylori*. N Engl J Med. 1995;332:139–42.

39. Malfertheiner P, Kirchner T, Kist M, et al. *Helicobacter pylori* eradication and gastric ulcer healing-comparison of three pantoprazole-based triple therapies. BYK Advanced Gastric Ulcer Study Group. Aliment Pharmacol Ther. 2003;17:1125–35.

40. Higuchi K, Fujiwara Y, Tominaga K, et al. Is eradication sufficient to heal gastric ulcers in patients infected with *Helicobacter pylori*? A randomized, controlled, prospective study. Aliment Pharmacol Ther. 2003;17:111–7.

41. Ray WA, Stein CM, Daugherty JR, et al. COX-2 selective non-steroidal anti-inflammatory drugs and risk of serious coronary heart disease. Lancet. 2002;360:1071–3.

42. Graham DJ, Campen D, Hui R, et al. Risk of acute myocardial infarction and sudden cardiac death in patients treated with cyclo-oxygenase 2 selective and non-selective non-steroidal anti-inflammatory drugs: nested case–control study. Lancet. 2005;365:475–81.

43. Hippisley-Cox J, Coupland C. Risk of myocardial infarction in patients taking cyclo-oxygenase-2 inhibitors or conventional non-steroidal anti-inflammatory drugs: population based nested case–control analysis. BMJ. 2005;330:1366.

44. Hernandez-Diaz S, Rodriguez LA. Association between nonsteroidal anti-inflammatory drugs and upper gastrointestinal tract bleeding/perforation: an overview of epidemiologic studies published in the 1990s. Arch Intern Med. 2000;160:2093–9.

45. Simon LS, Hatoum TH, Bittman RM, et al. Risk factors for serious nonsteroidal-induced gastrointestinal complications: regression analysis of the MUCOSA trial. Fam Med. 1996;28:204–10.

46. Lanza FL. A guideline for the treatment and prevention of NSAID-induced ulcers. Am J Gastroenterol. 1998;93:2037–46.

47. Soll AH. Medical treatment of peptic ulcer disease: practice guidelines. Practice Parameters Committee of the American College of Gastroenterology. JAMA. 1996;275:622–9.

48. Bhatt DL, Scheiman J, Abraham NS, et al. ACCF/ACG/AHA 2008 expert consensus document on reducing the gastrointestinal risks of antiplatelet therapy and NSAID use: a report of the American College of Cardiology Foundation Task Force on Clinical Expert Consensus Documents. J Am Coll Cardiol. 2008;52:1502–17.

49. Loke YK, Trivedi AN, Singh S. Meta-analysis: gastrointestinal bleeding due to interaction between selective serotonin uptake inhibitors and non-steroidal anti-inflammatory drugs. Aliment Pharmacol Ther. 2008;27:31–40.

50. Richy F, Bruyere O, Ethgen O, et al. Time dependent risk of gastrointestinal complications induced by non-steroidal anti-inflammatory drug use: a consensus statement using a meta-analytic approach. Ann Rheum Dis. 2004;63:759–66.

51. Kelly JP, Kaufman DW, Jurgelon JM, et al. Risk of aspirin-associated major upper-gastrointestinal bleeding with enteric-coated or buffered product. Lancet. 1996;348:1413–6.
52. Silverstein FE, Faich G, Goldstein JL, et al. Gastrointestinal toxicity with celecoxib vs. nonsteroidal anti-inflammatory drugs for osteoarthritis and rheumatoid arthritis. The CLASS study: a randomized controlled trial. JAMA. 2000;284:1247–55.
53. Battistella M, Mamdami MM, Juurlink DN, et al. Risk of upper gastrointestinal hemorrhage in warfarin users treated with nonselective NSAIDs or COX-2 inhibitors. Arch Intern Med. 2005;165:189–92.
54. Koch M, Dezi A, Ferrario F, et al. Prevention of nonsteroidal anti-inflammatory drug-induced gastrointestinal mucosal injury. A meta-analysis of randomized controlled clinical trials. Arch Intern Med. 1996;156:2321–32.
55. Lanza FL, Chan FK, Quigley EM. Guidelines for prevention of NSAID-related ulcer complications. Am J Gastroenterol. 2009;104:728–38.
56. Yeomans ND, Tulassay Z, Juhasz L, et al. A comparison of omeprazole with ranitidine for ulcers associated with nonsteroidal antiinflammatory drugs. N Engl J Med. 1998;338:719–26.
57. Hawkey CJ, Karrasch JA, Szczepanski L, et al. Omeprazole compared with misoprostol for ulcers associated with nonsteroidal antiinflammatory drugs. N Engl J Med. 1998;338:727–34.
58. Goldstein JL, Johanson JF, Hawkey CJ, et al. Clinical trial: healing of NSAID-associated gastric ulcers in patients continuing NSAID therapy – a randomized study comparing ranitidine with esomeprazole. Aliment Pharmacol Ther. 2007;26:1101–11.
59. Chan FK, Wong VW, Suen BY, et al. Combination of a cyclo-oxygenase-2 inhibitor and a proton-pump inhibitor for prevention of recurrent ulcer bleeding in patients at very high risk: a double-blind, randomised trial. Lancet. 2007;369:1621–6.
60. Papatheodoridis GV, Sougioultzis S, Archimandritis AJ. Effects of *Helicobacter pylori* and nonsteroidal anti-inflammatory drugs on peptic ulcer disease: a systematic review. Clin Gastroenterol Hepatol. 2006;4:130–42.
61. Malfertheiner P, Megraud F, O'Morain C, et al. Current concepts in the management of *Helicobacter pylori* infection: the Maastricht III Consensus Report. Gut. 2007;56:772–81.
62. McColl KE, el-Nujimi AM, Chittajallu RS, et al. A study of the pathogenesis of *Helicobacter pylori* negative chronic duodenal ulceration. Gut. 1993;34:762–8.
63. Lanas A, Remacha B, Sainz R, et al. Study of outcome after targeted intervention for peptic ulcer resistant to acid suppression therapy. Am J Gastroenterol. 2000;95:513–9.
64. Delchier JC, Isal JP, Eriksson S, et al. Double blind multicentre comparison of omeprazole 20 mg once daily versus ranitidine 150 mg twice daily in the treatment of cimetidine or ranitidine resistant duodenal ulcers. Gut. 1989;30:1173–8.
65. van Rensburg CJ, Louw JA, Girdwood AH, et al. A trial of lansoprazole in refractory gastric ulcer. Aliment Pharmacol Ther. 1996;10:381–6.

Chapter 11
Therapeutic Approach in Functional (Nonulcer) Dyspepsia

Arne Kandulski, Marino Venerito, and Peter Malfertheiner

Keywords: Functional dyspepsia, Therapy

INTRODUCTION

Functional dyspepsia (FD) is defined as the presence of dyspeptic symptoms thought to generate in the gastroduodenal region, in the absence of organic, systemic, or metabolic disease that is likely to explain the symptoms. The Rome III consensus conference defined two subentities of FD: the postprandial distress syndrome (PDS) and epigastric pain syndrome (EPS). The variation of symptoms due to different pathophysiological mechanisms complicates the therapeutic response [1, 2]. The selection of the therapeutic approach should be dependent on the predominant symptom (Table 11.1) [3–5].

THERAPEUTIC STRATEGIES IN DYSPEPSIA
Helicobacter pylori Eradication

Several studies validated "test-and-treat strategy" for *Helicobacter pylori* (*H. pylori*) as the first line option for young patients with chronic dyspeptic symptoms but without alarm symptoms [6–8], lately by the randomized placebo-controlled Canadian CADET-*Hp*

A. Kandulski (✉)
Department of Gastroenterology, Hepatology and Infectious Diseases, "Otto-von-Guericke" University, Magdeburg, Germany
e-mail: Arne.Kandulski@med.ovgu.de

143
M. Duvnjak (ed.), *Dyspepsia in Clinical Practice*,
DOI 10.1007/978-1-4419-1730-0_11,
© Springer Science+Business Media, LLC 2011

TABLE 11.1. Therapeutic options in the treatment of dyspepsia.

Therapeutic options in dyspepsia	
Acid suppressive therapy	Prokinetic drugs
H_2-receptor antagonists	Cisapride
Proton pump inhibitors	Domperidon
	Metoclopramide
H. pylori eradication	
Herbal preparations	5-HT_4 antagonist/dopaminergic drugs
Iberogast (*Iberis amaris*,	Tegaserod
peppermint, camomille)	
Peppermint/caraway oil	
Artichoke extract	
Cognitive behavioral therapy	Tricyclic antidepressants, selective
Hypnotherapy	serotonin reuptake inhibitors
	(SSRI)

trial on uninvestigated dyspeptic patients. This study showed a clear benefit in symptom relief for "test-and-treat" *H. pylori* compared to proton pump inhibitors (PPI) + placebo in the primary care setting [7]. According to the Maastricht III consensus guidelines, test-and-treat should be the strategy of first choice in patients under 45 years of age with dyspepsia [9]. In areas with low *H. pylori* prevalence (<20%) in the general population, empirical use of PPI alone is considered to be an equal option for symptom relief [10–12].

Acid Suppressive Therapy

Along with *H. pylori* eradication, empiric acid suppressive therapy has become the standard therapy, especially in areas with low *H. pylori* prevalence (<20%) [13]. Dependent on the predominant symptom and concomitant diseases, it is likely that patients respond to a trial of acid suppressive therapy [13, 14].

H_2 Receptor Antagonists

H_2 receptor antagonists were reported in a large meta-analysis of 22 studies to be over placebo. Due to further studies demonstrating PPI being superior over placebo or H_2 receptor antagonists, PPI therapy as acid suppressive therapy should be preferred and no further studies dealing H_2 receptor should be expected for the future [15, 16].

Proton Pump Inhibitors

In dyspeptic patients with epigastric pain and epigastric burning, pooled analysis of existing data predicts a better response to PPIs than placebo [14, 17]. Beyond symptomatic response, PPI therapy (esomeprazole, 40–80 mg/8 weeks) was evaluated as a diagnostic test in FD patients with negative findings in endoscopy [18]. Lately, the CADET-HN study randomized 512 (*H. pylori*-negative) patients to therapy with omeprazole, ranitidine, or cisapride for 4 weeks. The authors described a significant better response rate for omeprazole (31%) compared to ranitidine (21%), cisapride (13%), and to placebo (14%) [15]. Also, Moayyedi et al. described PPI therapy being superior over placebo (33% versus 23%; NNT 9; 95% CI 5–25; evaluating 6 clinical trials). No differences were found between different regimens of dosage [13].

Prokinetic Drugs

Although being an obvious therapeutic strategy for suspected dysmotility, the results of prokinetic drugs have been inconsistent due to heterogeneity of patients and small sample sizes. Cisapride has been withdrawn in most European countries and North America because of severe cardiac side effects. An advantage has been suggested for domperidone and cisapride superior over placebo (domperidone, OR of 7.0 (95% CI 3.6–16)) by several meta-analyses and systematic reviews. Veldhuyzen van Zanten et al. found both cisapride and domperidone to be efficacious in FD (cisapride OR: 2.9, 95% CI 1.5–5.8; domperidone OR: 7.0 95% CI 3.6–16). Also, Moayyedi and colleagues found prokinetic drugs being superior over placebo but were aware in the interpretation of the data due to publication bias or other heterogenecity-related issues [17, 19]. Itopride showed first promising results in a phase IIb study, but it was finally not superior over placebo in two similar placebo-controlled phase III trials [20, 21].

Other prokinetic drugs have been studied including serotonergic agents (tegaserod), motilin receptor agonists, and also grehlin receptor agonists (TZP101, mitemcinal) that still support the value of these agents in the management of dyspepsia [22–25].

As a different approach, the fundic relaxant agents 5-HT$_1$A receptor agonists (buspirone) and muscarinic receptor antagonists (acotiamide) were recently studied, but with inconsistent results, so far [26–28].

HERBAL PREPARATIONS

The results of studies dealing with herbal preparation supported a potential role in the therapy of FD, although most studies were too small to allow strict conclusions. One of the best evaluated preparations is Iberogast® (STW 5), a combination of herbal including *Iberis amaris*, peppermint, and chamomile, showing efficacy in a meta-analysis of 273 patients (OR 0.22, 95% CI 0.11–0.41, $P = 0.001$) [29–31]. Also, promising data were found for artichoke leaf extract demonstrating a significant improvement of symptoms in 247 patients compared to placebo [32]. Other agents, such as capsaicin – ingredient of red chili pepper and agonist of the vanilloid receptor (TRPV-1) – was studied in smaller series and found to improve epigastric pain and fullness compared to placebo [33–35].

ANTIDEPRESSANTS

In small clinical trials, amitriptyline (50 mg) was found to be effective in symptom improvement but did not correlate with physiological changes in balloon distension, suggesting central mediated effects [36, 37]. Although lower doses are used in the treatment of FD than typically necessary in the treatment of depression, also side effects can be expected (dry mouth, constipation) in some cases [38–40].

As in the central nervous system, selective serotonin reuptake inhibitors' (SSRI) increase has been shown to increase the level of synaptically released 5-HT also at the side of the enteric nervous system [39]. Paroxetine and sertaline do not alter the perception of gastric balloon distension but gastric accommodation in healthy volunteers [40, 41]. In this context, it needs to be stressed that antidepressant medications should be suggested for patients with psychological comorbidities (anxiety, depression) or long persistent symptoms that failed with more conventional therapies [42].

PSYCHOLOGICAL THERAPIES: COGNITIVE BEHAVIORAL THERAPY, HYPNOTHERAPY

Cognitive behavioral therapy and hypnotherapy are the best evaluated techniques in the treatment of functional gastrointestinal disorders [43, 44]. For irritable bowel disease and FD, hypnotherapy is effective compared to placebo and medical treatment [45]. In a multimodal approach of medical treatment along with psychotherapeutic support, Mine et al. showed a better outcome than medical treatment alone [46]. Despite these clinical benefits in different trials, inconsistent results were reported in a systematic review of psychological trials [47, 48].

ANTIALLERGIC MEDICATIONS

A new approach in the therapy of FD is gaining the eosinophilic infiltration that was found in the duodenum of dyspeptic patients

[49, 50]. In pediatric studies, eosinophilic infiltration was found in up to 70% of the patients. Therapy with histamine receptor antagonists lead to a reduction of eosinophilia and symptoms [51]. The association of FD with duodenal eosinophilia has been confirmed also in an adult population after adjusting for age, sex, and *H. pylori* status [52]. In particular, the prevalence of duodenal eosinophilia has been shown to be significantly higher in the subgroup of dyspeptic patients with postprandial distress syndrome than in controls (47.3%, $p < 0.04$) [49], but large randomized controlled trails are still warranted for montelukast in the treatment of FD.

CONCLUSIONS
FD is still a poorly understood entity but appears to be a highly heterogeneous disorder. Contributors to the pathogenesis of FD include genetic, environmental, pathological, and psychological factors. Progress in the understanding of the underlying pathogenetic mechanisms may result in a better management of these patients.

The first therapeutic approach in primary care setting should be the empirical prescription PPI medication. "Test-and-treat" strategy for *H. pylori* should be considered in areas with high *H. pylori* prevalence [53]. Also, concerning the long-term benefits of *H. pylori* eradication (preventing ulcer disease or risk reduction of gastric cancer), this approach remains an important strategy [54]. Especially in the area of dysmotility and hypersensitivity, new agents acting on muscle tone and coordination are still missing. In patients with persisting symptoms and psychological comorbidities (anxiety, depression), additional antidepressant therapy or psychotherapy should be considered.

References
1. Hunt RH, Fallone C, Veldhuyzen van Zanten S, et al. Etiology of dyspepsia: implications for empirical therapy. Can J Gastroenterol. 2002;16:635–41.
2. Kleibeuker JH, Thijs JC. Functional dyspepsia. Curr Opin Gastroenterol. 2004;20:546–50.
3. Bytzer P, Hansen JM, Rune S, et al. Identifying responders to acid suppression in dyspepsia using a random starting day trial. Aliment Pharmacol Ther. 2000;14:1485–94.
4. Madsen LG, Bytzer P. Reproducibility of a symptom response to omeprazole therapy in functional dyspepsia evaluated by a random-starting-day trial design. Aliment Pharmacol Ther. 2004;20:365–72.
5. Madsen LG, Wallin L, Bytzer P. Identifying response to acid suppressive therapy in functional dyspepsia using a random starting day trial – is gastro-oesophageal reflux important? Aliment Pharmacol Ther. 2004;20:423–30.

6. Tytgat G, Hungin AP, Malfertheiner P, et al. Decision-making in dyspepsia: controversies in primary and secondary care. Eur J Gastroenterol Hepatol. 1999;11:223–30.

7. Chiba N, Van Zanten SJ, Sinclair P, Ferguson RA, Escobedo S, Grace E. Treating *Helicobacter pylori* infection in primary care patients with uninvestigated dyspepsia: the Canadian adult dyspepsia empiric treatment-*Helicobacter pylori* positive (CADET-Hp) randomised controlled trial. BMJ. 2002;324:1012–6.

8. Talley NJ, Vakil N, Delaney B, et al. Management issues in dyspepsia: current consensus and controversies. Scand J Gastroenterol. 2004;39:913–8.

9. Malfertheiner P, Megraud PF, O'Morain C, et al. Current concepts in the management of *Helicobacter pylori* infection: the Maastricht III Consensus Report. Gut. 2007;56:772–81.

10. Spiegel BM, Vakil NB, Ofman JJ. Dyspepsia management in primary care: a decision analysis of competing strategies. Gastroenterology. 2002;122:1270–85.

11. Delaney BC, Qume M, Moayyedi P, et al. *Helicobacter pylori* test and treat versus proton pump inhibitor in initial management of dyspepsia in primary care: multicentre randomised controlled trial (MRC-CUBE trial). BMJ. 2008;336:651–4.

12. Ford AC, Moayyedi P, Jarbol DE, Logan RF, Delaney BC. Meta-analysis: *Helicobacter pylori* 'test and treat' compared with empirical acid suppression for managing dyspepsia. Aliment Pharmacol Ther. 2008;28:534–44.

13. Moayyedi P, Delaney BC, Vakil N, Forman D, Talley NJ. The efficacy of proton pump inhibitors in nonulcer dyspepsia: a systematic review and economic analysis. Gastroenterology. 2004;127:1329–37.

14. Talley NJ, Vakil N, Moayyedi P. American gastroenterological association technical review on the evaluation of dyspepsia. Gastroenterology. 2005;129:1756–80.

15. Veldhuyzen Van Zanten SJ, Chiba N, Armstrong D, et al. A randomized trial comparing omeprazole, ranitidine, cisapride, or placebo in helicobacter pylori negative, primary care patients with dyspepsia: the CADET-HN Study. Am J Gastroenterol. 2005;100:1477–88.

16. Armstrong D, Veldhuyzen Van Zanten SJ, Barkun AN, et al. White, Heartburn-dominant, uninvestigated dyspepsia: a comparison of 'PPI-start' and 'H2-RA-start' management strategies in primary care – the CADET-HR Study. Aliment Pharmacol Ther. 2005;21:1189–202.

17. Moayyedi P, Soo S, Deeks J, Delaney B, Innes M, Forman D. Pharmacological interventions for non-ulcer dyspepsia. Cochrane Database Syst Rev. 2006;CD001960.

18. Talley NJ, Vakil N, Lauritsen K, et al. Randomized-controlled trial of esomeprazole in functional dyspepsia patients with epigastric pain or burning: does a 1-week trial of acid suppression predict symptom response? Aliment Pharmacol Ther. 2007;26:673–82.

19. Moayyedi P, Soo S, Deeks J, et al. Systematic review: antacids, H_2-receptor antagonists, prokinetics, bismuth and sucralfate therapy for non-ulcer dyspepsia. Aliment Pharmacol Ther. 2003;17:1215–27.

20. Holtmann G, Talley NJ, Liebregts T, Adam B, Parow C. A placebo-controlled trial of itopride in functional dyspepsia. N Engl J Med. 2006;254:832–40.

21. Talley NJ, Tack J, Ptak T, Gupta R, Giguere M. Itopride in functional dyspepsia: results of two phase III multicentre, randomised, double-blind, placebo-controlled trials. Gut. 2008;57:740–6.

22. Chey WD, Howden CW, Tack J, Ligozio G, Earnest DL. Long-term tegaserod treatment for dysmotility-like functional dyspepsia: results of two identical 1-year cohort studies. Dig Dis Sci. 2010;55:684–97.

23. Vakil N, Laine L, Talley NJ, et al. Tegaserod treatment for dysmotility-like functional dyspepsia: results of two randomized, controlled trials. Am J Gastroenterol. 2008;103:1906–19.

24. Miner PB, Rodriguez-Stanley Jr S, Proskin HM, Kianifard F, Bottoli I. Tegaserod in patients with mechanical sensitivity and overlapping symptoms of functional heartburn and functional dyspepsia. Curr Med Res Opin. 2008;24:2159–72.

25. Yogo K, Onoma M, Ozaki K, et al. Effects of oral mitemcinal (GM-611), erythromycin, EM-574 and cisapride on gastric emptying in conscious rhesus monkeys. Dig Dis Sci. 2008;53:912–8.

26. Dinan TG, Mahmud N, Rathore O, et al. A double-blind placebo-controlled study of buspirone-stimulated prolactin release in non-ulcer dyspepsia – are central serotoninergic responses enhanced? Aliment Pharmacol Ther. 2001;15:1613–8.

27. Seto K, Sasaki T, Katsunuma K, Kobayashi N, Tanaka K, Tack J. Acotiamide hydrochloride (Z-338), a novel prokinetic agent, restores delayed gastric emptying and feeding inhibition induced by restraint stress in rats. Neurogastroenterol Motil. 2008;20:1051–9.

28. Tack J. Prokinetics and fundic relaxants in upper functional GI disorders. Curr Opin Pharmacol. 2008;8:690–6.

29. Von AU, Peitz U, Vinson B, Gundermann KJ, Malfertheiner P. STW 5, a phytopharmacon for patients with functional dyspepsia: results of a multicenter, placebo-controlled double-blind study. Am J Gastroenterol. 2007;102:1268–75.

30. Braden B, Caspary W, Borner N, Vinson B, Schneider AR. Clinical effects of STW 5 (Iberogast) are not based on acceleration of gastric emptying in patients with functional dyspepsia and gastroparesis. Neurogastroenterol Motil. 2009;21:632–8. e25.

31. Melzer J, Rosch W, Reichling J, Brignoli R, Saller R. Meta-analysis: phytotherapy of functional dyspepsia with the herbal drug preparation STW 5 (Iberogast). Aliment Pharmacol Ther. 2004;20:1279–87.

32. Holtmann G, Adam B, Haag S, Collet W, Grunewald E, Windeck T. Efficacy of artichoke leaf extract in the treatment of patients with functional dyspepsia: a six-week placebo-controlled, double-blind, multicentre trial. Aliment Pharmacol Ther. 2003;18:1099–105.

33. Rodriguez-Stanley S, Collings KL, Robinson M, Owen W, Miner Jr PB. The effects of capsaicin on reflux, gastric emptying and dyspepsia. Aliment Pharmacol Ther. 2000;14:129–34.

34. Bortolotti M, Coccia G, Grossi G. Red pepper and functional dyspepsia. N Engl J Med. 2002;346:947–8.

35. Bortolotti M, Coccia G, Grossi G, Miglioli M. The treatment of functional dyspepsia with red pepper. Aliment Pharmacol Ther. 2002;16:1075–82.

36. Otaka M, Jin M, Odashima M, et al. New strategy of therapy for functional dyspepsia using famotidine, mosapride and amitriptyline. Aliment Pharmacol Ther. 2005;21 Suppl 2:42–6.

37. Gorelick AB, Koshy SS, Hooper FG, Bennett TC, Chey WD, Hasler WL. Differential effects of amitriptyline on perception of somatic and visceral stimulation in healthy humans. Am J Physiol. 1998;275:G460–6.

38. Mertz H, Fass R, Kodner A, Yan-Go F, Fullerton S, Mayer EA. Effect of amitriptyline on symptoms, sleep, and visceral perception in patients with functional dyspepsia. Am J Gastroenterol. 1998;93:160–5.

39. Tack J, Lee KJ. Pathophysiology and treatment of functional dyspepsia. J Clin Gastroenterol. 2005;39:S211–6.

40. Tack J, Broekaert D, Coulie B, Fischler B, Janssens J. Influence of the selective serotonin re-uptake inhibitor, paroxetine, on gastric sensorimotor function in humans. Aliment Pharmacol Ther. 2003;17:603–8.

41. Ladabaum U, Glidden D. Effect of the selective serotonin reuptake inhibitor sertraline on gastric sensitivity and compliance in healthy humans. Neurogastroenterol Motil. 2002;14:395–402.

42. Saad RJ, Chey WD. Review article: current and emerging therapies for functional dyspepsia. Aliment Pharmacol Ther. 2006;24:475–92.

43. Haug TT, Wilhelmsen I, Svebak S, Berstad A, Ursin H. Psychotherapy in functional dyspepsia. J Psychosom Res. 1994;38:735–44.

44. Talley NJ, Owen BK, Boyce P, Paterson K. Psychological treatments for irritable bowel syndrome: a critique of controlled treatment trials. Am J Gastroenterol. 1996;91:277–83.

45. Calvert EL, Houghton LA, Cooper P, Morris J, Whorwell PJ. Long-term improvement in functional dyspepsia using hypnotherapy. Gastroenterology. 2002;123:1778–85.

46. Mine K, Kanazawa F, Hosoi M, Kinukawa N, Kubo C. Treating non-ulcer dyspepsia considering both functional disorders of the digestive system and psychiatric conditions. Dig Dis Sci. 1998;43:1241–7.

47. Soo S, Moayyedi P, Deeks J, Delaney B, Lewis M, Forman D. Psychological interventions for non-ulcer dyspepsia. Cochrane Database Syst Rev. 2005;CD002301.

48. Soo S, Forman D, Delaney BC, Moayyedi P. A systematic review of psychological therapies for nonulcer dyspepsia. Am J Gastroenterol. 2004;99:1817–22.

49. Walker MM, Salehian SS, Murray CE, et al. Implications of eosinophilia in the normal duodenal biopsy – an association with allergy and functional dyspepsia. Aliment Pharmacol Ther. 2010;31:1229–36.

50. Walker MM, Talley NJ, Prabhakar M, et al. Duodenal mastocytosis, eosinophilia and intraepithelial lymphocytosis as possible disease markers in the irritable bowel syndrome and functional dyspepsia. Aliment Pharmacol Ther. 2009;29:765–73.

51. Friesen CA, Neilan NA, Schurman JV, Taylor DL, Kearns GL, Abdel-Rahman SM. Montelukast in the treatment of duodenal eosinophilia

in children with dyspepsia: effect on eosinophil density and activation in relation to pharmacokinetics. BMC Gastroenterol. 2009;9:32.

52. Talley NJ, Walker MM, Aro P, et al. Non-ulcer dyspepsia and duodenal eosinophilia: an adult endoscopic population-based case–control study. Clin Gastroenterol Hepatol. 2007;5:1175–83.

53. Jarbol DE, Kragstrup J, Stovring H, Havelund T, Schaffalitzky de Muckadell OB. Proton pump inhibitor or testing for *Helicobacter pylori* as the first step for patients presenting with dyspepsia? A cluster-randomized trial. Am J Gastroenterol. 2006;101:1200–8.

54. Malfertheiner P, Sipponen P, Naumann M, et al. *Helicobacter pylori* eradication has the potential to prevent gastric cancer: a state-of-the-art critique. Am J Gastroenterol. 2005;100:2100–15.

Chapter 12
Prognosis

György Miklós Buzás

Keywords: Functional dyspepsia, Gastric cancer, *Helicobacter pylori*, Peptic ulcer, Prognosis

INTRODUCTION

Just like most of the functional gastrointestinal disorders, functional dyspepsia (FD) is a benign disorder. Its natural history is not marked by significant complications, such as peptic ulcer bleeding or perforation, and it has no mortality. In spite of this, FD is a chronic, long-lasting, and sometimes recurrent condition representing a significant symptomatic burden, causing impairment in the quality of life of the patients and high costs for society. In this chapter, natural course, prevalence, and risk of peptic ulcer and gastric cancer in FD will be analyzed.

NATURAL HISTORY OF FUNCTIONAL DYSPEPSIA

Most authors writing chapters on dyspepsia in textbooks agree that FD is a benign disorder [1–4]. In spite of its high prevalence and chronic nature, taking a closer look, there is a paucity of studies exploring the natural course of this disease. The reason for this is that most of the studies rather explored the incidence/prevalence of dyspepsia and the lack of a uniform definition of what we sometimes too easily call dyspepsia [5]. This is well illustrated

G.M. Buzás (✉)
Department of Gastroenterology, Ferencváros Health Service
Non-Profit Ltd, Budapest, Hungary
e-mail: drgybuzas@hotmail.com

M. Duvnjak (ed.), *Dyspepsia in Clinical Practice*,
DOI 10.1007/978-1-4419-1730-0_12,
© Springer Science+Business Media, LLC 2011

by the existence of more than 20 definitions of dyspepsia and 3 consecutive international classifications known as the Rome I–III criteria [6, 7]. Another further confusing factor is the existence of opposing forms of dyspepsia: uninvestigated vs. investigated, organic vs. functional (idiopathic), *Helicobacter pylori* (*H. pylori*) positive vs. negative, all with different outcome possibilities, i.e., a drug-induced dyspepsia will cease shortly after the cessation of the drug even without treatment, while an idiopathic FD could last several years either with or without treatment.

In this chapter, only the prognosis of idiopathic, functional dyspepsia will be discussed, focusing on prospective studies. The prognosis of organic dyspepsias is determined by their causes.

Talley et al. followed up 111 patients with essential dyspepsia for a mean term of 17 months. After endoscopy patients participated in telephone interviews every second month, it was found that patients with more pain at entry were more likely to have pain during the follow-up and about 20% of cases developed reflux symptoms. Demographic and environmental factors, length of dyspepsia history, and the history of peptic ulcer had no predictive value [8].

In the Swedish community, 1,290 patients aged 20–79 years were followed-up with a validated questionnaire at 0, 1, and 7 years. The prevalence of dyspepsia was 11.7% at entry and decreased to 8.1% during the follow-up, which suggests that the untreated symptoms persist over a long time, sometimes tending to decrease mainly in the elderly. In the meantime, however, symptoms of reflux disease increased from 6 to 11% and those of irritable bowel disease (IBS) from 15 to 18%. In about 10% of the cases, reflux patients changed to dyspepsia and/or IBS and vice versa [9]. In Finland, 201 dyspeptic patients were monitored for 7 years and divided in ulcer-like, reflux-like, dysmotility-like, unspecified, and IBS-like subgroups. There were no significant differences between mean age, gender, and *H. pylori* status. At the end of the follow-up, only 19.4% cases were asymptomatic (14.3% in dysmotility-like and 25% in the ulcer-like subgroup). Thirty percent of the patients consumed antacids, H_2 blockers, proton pump inhibitor (PPI), or prokinetics. There was a marked instability of dyspepsia subgroups, with 75% of the cases changing their subgroup during the follow-up [10].

A systematic review using sound methodology and minimizing publication bias included six prospective studies with a follow-up period of 1.5–10 years and reported an improvement of the symptoms in 30% to 70% of the cases. Some of the variations were caused by the timing of endoscopy (at entry or later), the local prevalence of *H. pylori*, and the use of different treatments. This work also reviewed seven retrospective studies in which the improved or symptom-free status was higher (48% to 80%) [11]. Lower educational level and higher symptom and psychological vulnerability scores predict a poorer prognosis in Sweden [12]. In a classic Danish study, the duration of dyspepsia was associated with a worse prognosis, contrasting with the recent data [11, 13].

Thus, it seems that the prognosis of FD, though benign, is difficult to define. A greater number of large and population-based studies is needed to examine the course of predefined forms (uninvestigated or investigated, *H. pylori* positive or negative forms, subgroups of dyspepsia according to the predominant symptom or Rome III criteria) [7]. Current trends suggest that the epidemiology of underlying causes of dyspepsia is changing: the incidence of reflux disease is increasing worldwide, while the prevalence of *H. pylori* infection is decreasing, at least in Western countries. Extended use of aspirin and other nonsteroidal anti-inflammatory drugs (NSAIDs) or the recent epidemic increase in diabetes mellitus with its gastrointestinal motility disorders are other factors for consideration.

Many therapies (H_2 receptor blockers, PPI, prokinetics, *H. pylori* eradication, herbal medicines, psychotherapy, etc.) could change the natural course of FD for variable periods; analysis of the symptomatic and economic benefits of these approaches is beyond the scope and size of this chapter. After ceasing, however, dyspeptic symptoms tend to reoccur in the majority of cases.

PREVALENCE AND RISK OF PEPTIC ULCER IN FUNCTIONAL DYSPEPSIA

With FD being a chronic and benign condition affecting the general population, there is a risk of developing organic digestive diseases. Studies performed in the pre-endoscopic and pre-*H. pylori* era showed that a distinct but variable proportion of unexplained dyspeptic patients will develop peptic ulcers, which, of course, will change the natural course of the disease. Interestingly, reassessing the problem after the introduction of endoscopy found much lower values (Table 12.1). It might be possible that in the early studies (1955–1972), the less accurate radiology examinations overestimated the ulcer prevalence, or, in the meantime, the epidemiology of peptic ulcer has been changed. In studies conducted during the endoscopic era, the low prevalence of new peptic ulcer

TABLE 12.1.   Incidence of peptic ulcer in patients with unexplained dyspepsia.

Year	Authors and ref. no	Country	No. of cases	Methods of investigation	Duration of follow-up (years)	% of peptic ulcer
1959	Barfred et al. [14]	Finland	235	X-ray	10	31
1959	Brummer et al. [15]	Finland	102	X-ray	5–6	12
1965	Krag [16]	Sweden	174	X-ray	7–27	40
1972	Gregory et al. [17]	United Kingdom	102	X-ray	6	3
1995	Lindell et al. [18]	Sweden	195	Endoscopy	10	2
2003	Heikinnen et al. [10]	Finland	79	Endoscopy, H. pylori testing	6–7	3.2
2009	Asfeldt et al. [19]	Norway	361	Endoscopy, H. pylori testing	17	6.9

in FD suggests that FD and H. pylori are only moderate risk factors for peptic ulcer. However, all studies come from Scandinavia and the UK, where both the prevalence of peptic ulcer and H. pylori infection has gradually decreased in past decades. The data are in agreement with the recent epidemiologic surveys. In a Danish group of 2,416 adults, interviewed between 1982 and 1994, the main risk factors for peptic ulcer were H. pylori infection, smoking, and the use of minor tranquillizers. While curiously, neither the intake of NSAIDs or previous dyspepsia affected the incidence of ulcers [20]. Interestingly enough, in this country, the improved medical treatment has not been accompanied by decreasing hospitalization and death rates from complicated peptic ulcers [21]. In the Dutch population, 3.5% duodenal and 2.4% gastric ulcers were found with 20,006 upper endoscopies [22]. In the United Kingdom, between 1997 and 2005, the incidence of uncomplicated peptic ulcers decreased from 1.1 to 0.52 cases/1,000 persons per year, while the proportion of H. pylori negative cases increased from 5% to 12% [23]. A recent systematic search of major databases confirmed a global 1-year prevalence rate of 0.12% to 1.50%, the majority of studies reported a decrease in the incidence/prevalence of peptic ulcers [24]. One may conclude from these data that the risk of peptic ulcer in FD is not higher than in the general population. Nevertheless, more prospective studies from more countries/populations are needed.

INCIDENCE AND RISK OF GASTRIC CANCER
IN FUNCTIONAL DYSPEPSIA

The most important factor determining mortality in FD is *H. pylori* infection, which can cause gastric cancer, associated with an increased risk of death. There is a health economy-driven tendency to omit endoscopy in patients <45 years in favor of a test-and-treat strategy, at least in cases without alarm symptoms. The importance of alarm symptoms was repeatedly emphasized, but in a recent meta-analysis, it was shown that they have limited value in the diagnosis of digestive cancers [25, 26]. However, a more detailed analysis of recent studies shows that in large series of dyspeptic patients, gastric cancer was detected in a sufficient proportion of patients, justifying a more careful investigation (Table 12.2).

TABLE 12.2. Incidence of gastric cancer in patients with dyspepsia.

Year	Author and ref. no	Country	No. of cases	Dyspeptic symptoms	Duration of study (years)	No. and % of gastric cancer
2001	Uemura et al. [27]	Japan	445	Nonulcer dyspepsia	4	21 (4.7)
2003	Boldys et al. [28]	Poland	880	No alarm symptoms	10	83 (9.7)
2005	Liou [29]		17,894	114 cases simple dyspepsia 111 cases alarm symptoms	5	225 (1.25)
2006	Bowrey [30]	United Kingdom	4,018	104 cases with alarm symptoms, 19 cases of "benign" dyspepsia	8	123 (3.0)
2007	Uehara et al. [31]	Peru	32,388	No alarm symptoms	5	285 (0.86)
2007	Muller et al. [32]	Brazil	2,019	Endoscopic screening for *H. pylori* infection in dyspeptic patients	9	23 (2.1)
2008	Sundar [33]	United Kingdom	11,145	Uncomplicated dyspepsia	4	109 (0.88)

In these studies, the incidence of gastric cancer in dyspeptic patients was higher than the background incidence of the disease in the respective countries [27–32, 34]. These high percentages could reflect merely the high proportion of cancer patients presenting with dyspepsia. Eradication of *H. pylori* prevents gastric cancer only if it is performed before the occurrence of intestinal metaplasia and gastric atrophy; to be efficient, we must prevent the precancerous lesions and not the cancer itself, by means of eradication early in the course of dyspepsia [35]. To achieve this goal, early detection of these mucosal changes by combined noninvasive methods (serum pepsinogen I and II, gastrin 17 and IgG/IgA antibodies against *H. pylori*) is of crucial importance [36].

CONCLUSIONS

Functional dyspepsia is a benign disease with a favorable long-term prognosis, without complications and mortality per se. Long-term follow-up studies showed that dyspeptic symptoms persist for years, have a tendency for spontaneous remission and relapse, and in a varying proportion of the cases, overlap with reflux or IBS symptoms. If untreated, the natural course of uninvestigated/investigated or *H. pylori* positive or negative dyspepsia or subgroups of FD is similar. There is a small, but sizable proportion of peptic ulcer and gastric cancer during the course of FD, which must be kept in mind either at primary care or specialist level; to have a preventive effect, early diagnosis of precancerous lesions and eradication of *H. pylori* infection is warranted.

References

1. Misiewicz JJ. Dyspepsia. In: Feldman M, Scharschmidt BF, editors. Sleisenger and Fordtran's gastrointestinal and liver disease. 5th ed. Philadelphia, PA: WB Saunders; 1993. p. 572–9.
2. McQuaid KR. Dyspepsia. In: Feldman M, Friedman LS, Sleisenger MH, editors. Sleisenger and Fordtran's gastrointestinal and liver disease. 7th ed. Philadelphia, PA: WB Saunders; 2002. p. 102–18.
3. Metz DV. Dyspepsia. In: Brand LJ, editor. Clinical practice of gastroenterology. 1st ed. Philadelphia, PA: Churchill Livingstone; 1999. p. 226–34.
4. Keller J, Layer P. Dyspepsie. In: Riemann JF, Fischbach W, Galle PR, Mössner J, editors. Gastroenterologie. 1st ed. Stuttgart: Georg Thieme; 2007. p. 505–14.
5. Vakil NB, Talley NJ. Dyspepsia. In: Talley NJ, Locke III RG, Saito YA, editors. GI epidemiology. 1st ed. Oxford: Blackwell Publishing; 2007. p. 143–8.
6. Bytzer P, Talley NJ. Dyspepsia. Ann Intern Med. 2001;134:815–22.

7. Tack J, Talley NJ, Camilleri M, et al. Functional gastroduodenal disorders. In: Drossman DA, editor. Rome III: the functional gastrointestinal disorders. 3rd ed. McLean, VA: Degnon Associates Inc.; 2006. p. 419–87.

8. Talley NJ, McNeil D, Hayden A, Colreavy C, Piper DW. Prognosis of chronic unexplained dyspepsia. A prospective study of potential predictor variables in patients with endoscopically diagnosed nonulcer dyspepsia. Gastroenterology. 1987;92:1060–6.

9. Agréus L, Svärdsudd K, Talley NJ, Jones MP, Tibblin G. Natural history of gastroesophageal reflux disease and functional abdominal disorders: a population-based study. Am J Gastroenterol. 2001;96:2905–14.

10. Heikkinnen M, Färkkilä M. What is the long-term outcome of the different subgroups of functional dyspepsia? Aliment Pharmacol Ther. 2003;18:223–9.

11. El-Serag HB, Talley NJ. Systemic review: the prevalence and clinical course of functional dyspepsia. Aliment Pharmacol Ther. 2004;19:643–54.

12. Sloth H, Jorgensen LS. Predictors for the course of chronic nonorganic upper abdominal pain. Scand J Gastroenterol. 1989;24:440–4.

13. Bonnevie O. Outcome of non-ulcer disease. Scand J Gastroenterol Suppl. 1982;79:135–8.

14. Thompson WG. Nonulcer dyspepsia. Can Med Assoc J. 1984;130:565–9.

15. Brummer P, Hakkinen I. X-ray negative dyspepsia: a follow-up study. Acta Med Scand. 1959;165:329–32.

16. Krag E. Pseudo-ulcer and true peptic ulcer. A clinical, radiographic and statistical follow-up study. Acta Med Scand. 1965;178:713–28.

17. Gregory DW, Davies GT, Evans KT, Rhodes J. Natural history of patients with X-ray-negative dyspepsia in general practice. Br Med J. 1972;4:519–20.

18. Lindell GH, Celebioglu F, Graffner HO. Non-ulcer dyspepsia in the long-term perspective. Eur J Gastroenterol Hepatol. 1995;7:829–33.

19. Asfeldt AM, Steigen SE, Løchen ML, et al. The natural course of *Helicobacter pylori* infection on endoscopic findings in a population during 17 years of follow-up: the Sørreisa gastrointestinal disorder study. Eur J Epidemiol. 2009;24:649–58.

20. Rosenstock S, Jørgensen T, Bonnevie O, Andersen L. Risk factors for peptic ulcer disease: a population based prospective cohort study comprising 2416 Danish adults. Gut. 2003;52:186–93.

21. Andersen IB, Bonnevie O, Jørgensen T, Sørensen TI. Time trends for peptic ulcer disease in Denmark, 1981–1993. Analysis of hospitalization register and mortality data. Scand J Gastroenterol. 1998;33:260–6.

22. Groenen MJ, Kuipers EJ, Hansen BE, Ouwendijk RJ. Incidence of duodenal ulcers and gastric ulcers in a Western population: back to where it started. Can J Gastroenterol. 2009;23:604–8.

23. Cai S, Garciá Rodriquez LA, Massó-González EL, Hernández-Diaz Z. Uncomplicatedpeptic ulcer in the UK: trends from 1997 to 2005. Aliment Pharmacol Ther. 2009;30:1039–48.

24. Sung JJ, Kuipers EJ, El-Serag HB. Systematic review: the global incidence and prevalence of peptic ulcer disease. Aliment Pharmacol Ther. 2009;29:938–46.

25. Maconi G, Manes G, Porro GB. Role of symptoms in diagnosis and outcome of gastric cancer. World J Gastroenterol. 2008;14:1149–55.
26. Vakil N, Moayyedi P, Fennerty MB, Talley NJ. Limited value of alarm features in the diagnosis of upper gastrointestinal malignancy: systematic review and meta-analysis. Gastroenterology. 2006;131:390–401.
27. Uemura N, Okamoto S, Yamamoto S, et al. *Helicobacter pylori* infection and the development of gastric cancer. N Engl J Med. 2001;345:784–9.
28. Boldys H, Marek TA, Wanczura P, Matusik P, Nowak A. Even young patients with no alarm symptoms should undergo endoscopy for earlier diagnosis of gastric cancer. Endoscopy. 2003;35:61–7.
29. Liou JM, Lin JT, Wang HP, et al. The optimal age threshold for screening upper endoscopy for uninvestigated dyspepsia in Taiwan, an area with a higher prevalence of gastric cancer in young adults. Gastrointest Endosc. 2005;61:819–25.
30. Bowrey DJ, Griffin SM, Wayman J, Karat D, Hayes N, Raimes SA. Use of alarm symptoms to select dyspeptics for endoscopy causes patients with curable esophagogastric cancer to be overlooked. Surg Endosc. 2006;20:1725–8.
31. Uehara G, Nago A, Espinoza R, et al. Optimal age for gastric cancer screening in patients with dyspepsia without alarm symptoms. Rev Gastroenterol Perú. 2007;27:339–48.
32. Muller LB, Fagundes RB, Moraes CC, Rampazzo A. Prevalence of *Helicobacter pylori* infection and gastric cancer precursor lesions in patients with dyspepsia. Arq Gastroenterol. 2007;44:93–8.
33. Sundar N, Muraleedharan V, Pandit J, Green JT, Crimmins R, Swift GL. Does endoscopy diagnose early gastrointestinal cancer in patients with uncomplicated dyspepsia? Postgrad Med J. 2006;82:52–4.
34. Crew KD, Neugut AI. Epidemiology of gastric cancer. World J Gastroenterol. 2006;21:354–62.
35. Ito M, Takata S, Tatsugami M, et al. Clinical prevention of gastric cancer by *Helicobacter pylori* eradication therapy: a systematic review. J Gastroenterol. 2009;44:365–71.
36. Leja M, Kupcinskas L, Funka K, et al. The validity of a biomarker method for indirect detection of gastric mucosal atrophy versus standard histopathology. Dig Dis Sci. 2009;54:2377–84.

Chapter 13
Quality of Life Issues

György Miklós Buzás

Keywords: Functional dyspepsia, *Helicobacter pylori*, Patient-reported outcome measures, Quality of life, Questionnaires, Randomized controlled trials

INTRODUCTION

Nowadays, the main method for assessing the efficiency of pharmacologic therapies are the randomized controlled trials (RCTs), which are regarded as an objective measure of the biologic response of the patients to a given treatment. However, beside quantifying therapeutic responses, there are many other subjective factors (emotional factors such as depression or anxiety, ability to perform daily activities at the workplace or at home, changes in eating/sleeping, social, familiar, and sexual habits), which are difficult to assess using quantitative methods. Both dyspepsia and quality of life (QoL) are ill-defined terms [1, 2]. Physicians traditionally prefer to use objective methods to diagnose and monitor treatment responses. However, many gastrointestinal diseases have a high symptom burden and enormous health-care costs but little objective evidence of the disease; this is especially true for the large group of functional disorders to which dyspepsia belongs [3, 4].

G.M. Buzás (✉)
Department of Gastroenterology, Ferencváros Health Service
Non-Profit Ltd, Budapest, Hungary
e-mail: drgybuzas@hotmail.com

M. Duvnjak (ed.), *Dyspepsia in Clinical Practice*,
DOI 10.1007/978-1-4419-1730-0_13,
© Springer Science+Business Media, LLC 2011

TABLE 13.1.   Aims and levels of QoL research in functional dyspepsia.

No.	Aim	Level of activity
1	Determination of incidence/ prevalence of FD in general or targeted populations	Primary care, epidemiologists
2	Clinical studies (RCTs, interventional/open trials)	Primary, secondary, or tertiary care, referral centers + pharmacologic companies
3	Quality control of health care	Health authorities
4	Cost-utility analysis	Health-care providers
5	Assessment of doctor– patient relationship	Primary care
6	Screening, evaluation, and follow-up of psychosocial problems occurring during therapy	Primary care
7	Work productivity analysis	Occupational medicine

AIMS OF QUALITY OF LIFE RESEARCH

Gastrointestinal diseases have been at the forefront of QoL research in the past 30 years. The aim of QoL assessment in functional dyspepsia (FD) is to unravel several aspects of patients' health related to daily life/activities, which usually remain hidden during the conventional doctor–patient interaction. The aims of QoL assessment in FD are presented in Table 13.1, along with the proposed level of these activities.

DEVELOPMENT OF QUALITY OF LIFE QUESTIONNAIRES IN FUNCTIONAL DYSPEPSIA

Dedicated questionnaires are the main instruments of QoL research. Generic questionnaires were developed in the 1980s (Sickness Impact Profile, Nottingham Health Profile, Medical Outcome Study SF36, and its short-form MOS-SF8), all of which have been used extensively in gastrointestinal studies. It quickly became clear that generic questionnaires do not cover the specific aspects of most diseases, and to overcome this, disease-specific questionnaires were developed. A large variety of instruments were elaborated that allow patients to describe their symptoms, overall state of health, or the effect of therapeutic measures; if used in primary/specialist care, they improve the physician's understanding of diseases. The standardized instruments for assessment of health status could be classified as generic, disease-specific symptom, and QoL or treatment-specific questionnaires [3]. Taken together, these instruments were defined recently as patient-related outcome measures (PRO); thus QoL questionnaires constitute only a part of them.

Developing and testing a questionnaire is more difficult than using it, taking months of hard work and collective effort. Before addressing the work, it is advisable to see whether an appropriate instrument exists; it is easier to translate/adapt and locally validate a still existing questionnaire than prepare a new one [5]. Developing a questionnaire is a multiphase process. The items of PRO instruments should be generated by interviewing focus groups or by surveying literature: physicians, nurses, and psychologists must be involved in this process. The interviewers have to be trained to carry out the questionnaire, either face-to-face, by phone, or in writing (letter or e-mail). The responses can be interpreted optionally on a Likert-scale, visual-analog scale, score system, or simply on a yes/no basis. Before deploying them in practice, the questionnaires need to obtain an appropriate validation. The reliability of an instrument is checked using the test-retest method and measuring internal consistency. The face, convergent, divergent, and content validity as well as responsiveness must be tested as appropriate; the statistical methodology is described in the literature and is available in different software packages [1, 6]. Use of unevaluated, in-house questionnaires is strongly discouraged.

Language constitutes a particular problem. For international use, questionnaires must be translated and validated in the target languages. Translation involves the forward–backward method and professional translators, native speakers of the original and fluent in the target language, and vice versa. Validating the translated questionnaire for the target population (both healthy persons and patients) is essential and must be followed by cognitive debriefing. Finally, international harmonization is needed especially where the populations have different lifestyles/habits, and wide conceptual differences are expected.

Some of the questionnaires are free for use, and others are subject to copyright/permission from their authors. Fees for use may be requested by some specialized companies/institutions.

QoL questionnaires developed for the study of FD are presented in Table 13.2. There is no perfect questionnaire, covering all QoL/PRO aspects of any given disease [7–24]. The simultaneous use of a generic, a disease-specific symptom scale, and QoL questionnaire would be optimal, although it is time-consuming

TABLE 13.2. Features of quality of life questionnaires used in evaluating functional dyspepsia.

Instrument name, ref. no	Year	Structure	Evaluation	Original and target languages
Gastrointestinal Symptoms Rating Scale (GSRS) [8]	1995	15 Questions in 5 dimensions	7-Point Likert scale	English, German, French
Glasgow Dyspepsia Severity Score (GDSS) [9]	1995	15 Questions in 5 dimensions	5-Point Likert scale	English
Leeds Dyspepsia Questionnaire (LDQ) [10]	1998	8 Items with 2 stems relating to symptom frequency and severity	Score from 0 to 40	English
Quality of Life in Reflux and Dyspepsia (QoLRAD) [11]	1998	36 Questions in 6 dimensions	5-Point Likert scale	English
Domestic/International Gastroenterology Surveillance Study (DIGEST) [12]	1999	38 Items assessing the frequency/severity of symptoms	Yes/no	English, Italian Japanese, German, French
Functional Digestive Disease Quality of Life Questionnaire [13]	1999	48 Items in 8 dimensions	5-Point Likert scale	French, English, German, Hungarian
Nepean Dyspepsia Index (NDI) [14, 20]	1999	42 Items in 17 dimensions	5-Point Likert scale	English, German, French, Chinese, Korean, Malay
Quality of Life in Peptic Ulcer Disease [15]	1999	30 Items	Variable Likert scale	Italian, English, German
Multidimensional Measure of Dyspepsia-Related Health [16]	1999	25 Items in 5 dimensions	5-point Likert scale	English

Dyspepsia Symptom Severity Index (DSSI) [17]	2000	20 Items in 3 dimensions	Score from 0 to 5	English
Nepean Dyspepsia Index short form (NDI-SF) [18]	2001	10 Items	5-Point Likert scale	English
Severity of Dyspepsia Assessment (SODA) [19]	2001	24 Items	5-Point Likert scale	English
Gastrointestinal Symptom Score (GISS) [21]	2005	10 Dyspepsia-specific items	5-Point Likert scale	English, German
Global Overall Symptom Scale (GOS) [21]	2006	10 Dyspepsia-specific items	7-Point Likert Scale	English
Functional Dyspepsia-Related Quality of Life (FD-QoL) [22]	2006	33 Items in 7 dimensions	5-Point Likert scale	Korean
Euroqol (EQ-5D) [23]	2009	5 Items	3 Grades of severity	English, Malay

and troublesome for the patients, which reduces compliance. QoL research requires dedicated, trained, and paid personnel for their effort: this is frequently not the case in busy practices. Funds must be raised because QoL assessment is not covered by health insurance companies.

USE OF QUALITY OF LIFE ASSESSMENT IN FUNCTIONAL DYSPEPSIA

QoL instruments have successfully been used in assessing the prevalence and severity of FD and evaluating novel therapies.

The prevalence of FD is between 7 and 40% in Western countries, with large differences according to the definition of FD, target populations, methods of data collection, and the duration of observation. Most of the studies used the Rome I and II criteria of functional gastrointestinal disorders; although received with enthusiasm, the Rome III criteria have yet to stimulate new research in FD [24]. Studies performed in general populations revealed that the prevalence of FD is higher when the QoL instruments are incorporated in the evaluation of the patients: this was observed when validation of Nepean Dyspepsia Index (NDI), where the prevalence of FD was 32% at primary care level and 55% according to gastroenterologists [18]. In the Leeds HELP Study, combined use of Psychological General Well Being (PGWB) and Leeds Dyspepsia Questionnaire (LDQ) detected dyspepsia in 3,177 patients from 8,407 persons participating in a population survey (38%) [25, 26]. An international survey on 5,581 patients from Canada, Italy, Japan, the Netherlands, Switzerland, and the USA using PGWB and Domestic/International Gastroenterology Surveillance Study (DIGEST) instruments reported dyspeptic symptoms in 46.4% of responders with the highest level in the USA (65.3%) and the lowest in Switzerland (14.9%) [13]. A recent survey of 2,025 Belgian subjects found dyspeptic symptoms in 417 persons (20.6%) and overlapping reflux symptoms in 141 patients (33.8%) [27]. Thus, it is advisable to determine the prevalence of FD in each population using QoL instruments.

QoL instruments are able to recognize differences between healthy individuals and FD patients and other diseases. Moreover, they can assess the severity of the disease. The QoL of dyspeptic patients is worse than that of healthy subjects [12–17, 28, 29]. Variable degrees of impairment of daily activities, social functions, eating/sleeping/sexual habits, and health perceptions all occur and can enhance anxiety and depression. The QoL with FD could be worse than with peptic ulcer, reflux, or irritable bowel syndrome [12, 13, 29]. The worsening of QoL is similar in subclasses of FD (ulcer-like, reflux-like, dysmotility, or mixed type) [29]. No consistent differences in QoL were identified in uninvestigated vs. investigated FD [21]. Life events (loss of job, financial crisis, death of family members/friends, divorce, etc.) adversely affect QoL. Associated diseases (diabetes, hypertension, chronic liver disease) lead to further impairment but could cause confusion in the assessment of QoL [1, 30]. The impairment varies between populations: the NDI showed different dyspepsia scores in Australian, Canadian, Chinese, Malay, or Korean subjects [12, 18, 20, 22, 23].

Few studies addressed the role of pathogenetic factors in relation to the QoL in FD. The impairment of QoL is similar in *Helicobacter pylori* (*H. pylori*) positive and negative patients as measured by Functional Dyspepsia-Related Quality of Life (FD-QoL) [29]. Measurements using short-form 36 (SF36) and NDI in 864 patients showed that delayed gastric emptying do not explain the impairment of QoL [31]. The role of acid secretion, gastric accommodation, myoelectric activity and hypersensitivity, autonomic dysfunction, and hormonal changes (gastrin, pancreatic polypeptide, cholecystokinin) has not yet been studied.

THERAPEUTIC STUDIES

Traditionally, FD was successfully treated with antacids, H_2 receptor blockers, proton pump inhibitors (PPIs), and prokinetics, but QoL studies have not been systematically conducted during their development. PRO/QoL assessment was gradually incorporated into the methodology of RCTs, making substantial contribution to the interpretation of results. Table 13.3 presents the most recent studies [29, 32–42]. Cisapride was useful in improving QoL in some studies but was withdrawn because of side-effects [29, 32]. The use of PPIs is supported by their favorable effect on QoL [32–34]. More studies are needed to confirm the efficiency of novel prokinetics, antidepressants, and tegaserod, while other compounds such as motilin antagonists, fedotozin, capsaicin, and dezloxiglumide still await further evaluation. Recent data suggest that herbal medicines – artichoke leaf, iberogast, standardized Japanese preparations – are useful in improving FD symptoms [32, 42, 43].

The most controversial topic is the effect of *H. pylori* eradication on the QoL in FD. Current recommendations include *H. pylori* positive FD as a possible option for eradicating the infection [43]. Studies performed in different populations lead to equivocal results. An updated, high-quality meta-analysis including 21 RCTs

TABLE 13.3.   Quality of life assessment in randomized controlled trials in functional dyspepsia.

Authors	Year	Investigational/control drug	No. of patients	QoL/PRO instrument	Comments
Holtmann et al. [32]	2003	Artichoke leaf vs. placebo	247	NID	Artichoke leaf was superior to placebo
Veldhuyzen van Zanten et al. [33]	2005	Omeprazole vs. ranitidine, cisapride, or placebo	512	GOS	Omeprazole was superior to ranitidine, cisapride, or placebo in *H. pylori* negative dyspepsia
Holtmann et al. [34]	2006	Itopride vs. placebo	524	LDQ	Itopride significantly improved FD symptoms
Veldhuyzen van Zanten et al. [35]	2006	Esomeprazole vs. placebo	502	GOS	Esomeprazole was more effective than placebo at 4 weeks
Raedsch et al. [36]	2007	Phytopharmacon STW5 vs. metoclopramide	961	GISS	Phytotherapy was superior to prokinetic
Talley et al. [37]	2008	Itopride vs. placebo	1,170	LDQ	Itopride was not superior to placebo
Vakil et al. [38]	2008	Tegaserod vs. placebo + continuous PPI	101	NDI-SF	Tegaserod was not superior to placebo
Van Kerkhoven et al. [39]	2008	Venlaflaxine vs. placebo	160	GSRS, LDQ	Venlafaxine was not more effective than placebo

	Year	Intervention	N	Measures	Result
Miwa et al. [40]	2009	Tandospirone vs. placebo	144	GSRS, MOS-SF8, State-Trait Anxiety Inventory	Tandospirone was superior to placebo
Park et al. [41]	2009	Six-point vs. nondefined-point acupuncture	68	NDI	Both acupunctures improved FD symptoms
Braden et al. [42]	2009	Iberogast (STW 5) vs. placebo	103	GISS	Iberogast was superior to placebo

and 3,566 patients showed that eradicating the infection reduced the relative risk of dyspepsia by 10% compared to placebo, with the number needed to treat to cure one case of dyspepsia being 14. The benefit is small but statistically significant and cost-effective [44, 45]. Timely eradication is useful in preventing peptic ulcers, precancerous lesions, and gastric cancer, and it reduces the infectious burden of the general population. Clearly, more studies in different populations/settings are needed for a definitive answer and this topic deserves a separate chapter.

CONCLUSIONS

Several instruments for measuring PRO were prepared in the past decades. QoL questionnaires were progressively implemented into the methodology of clinical trials. The study of QoL in FD revealed several aspects of this highly prevalent condition, which remained hidden during the traditional patient–physician relationship. Developing a validated questionnaire, however, is a difficult task. In FD patients, several dimensions of the QoL are impaired (daily activities, eating/sleeping, anxiety, coping with disease). Incorporating PRO measurement in recent RCTs showed an improvement of QoL in FD under several therapies (PPIs, cisapride, itopride, phytotherapy, acupuncture), while others (tegaserod, venlafaxine) provided no benefit over placebo. *H. pylori* eradication leads to a modest yet significant and cost-effective reduction of dyspeptic symptoms in some populations.

Acknowledgments   The author is indebted to Douglas Arnott (EDMF Translation Bureau, Etyek, Hungary) for correcting the English manuscript for this chapter and chapter "Prognosis." The secretarial help of Mrs. Jolán Józan (Semmelweis University, Department of Physiology, Budapest, Hungary) is highly appreciated.

References

1. Fayer PM, Machin D, editors. Quality of life. Assessment, analysis and interpretation. Chichester: Wiley; 2000.
2. Bytzer P, Tally NJ. Dyspepsia. Ann Intern Med. 2001;134:815–22.
3. Wiklund I. Patient-reported outcomes. In: Talley NJ, Locke III GR, Saito YA, editors. GI epidemiology. Oxford: Blackwell; 2006. p. 24–30.
4. Creed F, Levy RL, Bradley LA, et al. Psychosocial aspects of functional gastrointestinal disoders. In: Drossman DA, Corazziari E, Spiller RC, Thompson WG, editors. The functional gastrointestinal disorders, Rome III. McLean, VA: Degnon Associates; 2006. p. 313–4. 318–21, 346–7.
5. Locke III GR. GI questionnaires. In: Talley NJ, Locke III GR, Saito YA, editors. GI epidemiology. Oxford: Blackwell; 2006. p. 30–4.

6. Borenstein M, Hedges LV, Higgins JPT, Rothstein HR, editors. Introduction to meta-analysis. Chichester: Wiley; 2009.

7. Yacavone RF, Locke 3rd GR, Provenzale DT, Eisen GM. Quality of life measurement in gastroenterology: what is available? Am J Gastroenterol. 2001;96:285–97.

8. Dimenas E, Glise H, Hallerback B, Hernquist H, Svedlund J, Wiklund I. Well-being and gastrointestinal symptoms among patients referred to endoscopy owing to suspected duodenal ulcer. Scand J Gastroenterol. 1995;30:1046–52.

9. el-Omar EM, Banerjee S, Wirz A, McColl KE. The Glasgow Dyspepsia Severity Score: a tool for the global measurement of dyspepsia. Eur J Gastroenterol Hepatol. 1996;8:967–71.

10. Moayyedi P, Duffett S, Braunholtz D, et al. The Leeds Dyspepsia Questionnaire: a valid tool for measuring the presence and severity of dyspepsia. Aliment Pharmacol Ther. 1998;12:1257–62.

11. Wiklund I, Junghard O, Grace E, et al. Quality of Life in Reflux and Dyspepsia patients. Psychometric documentation of a new disease-specific questionnaire (QOLRAD). Eur J Surg Suppl. 1998; 583:41–9.

12. Enck P, Dubois D, Marquis P. Quality of life in patients with upper gastrointestinal symptoms: results from the Domestic/International Gastroenterology Surveillance Study (DIGEST). Scand J Gastroenterol Suppl. 1999;231:48–54.

13. Chassany O, Marquis P, Scherrer B, et al. Validation of a specific quality of life questionnaire for functional digestive disorders. Gut. 1999;44:527–33.

14. Talley NJ, Haque M, Wyeth JW, et al. Development of a new dyspepsia impact scale: the Nepean Dyspepsia Index. Aliment Pharmacol Ther. 1999;13:225–35.

15. Bamfi F, Oliveri A, Arpinelli F, et al. Measuring quality of life in dyspeptic patients: development and validation of a new specific health status questionnaire: final report from the Italian QPD project involving 4000 patients. Am J Gastroenterol. 1999;94:730–8.

16. Cook KF, Rabeneck L, Campbell CJ, Wray NP. Evaluation of a multidimensional measure of dyspepsia-related health for use in a randomized clinical trial. J Clin Epidemiol. 1999;52:381–92.

17. Leidy NK, Farup C, Rentz AM, Ganoczy D, Koch KL. Patient-based assessment in dyspepsia:development and validation of Dyspepsia Symptoms Severity Index (DSSI). Dig Dis Sci. 2000;45:1172–9.

18. Talley NJ, Verlinden M, Jones M. Quality of life in functional dyspepsia: responsiveness of the Nepean Dyspepsia Index and development of a new 10-item short form. Aliment Pharmacol Ther. 2001;15:207–16.

19. Rabeneck L, Cook KF, Wristers K, Souchek J, Menke T, Wray NP. SODA (severity of dyspepsia assessment): a new effective outcome measure for dyspepsia-related health. J Clin Epidemiol. 2001;54:755–65.

20. Tian XP, Li Y, Liang FR, et al. Translation and validation of the Nepean Dyspepsia Index for functional dyspepsia in China. World J Gastroenterol. 2009;15:3173–7.

21. Veldhuyzen van Zanten SJ, Chiba N, Amstrong D, et al. Validation of a 7-point Global Overall Symptom scale to measure the severity

of dyspepsia symptoms in clinical trials. Aliment Pharmacol Ther. 2006;23:521–9.

22. Lee EH, Hahm KB, Lee HJ, et al. Development and validation of a functional dyspepsia-related quality of life (FD-QOL) scale in South Korea. J Gastroenterol Hepatol. 2006;21:268–74.

23. Mahadeva S, Wee HL, Goh KL, Thumboo L. The EQ-5D (Euroqol) is a valid generic instrument for measuring quality of life in patients with dyspepsia. BMC Gastroenterol. 2009;9:20.

24. Talley NJ, Ruff K, Jiang X, Jung HK. The Rome III Classification of dyspepsia: will it help research? Dig Dis Sci. 2008;26:203–9.

25. Moayyedi P, Forman D, Braunholz D, et al. The proportion of upper gastrointestinal symptoms in the community associated with *Helicobacter pylori*, lifestyle factors, and nonsteroidal anti-inflammatory drugs. Leeds HELP Study Group. Am J Gastroenterol. 2000;95:1448–55.

26. Moayyedi P, Feltbower L, Brown J, et al. Effect of population screening and treatment for *Helicobacter pylori* on dyspepsia and quality of life in the community: a randomised controlled trial. Leeds HELP Study Group. Lancet. 2000;355:1665–9.

27. Piessevaux H, De Winter B, Louis E, et al. Dyspeptic symptoms in the general population: a factor and cluster analysis of symptom groupings. Neurogastroenterol Motil. 2009;21:378–88.

28. Meineche-Schmidt V, Talley NJ, Pap Á, et al. Impact of functional dyspepsia on quality of life and health care consumption after cessation of antisecretory treatment. A multicentre 3-month follow-up study. Scand J Gastroenterol. 1999;34:566–74.

29. Buzás GM. Quality of life in patients with functional dyspepsia: short- and long- term effect of *Helicobacter pylori* eradication with pantoprazole, amoxicillin, and clarithromycin or cisparide therapy: a prospective, parallel-group study. Curr Ther Res. 2006;67:305–20.

30. Haag S, Senf W, Häuser W, et al. Impairement of health-related quality of life in functional dyspepsia and chronic liver disease: the influence of depression and anxiety. Aliment Pharmacol Ther. 2008;27:561–71.

31. Talley NJ, Locke III GR, Lahr BD, et al. Functional dyspepsia, delayed gastric empyting and impaired quality of life. Gut. 2006;55:933–9.

32. Holtmann G, Adam B, Haag S, Collet W, Grünewald E, Windeck T. Efficacy of artichoke leaf extract in the treatment of patients with functional dyspepsia: a six-week placebo-controlled, double-blind, multicentre trial. Aliment Pharmacol Ther. 2003;18:1099–105.

33. Veldhuyzen van Zanten SJ, Chiba N, Armstrong D, et al. A randomized trial comparing omeprazole, ranitidine, cisapride, or placebo in *Helicobacter pylori* negative, primary care patients with dyspepsia: the CADET-HN Study. Am J Gastroenterol. 2005;100:1477–88.

34. Holtmann G, Talley NJ, Liebregtd T, Adam B, Parow C. A placebo-controlled trial of itopride in functional dyspepsia. N Engl J Med. 2006;354:832–40.

35. van Zanten SV, Armstrong D, Chiba N, et al. Esomeprazole 40 mg once a day in patients with functional dyspepsia: the randomized placebo-controlled "ENTER" trial. Am J Gastroenterol. 2006;101:2096–106.

36. Raedsch R, Hanisch J, Bock P, Sibaev A, Vinson B, Gundermann KJ. Assessment of the efficacy and safety of the phytopharmacon STW 5 versus metoclopramide in functional dyspepsia: a retrolective cohort study. Z Gastroenterol. 2007;45:1041–8.

37. Talley NJ, Tack J, Ptak K, Gupta R, Giguère M. Itopride in functional dyspepsia: results of two phase III multicentre, randomised, double-blind, placebo-controlled trials. Gut. 2008;57:740–6.

38. Vakil N, Kianifard F, Bottoli I. Exploratory study of tegaserod for dyspepsia in women receving ppis for heartburn. Arch Drug Inf. 2008;1:79–88.

39. van Kerkhoven LA, Laheij RJ, Aparicio N, et al. Effect of the antidepressant venlafaxine in functional dyspepsia: a randomized, double-blind, placebo-controlled trial. Clin Gastroenterol Hepatol. 2008;6:746–52.

40. Miwa H, Nagahara A, Tominaga K, et al. Efficacy of the 5-HT1A agonist tandospirone citrate im improving symptoms of patients with functional dyspepsia: a randomized controlled trial. Am J Gastroenterol. 2009;104:2779–87.

41. Park YC, Kang W, Choi SM, Son CG. Evaluation of manual acupuncture at classical and nondefined points for treatment of functional dyspepsia: a randomized-controlled trial. J Altern Complement Med. 2009;15:879–84.

42. Braden B, Caspary W, Börner N, Vinson B, Schneider AR. Clinical effects of STW 5 (Iberogast) are not based on acceleration of gastric emptying in patients with functional dyspepsia and gastroparesis. Neurogastroenterol Motil. 2009;21:632–8.

43. Suzuki H, Inadomi JM, Hibi T. Japanese herbal medicine in functional gastrointestinal disorders. Neurogastroenterol Motil. 2009;21:688–96.

44. Malfertheiner P, Mégraud F, O'Morain C, et al. Current concepts in the management of *Helicobacter pylori* infection: the Maastricht III Consensus Report. Gut. 2007;56:772–81.

45. Moayyedi P, Soo S, Deeks J, et al. Eradication of *Helicobacter pylori* for non-ulcer dyspepsia. Cochrane Database Syst Rev. 2006;CD002096.

Chapter 14
Economic Analyses of Present Management Strategies and Nonprescription Therapy in Treatment of Dyspepsia

Mattijs E. Numans

Keywords: Dyspepsia, Cost-effectiveness, Diagnosis, Treatment strategies

INTRODUCTION

Although pharmaceutical as well as healthcare developments move forward, the initial management of dyspepsia, which usually starts off in primary care, still remains difficult to decide on. An average primary care physician deals with dyspepsia almost daily, and it accounts for major healthcare budgets in most countries. Unfortunately, evidence on which to base the best initial management strategy is still inconclusive. Most studies to date have reported on single drug comparisons or on comparison with prompt endoscopy and mainly involved patients either with persisting dyspeptic symptoms or with predominantly reflux-like

M.E. Numans (✉)
Professor Innovation & Quality Academic Primary Care,
Amsterdam Free University Medical Center
and
Coordinator Julius Primary Care Network,
University Medical Center Utrecht, Utrecht, The Netherlands
e-mail: m.e.numans@umcutrecht.nl

M. Duvnjak (ed.), *Dyspepsia in Clinical Practice*,
DOI 10.1007/978-1-4419-1730-0_14,
© Springer Science+Business Media, LLC 2011

symptoms, referred to secondary care. Several meta-analyses and reviews have been done to address important questions concerning treatment strategies for patients with dyspeptic symptoms. The Cochrane review on initial management of dyspepsia showed that only a few studies, mostly of inadequate methodology, dealt with this subject, and this Cochrane review was recently withdrawn [1]. Investigators concluded that large gaps in knowledge on the most cost-effective management strategy for uninvestigated dyspepsia still exist. Although new research was published, the final verdict on factors to be involved in the initial decision has still not been reached. Consequently, current guidelines for management of dyspepsia are inconsistent, and the cost-effectiveness of chosen strategies has substantial unknown variance depending on cultural and economical context.

The American Gastroenterological Association (AGA) and Canadian guidelines recommend empirical proton pump inhibitor (PPI) treatment for patients with predominant gastroesophageal reflux disease (GERD), and for all others, *Helicobacter pylori* (*H. pylori*) test-and-treat followed by empirical PPI treatment [2, 3]. According to the AGA guidelines, empirical PPI treatment is also an initial option in a population with low *H. pylori* prevalence. UK guidelines state that there is currently insufficient evidence to guide which of these two options should be offered first [4]. Scottish guidelines adopt the ROME II definition for dyspepsia, necessitating initial endoscopy for diagnosis. They advise treating functional dyspepsia with antacids or histamine 2 receptor-antagonists (H2RAs), followed by *H. pylori* test-and-treat when symptoms persist [5]. By contrast, Dutch guidelines since 1993 still recommend a step-up empirical treatment strategy with antacids or H2RAs for all patients with new onset dyspepsia, and reserve PPI treatment for patients with persistent predominantly GERD symptoms, and *H. pylori* test-and-treat for all other "nonreflux" patients with persistent symptoms [6]. Direct endoscopic diagnosis does not seem the most cost-effective measure upfront and is therefore only indicated for patients presenting with alarm symptoms, although safe selection of alarm symptoms seems very difficult [7]. Following study results published in widely accessible medical journals, initial treatment with PPIs is used widely because of its presumed superior cost-effectiveness. However, a step-up approach might be the most cost-effective in reality. When properly followed up, it enables physicians to go along with the natural course of dyspepsia, which is that 80% of the patients are free of symptoms after 1 year, independent of the intervention chosen [8, 9].

INITIAL PRIMARILY DIAGNOSTIC STRATEGIES

Considering symptoms, medical history, and the results of physical examination, physicians hypothesize that the patient is suffering from dyspepsia during the first consultation. Usually, prompt endoscopy, *H. pylori* testing (followed by treatment), and in rare cases, radiology with barium meal are the first diagnostic options. Advantages of these diagnostic strategies and kicking off with empirical treatment without confirmed diagnosis have to be evaluated. Although with various methodology, efficacy studies of all diagnostic strategies compared with each other or with empirical treatment have been reported in the literature.

PROMPT INVESTIGATION VERSUS SHORT-TERM TREATMENT WITH PPI OR H2RAS

One of the first landmark studies on cost-effectiveness of prompt investigation versus empirical treatment was the Danish study comparing prompt endoscopy with empirical H2RA therapy, published in the Lancet in 1994 [10]. The population that was studied in the pre-*H. pylori* era had relatively high peptic ulcer prevalence, in which after 1 year, they found no differences in symptoms or quality of life measures between both groups. The empirical treatment strategy in dyspepsia was associated with higher costs due mainly to a higher number of sick-leave days and cost of ulcer drug use. Although a meta-analysis on the effect of prompt initial investigation with gastroscopy, published a couple of years later, did not quite reach statistical significance at the 95% level. It seems that the summary of the results of these trials suggests that initial investigation is associated with a reduction in the number of patients who are still symptomatic after 1 year compared with empirical acid suppression [11]. This difference is due to enabling relatively early treatment of a treatable disease diagnosed with endoscopy that does not improve sufficiently with empirical acid suppression (e.g., *H. pylori* – or nonsteroidal antiinflammatory drugs (NSAIDs) – related severe ulcers, early gastric cancer, or obstructive disease that can be treated otherwise) or a disease diagnosed by other tests after endoscopic exclusion of gastroesophageal disorders (e.g., gallstones).

Detailed cost data are only available from few studies comparing early investigation, either with barium meal or with prompt gastroscopy, with acid suppression. Although early endoscopy seems to have some clinical advantages over empirical treatment, depending on local costs of performing endoscopy (even varying from as low as €50 in Southern or East Europe to €600 in the USA), it is usually the more expensive option. This is especially in cases when generically produced PPIs cost only €0.05 per day, which is currently the situation in most countries. Loss of information in initial double contrast barium meal investigation and substantial amounts of follow-up endoscopies to confirm doubtful findings do reduce the potential advantages of the lower price of radiologic investigation (€10–20).

H. PYLORI TEST-AND-TREAT VERSUS SHORT-TERM TREATMENT WITH PPI OR H2RA

Only few trials have been published in this area since it was stated in current guidelines that the knowledge of a positive *H. pylori* status automatically leads to eradication. In contrast to the comparison with endoscopy-based management, there appears to be a difference in effectiveness in favor of test-and-treat, whereas costs are similar (Table 14.1). This may be because *H. pylori* eradication therapy prevents the recurrence of peptic ulcers as well as future ulcers in patients that might develop them. The CADET-HP trial showed that

TABLE 14.1. Number of individual dyspepsia-related resources used, following initial intervention and weighted mean difference in their use for "test-and-treat" compared to empirical PPI therapy in an individual patient data meta-analysis (reproduced with permission [15]).

	Total number in "test-and-treat" arm ($n = 750$)	Total number in empirical PPI arm ($n = 724$)	Weighted mean difference in use	95% Confidence interval
Primary care physician visits	1,049	980	0.01	−0.17 to 0.20
Out-patient visits	59	71	−0.02	−0.08 to 0.03
In-patient days	29	35	−0.01	−0.03 to 0.01
Upper GI endoscopies	163	191	−0.06	−0.13 to 0.02
Ultrasound scans	13	18	−0.01	−0.03 to 0.01
13Carbon-urea breath tests	1	9	−0.01	−0.03 to 0
Defined daily dose (DDD) of PPIs	34,161	28,535	6.08	−1.75 to 13.90
DDD of H2RAs	8,778	4,819	2.63	−0.36 to 5.63
DDD of prokinetics	304	532	−0.38	−1.06 to 0.31
Courses of eradica-tion therapy	11	32	−0.03	−0.05 to −0.01

the incremental cost-effectiveness ratio of *H. pylori* eradication was €290 per treatment success, indicating a lower cost with treatment success compared with PPI treatment alone [12]. In a later study in the primary care setting, *H. pylori* test-and-treat and acid suppression were found to be equally cost effective in the initial management of dyspepsia [13]. Empirical acid suppression was considered an appropriate initial strategy in a low *H. pylori* prevalence environment. As costs are similar overall, general practitioners should discuss with patients at which point to consider *H. pylori* testing. The overall efficacy of an *H. pylori* test-and-treat strategy seems limited [14]. There has been an ongoing debate whether *H. pylori* eradication may worsen heartburn symptoms. However, the CADET-HP study (comparing *H. pylori* eradication with placebo) reported a subgroup analysis, based on predominant symptom at entry, which showed comparable differences of effectiveness in patients with predominantly heartburn symptoms as in those without [12].

In practice, any benefit of *H. pylori*-driven treatment strategies will be limited to the proportion of patients testing positive for *H. pylori*, and the proportion of patients testing *H. pylori* positive actually suffering from peptic ulcer disease. So the real impact of the strategy will depend on true *H. pylori* prevalence in the population the physician is treating. This might lead to the conclusion that cost-effectiveness of short-term treatment with acid-reducing medication is higher at least in current Western populations with a relatively low *H. pylori* prevalence [15].

HELICOBACTER PYLORI TEST-AND-TREAT VERSUS PROMPT ENDOSCOPY

Again, a Danish study on this comparison was published in the Lancet in 2000 [16]. The authors concluded that *H. pylori* test-and-treat strategy is as efficient and safe as prompt endoscopy for management of dyspeptic patients in primary care. However, fewer patients were satisfied with their treatment. The overall cost-effectiveness of this comparison can be studied based on an individual patient data (IPD) meta-analysis (Ford et al. 2005), which consists of six randomized controlled trials (RCTs) including the Danish study [17]. The effect found on symptom reduction was equivalent to an absolute difference of 5% in favor of endoscopy-based management. However, even if there is a small effect on symptoms in favor of endoscopy, it is still not cost effective. The principal effect of *H. pylori* test-and-treat rather than endoscopy is a highly significant two-thirds reduction in the number of endoscopies performed. This reduction applied

TABLE 14.2. Weighted mean difference in costs for prompt endoscopy versus "test-and-treat" (after Ford et al. 2005) [17].

Cost (€2010)	Weighted mean difference	95% Confidence interval
Total cost	295	209 to 380
Primary care costs	–21	–50 to 8
Secondary care costs	8	–7 to 228
Investigation costs	241	216 to 265
Drug costs	36	–18 to 91

in secondary care studies as well as in the primary care trial suggests that the effect might be transportable from secondary to primary care. Even by allowing *H. pylori* tests-and-treat to be costly, it is likely that significant cost reductions would accrue by the reduced amount of endoscopies (Table 14.2).

In the international context, countries with high rates of *H. pylori* infection, high rates of peptic ulcer disease, high availability of noninvasive tests for *H. pylori*, and high costs for endoscopy are likely to find that test-and-treat is more cost effective than endoscopy-based management. Of these, the cost of endoscopy is the most significant, varying from €600 in the US to €400 in the UK and only €60 in Southern European countries. Although the health systems differ, they all operate in the context of the patient being managed by a primary care physician and referred for endoscopy. The IPD meta-analysis of net monetary benefit showed highly significant savings using *H. pylori* test-and-treat rather than endoscopy [17]. A sensitivity analysis of altering the unit cost of endoscopy did not find a point at which endoscopy-based management became more cost effective. So again, even in current Western societies with a relatively low *H. pylori* prevalence, prompt endoscopy seems the more expensive option.

INITIAL SHORT-TERM TREATMENT STRATEGIES

Effect and cost-effectiveness of short-term treatment strategies for dyspepsia largely depend on the accepted definition of symptoms for dyspepsia diagnosis. The Rome working parties have recommended that patients with predominant reflux-type symptoms are excluded from the definition of dyspepsia and diagnosed as GERD. The original Rome criteria based on symptom patterns did not prove to have adequate predictive value. The revised Rome II and Rome III criteria, based on "predominant" symptoms, have yet to be tested further, especially in primary care populations [18]. The symptom-based Rome classification of functional dyspepsia seems not to lead to an easily applicable and consistent system that is useful in clinical practice nor in scientific research. Further studies testing the effect and usefulness of tighter symptom definitions are required.

PROTON PUMP INHIBITORS

In patients presenting with dyspepsia and without an initial diagnosis, starting off with PPIs is considered significantly more effective than starting off with either antacids or H2RAs in the first 4 weeks. Summary results of RCTs show that approximately 40% of patients improve with an H2RA or antacid and an additional 20% improves with PPI. In case of predominating heartburn symptoms among patients with dyspepsia (according to strict definitions these patients might be classified as patients with reflux symptoms or reflux disease), effects are slightly better [19]. With a similar control event rate, the benefit with PPI was seen for global symptoms, heartburn, and epigastric pain (with the exception of PPI versus antacids). The benefit on heartburn was greater than for epigastric pain alone, as expected due to biological plausibility of the effect [11].

HISTAMINE 2 RECEPTOR-ANTAGONISTS

Differences between H2RA and PPI treatment effects are of importance, since H2RAs are cheaper than PPIs, even after expiration of patents, and more convenient than taking huge amounts of antacids to produce the same effect. Based on a meta-analysis of short term treatment of GERD, the advantage of PPIs over H2RA in empirical treatment effect seems greater when the prior chance of erosive lesions is larger [19]. This will be the case in patients with longstanding relatively heavy symptomatology, selected for endoscopy or referral. Patients presenting with a new episode of dyspepsia in primary care might be at least equally effectively treated with the more easily available and cheaper H2RAs. This might be the reason that in a recent primary care-based trial of step-up versus step-down treatment of dyspepsia in the Netherlands, cost-effectiveness of both strategies was comparable [9].

ANTACIDS

Antacids usually are passed by physicians prescribing therapy for dyspepsia. Whether this is justified depends on local circumstances, availability, and perceived effectiveness. In the absence of true placebo-controlled trials, one can conclude that, in terms of short-term symptom relief, PPIs as well as H2RAs usually are more effective than antacids at least in patients with relatively more heartburn symptoms. PPIs might be also more acceptable to patients than antacids but are more costly. Therefore, in primary care, H2RAs might be a more adequate first empirical treatment step induced by physicians in most cases. There are no long-term treatment trials, which is important as dyspepsia is considered to be a chronic and relapsing condition. It is possible that intermittent use of a PPI or H2RA or even antacids may be equally effective at less cost than continuous therapy. However, no other solid

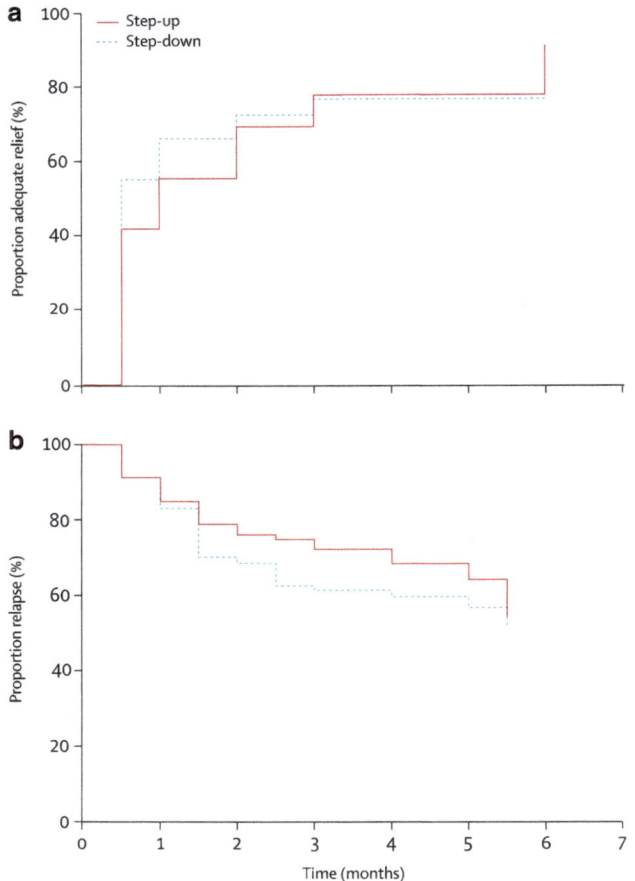

FIG. 14.1 Relief and relapse in step-up versus step-down in dyspepsia [9].

evidence on a choice for prescription of antacid can be presented except one that was part of the Dutch step-up versus step-down trial. In both arms, approximately a third of the patients ended up in step 3, so they experienced equal symptom reduction while either using PPI or antacids (Fig. 14.1) [9].

PROKINETICS
The use of motility-influencing agents and more advanced prokinetic drugs in clinical practice was significantly constrained by serious adverse reactions to cisapride, registered in the late nineties of the twentieth century. The last primary care study carried out with cisapride showed no relevant differences in effect compared with H2RAs among mainstream patients with dyspepsia [8]. There are virtually no studies that substantiate the efficacy of domperidone. Given the limited therapeutic options, in this group of patients, additional use of domperidone may be considered when dysmotility symptoms prevail, but no cost-effectiveness studies are available to support an initial choice for this strategy.

NONPRESCRIPTION THERAPY AND MEDICAL ADVICE
Patients with dyspepsia symptoms are often accompanied with nonmedical side opinions and nonevidence-based medical advice. Patients themselves are often under the assumption that their symptoms are associated with smoking, obesity, posture, and certain foods, which generally can be considered as true. However, evidence on efficacy or cost-effectiveness of any of the advices given is lacking.

SCIENTIFIC SUPPORT
Several researches on the effect of nondrug advice in dyspepsia and reflux patients were conducted in healthy subjects. The intensity of the pattern of complaints was seldom considered. Usually, the lower esophageal sphincter (LES) pressure or the acidity in the esophagus was taken as an outcome measure. A couple of comparative studies with small numbers of patients can be found in literature.

NUTRITION
Studies in healthy subjects show that pressure in the LES and/or the acidity in the esophagus can be influenced by coffee, alcohol,

high quantity food intake, high fat meals, carbonated beverages, and peppermint [20–22].

SMOKING
Smoking seems to be associated with severe symptoms of dyspepsia as well as reflux. However, any effect of stop smoking advice has not been reported.

OVERWEIGHT
Although a relationship of GERD symptoms with overweight is evident, a couple of methodologically poor intervention studies have shown mixed results. Only one study suggested that only positive effect on symptoms was seen in patients with an exceptionally large weight loss [23].

STRESS AND OTHER PSYCHOLOGICAL FACTORS
Even though many studies illustrate that dyspeptic patients have a higher burden of psychosocial and psychiatric comorbidity, the causal contribution of psychiatric and psychological factors to (functional) dyspepsia remains unclear [24]. Results from studies with binary data show that dyspeptic patients have an increased risk of having a psychiatric disorder, particularly depression. Combined data from several studies show an increased presence of psychiatric and personality disturbances in patients with dyspepsia. Moreover, it demonstrates marked differences in frequency of major life events and coping behavior between dyspeptic patients and healthy controls. Recently, we reported that younger patients in primary care consulting with dyspepsia have higher levels of depression and somatization [25]. Psychological morbidity and coping style contribute to dyspepsia symptom severity. More population-based, well-designed, prognostic studies that address psychological factors as well as different treatment strategies for dyspepsia are needed. That way, more detailed conclusions could be drawn and, hopefully, it would help the clinician.

OVER-THE-COUNTER MEDICATION
Currently, in many countries, antacids, H2RAs, and PPIs are available in low dosage without prescription. This means that cost-effectiveness considerations mentioned in the paragraph

on strategies with initial prescription of short-term treatment with these drugs should be translated to their over-the-counter availability. This, however, has not been done in literature until now.

CONCLUSIONS

Reviewing cost effectiveness of the options studied in this chapter, among the primarily diagnostic strategies, endoscopy-based management appears to be slightly more effective than strategies kicking off with a noninvasive *H. pylori* test-and-treat when positive. Although endoscopy has many clinical advantages, especially in selected and referred populations, prompt endoscopy is not cost effective, either in comparison with *H. pylori* test-and-treat or with empirical PPI treatment. *H. pylori*-driven strategies seem more cost effective than empirical treatment only in populations with relatively high *H. pylori* prevalence. *H. pylori* test-and-treat may be as effective but is cheaper than endoscopy in patients not at risk of malignant diseases, particularly in younger patients in populations with relatively high *H. pylori* prevalence. When endoscopy becomes cheaper, more accessible, or even available on-site in primary care settings, cost-effectiveness of prompt endoscopy might increase.

Among strategies starting with short-term treatment, a step-up approach seems the most cost-effective and adequate approach in primary care populations with low-risk dyspepsia, by definition with low to moderate heartburn symptomatology and no alarm symptoms. With the costs of the PPIs decreasing, the cost-effectiveness of a step-down approach might be of more interest to populations with a relatively high proportion of patients with reflux-like symptoms that might be caused by food habits, overweight, or other factors.

References

1. Delaney B, Ford AC, Forman D, Moayyedi P, Qume M. WITHDRAWN: initial management strategies for dyspepsia. Cochrane Database Syst Rev. 2009;CD001961
2. Talley NJ. American Gastroenterological Association medical position statement: evaluation of dyspepsia. Gastroenterology. 2005;129:1753–5.
3. Veldhuyzen van Zanten SJ, Bradette M, Chiba N, et al. Evidence-based recommendations for short- and long-term management of uninvestigated dyspepsia in primary care: an update of the Canadian Dyspepsia Working Group (CanDys) clinical management tool. Can J Gastroenterol. 2005;19:285–303.

4. National Institute for Clinical Excellence (NICE). Dyspepsia: management of dyspepsia in adults in primary care, Clinical guideline, vol. 17. London: National Institute for Clinical Excellence; 2004.

5. Scottish Intercollegiate Guidelines Network. Dyspepsia: a national clinical guideline. Report no 68. Edinburgh: Scottish Intercollegiate Guidelines Network; 2003.

6. Dutch Institute for Healthcare Improvement (CBO), Dutch College of General Practitioners (NHG). Multidisciplinary guideline "dyspepsia". Alphen aan den Rijn, Netherlands: Dutch Institute for Healthcare Improvement and Dutch College of General Practitioners; 2004 (in Dutch).

7. Numans ME, van der Graaf Y, de Wit NJ, de Melker RA. How useful is selection based on alarm symptoms in requesting gastroscopy? An evaluation of diagnostic determinants for gastro-oesophageal malignancy. Scand J Gastroenterol. 2001;36:437–43.

8. Quartero AO, Numans ME, de Melker RA, Hoes AW, de Wit NJ. Dyspepsia in primary care: acid suppression as effective as prokinetic therapy. A randomized clinical trial. Scand J Gastroenterol. 2001;36:942–7.

9. van Marrewijk CJ, Mujakovic S, Fransen GAJ, et al. Effect and cost-effectiveness of step-up versus step-down treatment with antacids, H2-receptor antagonists, and proton pump inhibitors in patients with new onset dyspepsia (DIAMOND study): a primary care based randomised controlled trial. Lancet. 2009;373:215–25.

10. Bytzer P, Hansen JM, Schaffalitzky de Muckadell OB. Empirical H2-blocker therapy or prompt endoscopy in management of dyspepsia. Lancet. 1994;343:811–6.

11. Delaney B, Moayyedi P, Deeks J, et al. The management of dyspepsia: a systematic review. Health Technol Assess. 2000;4:1–189.

12. Chiba N, Veldhuyzen Van Zanten SJ, Escobedo S, et al. Economic evaluation of *Helicobacter pylori* eradication in the CADET-Hp randomized controlled trial of *H. pylori*-positive primary care patients with uninvestigated dyspepsia. Aliment Pharmacol Ther. 2004;19:349–58.

13. Delaney BC, Qume M, Moayyedi P, et al. *Helicobacter pylori* test and treat versus proton pump inhibitor in initial management of dyspepsia in primary care: multicentre randomised controlled trial (MRC-CUBE trial). BMJ. 2008;336:651–4.

14. Moayyedi P, Soo S, Deeks J, et al. Systematic review and economic evaluation of *Helicobacter pylori* eradication treatment for non-ulcer dyspepsia. Dyspepsia Review Group. BMJ. 2000;321:659–64.

15. Ford AC, Moayyedi P, Jarbol DE, Logan RF, Delaney BC. Meta-analysis: *Helicobacter pylori* 'test and treat' compared with empirical acid suppression for managing dyspepsia. Aliment Pharmacol Ther. 2008;28:534–44.

16. Lassen AT, Pedersen FM, Bytzer P. Schaffalitzky de Muckadell OB. Helicobacter pylori test-and-eradicate versus prompt endoscopy for management of dyspeptic patients: a randomised trial Lancet. 2000;356:455–60.

17. Ford AC, Qume M, Moayyedi P, et al. *Helicobacter pylori* "test and treat" or endoscopy for managing dyspepsia: an individual patient data meta-analysis. Gastroenterology. 2005;128:1838–44.
18. van Kerkhoven LA, Laheij RJ, Meineche-Schmidt V, Veldhuyzen-van Zanten SJ, de Wit NJ, Jansen JB. Functional dyspepsia: not all roads seem to lead to rome. J Clin Gastroenterol. 2009;43:118–22.
19. van Pinxteren B, Numans ME, Lau J, de Wit NJ, Hungin AP, Bonis PA. Short-term treatment of gastroesophageal reflux disease. J Gen Intern Med. 2003;18:755–63.
20. Pehl C, Pfeiffer A, Wendl B, Kaess H. Different effects of white and red wine on lower esophageal sphincter pressure and gastroesophageal reflux. Scand J Gastroenterol. 1998;33:118–22.
21. Nebel OT, Castell DO. Inhibition of the lower oesophageal sphincter by fat – a mechanism for fatty food intolerance. Gut. 1973;14:270–4.
22. Salmon PR, Fedail SS, Wurzner HP, Harvey RF, Read AE. Effect of coffee on human lower oesophageal function. Digestion. 1981;21:69–73.
23. Mathus-Vliegen LM, Tytgat GN. Twenty-four-hour pH measurements in morbid obesity: effects of massive overweight, weight loss and gastric distension. Eur J Gastroenterol Hepatol. 1996;8:635–40.
24. Soo S, Moayyedi P, Deeks J, Delaney B, Lewis M, Forman D. Psychological interventions for non-ulcer dyspepsia. Cochrane Database Syst Rev. 2005;CD002301.
25. Mujakovic S, de Wit NJ, van Marrewijk CJ, et al. Psychopathology is associated with dyspeptic symptom severity in primary care patients with a new episode of dyspepsia. Aliment Pharmacol Ther. 2009;29:580–8.

Chapter 15
Dyspepsia in Children: Epidemiology, Clinical Presentation, and Causes

Oleg Jadrešin

Keywords: Dyspepsia, Children, Epidemiology, Clinical presentation

INTRODUCTION

Chronic abdominal pain is the most common gastrointestinal symptom in children. According to the definition of Apley and Nash, recurrent abdominal pain occurs in more than three episodes over more than 3 months and is severe enough to affect daily activities of a child [1]. As in majority of children with chronic abdominal pain no clear structural or biochemical pathology can be found, the term "pain-related functional gastrointestinal disorders" has replaced the old term "chronic abdominal pain" [2, 3]. After the original definition, subgroups of the disorder have been described and according to the "Rome III" criteria a clinician can differentiate between functional dyspepsia (FD), irritable bowel syndrome, abdominal migraine, and functional abdominal pain (syndrome) (Table 15.1) [2]. Visceral sensation, hormonal changes, inflammation, motility disturbances, and psychological factors have all been suggested as contributory factors [3]. Despite the fact that disorders are by definition functional, symptoms may persist for years and the reported quality of life of children may be similar to children with inflammatory bowel disease or gastroesophageal reflux disease (GERD) [4].

O. Jadrešin (✉)
Department of Pediatric Gastroenterology and Nutrition,
University Children's Hospital Zagreb, Zagreb, Croatia
e-mail: oleg.jadresin@yahoo.com

M. Duvnjak (ed.), *Dyspepsia in Clinical Practice*,
DOI 10.1007/978-1-4419-1730-0_15,
© Springer Science+Business Media, LLC 2011

TABLE 15.1   Pain-related functional gastrointestinal disorders (Rome III criteria) [2].

Functional dyspepsia	Persistent or recurrent pain or discomfort centered in the upper abdomen
	Not relieved by defecation or associated with the onset of a change in stool frequency or stool form
	No evidence of an inflammatory, anatomic, metabolic, or neoplastic process
	Duration at least 2 months
Irritable bowel syndrome	Abdominal discomfort or pain associated (at least 25% of time) with two of following:
	Improvement with defecation
	Change in stool frequency
	Change in stool form
Functional abdominal pain	Episodic or continuous abdominal pain at least once a week for a minimum of 2 months
Functional abdominal pain syndrome	Functional abdominal pain accompanied by headaches, limb pain or difficulty in sleeping
Abdominal migraine	Paroxysmal episodes of intense, acute periumbilical pain
	Lasts from one hour to days, separated by asymptomatic periods
	Often accompanied by nausea, vomiting, anorexia, photophobia, pallor or headaches

DEFINITION AND CLINICAL PRESENTATION OF DYSPEPSIA IN CHILDREN

Dyspepsia refers to persistent or recurrent pain or discomfort in the upper abdomen that is not relieved by defecation or associated with the onset of a change in stool frequency or stool form. According to Rome III criteria for FD, the symptoms should occur at least once a week during 2 months and there is no evidence of an inflammatory, anatomic, metabolic, or neoplastic process that explains the subject's symptoms. The pain may be accompanied with nausea, vomiting, epigastric fullness, bloating, or early satiety. Dyspeptic symptoms may follow a viral illness [2, 5].

Children with recurrent abdominal pain are also more likely to have headache, joint pain, anorexia, excessive gas, and altered bowel symptoms. However, none of these associated symptoms has been reported to distinguish between organic and functional abdominal pain. Frequency, severity, or timing of pain is not helpful either [6]. The presence of alarm symptoms and signs suggests a higher probability or prevalence of organic disease and may justify the performance of diagnostic tests. Alarm symptoms

TABLE 15.2. Alarm symptoms and signs in children and adolescents with abdominal pain-related functional gastrointestinal disorders [2].

Persistent right upper or right lower quadrant pain
Dysphagia
Persistent vomiting
Gastrointestinal blood loss
Nocturnal diarrhea
Pain that awakes the child
Family history of inflammatory bowel disease, celiac disease or peptic ulcer disease
Arthritis
Perianal disease
Unexplained fever
Involuntary weight loss
Deceleration of linear growth
Delayed puberty

and signs include involuntary weight loss, deceleration of linear growth, gastrointestinal blood loss, persistent vomiting, nocturnal diarrhea, persistent right upper or right lower quadrant pain, dysphagia, unexplained fever, delayed puberty, arthrtitis, perirectal disease, and family history of inflammatory bowel disease, celiac disease, or peptic ulcer disease (Table 15.2) [2, 6].

EPIDEMIOLOGY

The reported prevalence of chronic abdominal pain in Western countries is 0.3% to 19% and most (over 90%) of the children have no identifiable organic cause for pain [7–9]. Chronic abdominal pain seems to account for 2% to 4% of all pediatric office visits [10]. In a primary pediatric setting, organic disease is found only in 5% of children with chronic abdominal pain. In pediatric gastroenterology departments, approximately 40% children have an underlying pathology [11]. There are two age peaks in the prevalence of chronic abdominal pain: at 4–6 years of age and early adolescence. Chronic abdominal pain is uncommon under the age of 4 [1, 12–14]. Gender differences manifest around puberty with a slight female predominance [12, 15].

The prevalence of dyspepsia in children varies between 3.5% and 27% according to gender and country of origin [16, 17]. Approximately 5% to 10% of otherwise healthy adolescents have had symptoms of nausea and heartburn within the past year and 20% of adolescents have noted upper abdominal pain at some time during the previous year [18]. According to the study of

Hyams et al., 62% of symptomatic adolescents who undergo an upper endoscopy have no organic or mucosal abnormalities and are considered to have FD [16]. Seventy percent of children with FD were asymptomatic or much improved after a follow-up period of 6 months to 2 years and 85% of them were receiving no therapy [16].

The prevalence increases with age, from 2.5% in children between 3 and 9 years of age to 8.5% in children between 10 and 17 years of age [19].

CAUSES OF DYSPEPSIA IN CHILDREN

FD probably develops as a result of interaction of biological, psychological, and social factors. Biological factors are inflammation, hypersensitivity to gastric distension, impaired accommodation to meal, delayed gastric emptying, altered antroduodenal motility, and gastric dysrhythmias [20–22]. In conclusion, 47% to 68% of children with FD have delayed gastric emptying (measured by ultrasound or scintigraphy) and 50% to 64% have abnormalities of gastric rhythm seen on electrogastrography [23–25]. Symptoms such as bloating and abdominal pain may be associated with abnormal gastric and small bowel transit. Children with fast gastric emptying and slow small bowel transit were more likely to report bloating; abdominal pain was associated with slow small bowel transit [26].

Visceral hypersensitivity is a conscious perception of visceral stimulation independent of the intensity of stimulation. Adult patients with FD may have lower discomfort thresholds to gastric distension [27]. Reduced gastric accommodation, hypersensitivity to distension, and impaired gastric emptying have been reported in adolescents with FD [23, 27, 28].

Inflammation influences gastric emptying, as demonstrated in electrogastrography studies of *Helicobacter pylori* gastritis, celiac disease and food allergy [20, 29–31]. Increased mast cell density and eosinophil activation have been reported in celiac disease [32]. Mast cells have also been implicated in stress-induced delays in gastric emptying and visceral hyperalgesia [33, 34].

Patients with recurrent abdominal pain have more symptoms of anxiety and depression than healthy community controls and are at risk of later emotional symptoms and psychiatric disorders. There is also evidence that parents of patients with recurrent abdominal pain have more symptoms of anxiety, depression, and somatization than parents of community controls or parents of other pediatric patients [6]. Main conditions that should be considered in the differential diagnosis of FD in childhood and adolescence are listed in Table 15.3.

TABLE 15.3. Differential diagnosis of dyspepsia in children.

Gastroesophageal reflux disease
Eosinophilic esophagitis/gastritis
Drug-induced gastropathy
Peptic ulcer disease
Inflammatory bowel disease
Henoch–Schoenlein purpura
Gallbladder disease
Recurrent acute/chronic pancreatitis
Gastroparesis
Biliary dyskinesia
Chronic intestinal pseudoobstruction
Abdominal migraine
Psychiatric disorders

Helicobacter pylori Infection

Approximately 50% of the world's population is infected with *Helicobacter pylori* (*H. pylori*) [35]. The prevalence rates vary in different parts of the world and may be as high as high as 80% by the age of 10 years in developing countries [36–40]. The prevalence is much lower in developed countries (10% by age of 10 years in the USA, 2% in children of Swedish parents in Sweden), but even in these countries more than 50% of children living in poor socio-economic conditions may be infected [41–43]. Children with an infected family member (most often mother or an older sibling), residing under crowded conditions, with two or more siblings or having poor hygiene are at increased risk for infection [43–46]. Infection with *H. pylori* is a risk factor for developing peptic ulcer disease, gastric adenocarcinoma, and mucosa-associated lymphoid tissue (MALT) lymphoma [39, 47, 48]. The infection is usually acquired in childhood but children rarely develop serious complications [17]. Children are most at risk for acquiring infection prior to the age of 3 years, mostly between 12 and 24 months of age, and the risk decreases after the age of 5 years [46]. Children under the age of 5 years may be at risk for recurrent infection [49].

The association between non-ulcer dyspepsia and *H. pylori* infection has been controversial. Prevalence of *H. pylori* infection in children with and without recurrent abdominal pain is similar, and no supporting evidence was found for a role of *H. pylori* infection in recurrent abdominal pain in childhood [16, 41, 50, 51]. Most people who acquire *H. pylori* infection in childhood develop chronic gastritis without symptoms, but the chronic infection may progress to complications in both symptomatic and asymptomatic patients [51]. There is no evidence that *H. pylori* gastritis causes symptoms in the absence of duodenal ulcer disease and its eradication is consistently associated with improved symptoms only in children with duodenal ulcer disease [41, 50, 52].

Nodularity of the antral mucosa has been described in association with *H. pylori* gastritis in children [53]. Chronic inflammatory reaction with the infiltration of lymphocytes and plasma cells is usually found in the superficial parts of gastric mucosa. Atrophy of gastric mucosa is extremely rare in children from Western countries but has been reported in Japan [41, 54, 55]. Intestinal metaplasia is common in adults with chronic gastritis with a longer duration of the disease and has also been reported in Japanese children, with or without *H. pylori* infection [55].

Anatomic location of gastric inflammation and degree of gastric acid production are associated with a diverse outcome. Antral-predominant gastritis with increased acid production predisposes to ulcer-related disease (mainly duodenal ulcers) and pan or corpus-predominant gastritis with decreased acid production to gastric atrophy, intestinal metaplasia, and gastric adenocarcinoma [56, 57]. IL-1 gene cluster polymorphisms, possibly enhancing production of IL-1b, are associated with an increased risk of hypochlorhydria and gastric cancer in persons infected with *H. pylori* [58–60].

H. pylori infection has also been associated with many extraintestinal conditions, but stronger association has been found only for iron deficiency anemia. Iron absorption is thought to be decreased due to pangastritis, hypochlorhydria, and the inhibition of the reduction of iron to its ferrous state. *H. pylori* may also sequester iron or use it for growth [61–63].

Gastritis and Peptic Ulcer Disease

Acid-peptic disease in childhood develops as a consequence of imbalance between mucosal defensive and aggressive factors and may present as gastritis, duodenitis, mucosal erosion, or ulceration [64]. Gastric secretion becomes close to adult values by 3–4 years of age and is stimulated through neuroendocrine (acetylcholine and vagus), endocrine (gastrin and pepsin), and paracrine ways (histamine) [65]. In *H. pylori* infection, elevated levels of serum pepsinogen I have been demonstrated as a result of antral inflammation [66]. Disturbances in bicarbonate secretion (due to nonsteroidal anti-inflammatory drugs, NSAIDs), mucosal blood flow, or the mucus layer are also important in the pathogenesis of acid-peptic disease [64].

Peptic ulcer is a rare disease in childhood with the reported incidence of 1 case per 2,500 hospital admissions to a university hospital [67]. Primary (idiopathic) peptic ulcers are diagnosed in 1.8% to 3.6% of the total number of upper endoscopies in children [68]. Secondary peptic ulcer disease develops as a reaction to acute stress, severe systemic illness, or due to the intake of drugs. In children, duodenal ulcers are more common than gastric ulcers. Primary duodenal ulcers are rare in children under 10 years of age but the prevalence increases in adolescence. Gastric ulcers in children are almost always secondary [53, 69]. *H. pylori* infection is found in almost 90% of children with primary duodenal ulcer disease [70]. Eradication of the bacteria prevents the ulcer relapse [71]. *H. pylori* infection of the antral mucosa and gastric metaplasia of the duodenum have been found to be risk factors for duodenal ulceration [72]. An increase in the proportion of *H. pylori*-negative peptic ulcers is observed in adults and children, possibly due to the decreasing prevalence of the *H. pylori* infection [68, 73].

The most frequent presentation of peptic ulcer disease in children is abdominal pain and acute gastrointestinal bleeding. Primary duodenal ulcer is associated with chronic or recurrent symptoms and most children present with episodic epigastric pain, frequently associated with vomiting and nocturnal awakening [74,75]. Other possible symptoms are anemia, early satiety, and weight loss. Children older than 8 years may have symptoms as adults, such as pain or discomfort that exacerbates with meal. Younger children may not be able to localize the pain and may present with anorexia and irritability. Up to 25% of children with duodenal ulcer present only with painless gastrointestinal bleeding or anemia [75].

Primary infectious gastritis may be caused by other agents, apart from *H. pylori* (*Helicobacter heilmannii*, Cytomegalovirus, Herpes simplex, Influenza A, *Candida albicans*, *Giardia lamblia*). *H. heilmannii* can be transmitted from cats and causes chronic active gastritis in children and adults [76].

Hypersecretory states (Zollinger–Ellison syndrome and antral G-cell hyperplasia) are rarely found in children and should be suspected in severe or recurrent duodenal and gastric ulcers, resistance to proton pump inhibitor (PPI) treatment, multiple ulcers or ulcers in different locations. Other conditions with acid hypersecretion in childhood are systemic mastocytosis, short bowel syndrome first year after surgical resection, hyperparathyroidism, renal failure, and cystic fibrosis [77].

The most common drugs associated with drug-induced gastropathy and ulcers are NSAIDs. NSAIDs inhibit cyclooxygenase-1 enzyme (COX-1) and reduce prostaglandin synthesis; consequently gastric mucosal blood flow is diminished as well as production of the mucus–bicarbonate barrier [78]. Concurrent use of anticoagulants, corticosteroids, or coagulopathy increases the risk of complications [79].

Gastritis and gastric ulcerations are found in 46% to 75% of children with Crohn's disease (CD) and are mostly localized in gastric corpus. Although most commonly found in CD, granulomatous gastritis has been also described in *H. pylori* infection, sarcoidosis, infectious gastritides, and other rare conditions [80].

Ménétrier's disease is a rare disorder characterized by giant hypertrophy of the mucosal folds in stomach. Cytomegalovirus and *H. pylori* are the most frequently found pathogens associated with this condition. The disease manifests with vomiting, abdominal pain, anorexia, and the signs of protein loss [81].

Lymphocytic gastritis, characterized by an intense lymphocytosis of the foveolar and surface epithelium and chronic inflammation in the lamina propria, is reported in association with celiac disease, *H. pylori* gastritis, and chronic varioliform gastritis [80]. Celiac disease may manifest with dyspeptic symptoms and histological changes normalize after gluten withdrawal [82, 83].

Eosinophil-mediated gastritis may be a presentation of food allergy or be a primary disease (primary eosinophilic gastritis). Gastric eosinophilia may also occur in hypereosinophilic syndrome, infectious gastritis, celiac disease, inflammatory bowel disease, drug hypersensitivity, and other conditions. Allergic gastritis mainly affects young infants with cow's milk protein allergy but multiple food intolerances may also occur (egg, soy, cereals, vegetables, poultry) [80]. Any eosinophilic infiltration in the stomach is pathological, and in the duodenum, more than 20 eosinophils per high power field is suggestive of eosinophilic disease [84].

Primary eosinophilic gastritis may manifest at any age and may affect any part of the gastric wall. In mucosal form, children may present with vomiting, abdominal pain, and gastric blood loss, and motility disturbances and gastric outlet obstruction may occur if muscular layer is affected [85, 86]. Serosal forms produce eosinophilic ascites [80, 87]. Swollen gastric mucosal folds, nodules, and polyps may be found on endoscopy but the eosinophilic infiltration may not be seen histologically if mucosa is not affected [81]. Eosinophilic gastritis may also be a part of the eosinophilic gastroenteritis and may present with abdominal pain, vomiting, diarrhea, malabsorption, occult blood loss, or protein-losing enteropathy [80]. Main causes of gastritis and gastropathy of childhood are listed in Table 15.4.

TABLE 15.4. Main causes of gastritis and gastropathy in childhood and adolescence.

Infection
   Helicobacter pylori/*H. heilmannii* and other bacteria
   Viruses
   Parasites
Drug-induced (NSAIDs, corticosteroids, valproate, potassium chloride)
Corrosive
Radiation
Granulomatous
   Mycobacteria and other infectious agents
   Crohn's disease
   Chronic granulomatous disease
   Sarcoidosis
   Vasculitis-associated
Eosinophil-mediated
Lymphocytic
   CMV infection
   H. pylori infection
   Celiac disease
Vascular (portal hypertensive gastropathy)
Autoimmune
   Henoch-Schoenlein purpura
   Autoimmune polyendocrine syndrome type 3
Other
   Collagenous
   Menetrier's disease
   Zollinger-Ellison syndrome
   Uremic gastropathy

Gastroesophageal Reflux Disease

Gastroesophageal reflux (GER) is the passage of gastric contents into the esophagus with or without regurgitation or vomiting. GER is a physiologic event, occurring in healthy infants, children, and adults with mostly short, postprandial reflux episodes and with no or few symptoms. Gastroesophageal reflux disease (GERD) develops when the reflux causes frequent symptoms and/or complications [88]. Reflux episodes occur mostly during transient relaxations of the lower esophageal sphincter unaccompanied by swallowing [89]. Neurological impairment, obesity, esophageal atresia, chronic lung disease, and a history of prematurity are risk factors for development of GERD [88].

Symptoms and signs of reflux disease in childhood vary with age (Table 15.5) [88,89]. Esophagitis, erosions, exudate, ulcers,

TABLE 15.5. Symptoms of gastroesophageal reflux disease (GERD) in childhood.

Infants and small children	Older children and adolescents
Recurrent regurgitation and/or vomiting	Heartburn
Weight loss or poor weight gain	Chest pain
Hematemesis	Chronic cough due to laryngeal/ pharyngeal inflammation
Irritability	Dental erosions
Wheezing or stridor	
Cough	
Horseness	
Apparent life threatening events (ALTE)	

strictures, hiatal hernia, areas of possible esophageal metaplasia, and polyps may be found in GERD when endoscopy is performed [88]. Reflux esophagitis is defined as the presence of endoscopically visible breaks in the esophageal mucosa at or immediately above the gastroesophageal junction [90,91]. The presence of endoscopically normal esophageal mucosa does not exclude nonerosive gastroesophageal reflux disease (NERD). Esophageal eosinophilia, elongation of papillae, basal hyperplasia, and dilated intercellular spaces are seen in reflux esophagitis and may also be found in other sorts of esophagitis or in healthy individuals. Barrett's esophagus is present when cardiac-type mucosa is found in esophageal biopsies (with or without intestinal metaplasia) and is seen mostly in children with high risk for GERD [88].

Eosinophilic Esophagitis

Eosinophilic esophagitis (EE) is a disease of increasing prevalence and often presents with symptoms that suggest presence of GERD [92, 93]. Older children and adults with EE may develop dysphagia and food impaction, while food refusal and failure to thrive may manifest in infants [92, 94]. EE is found more commonly in males (often teenagers) and is often associated with other atopic diseases [95]. Aeroallergens may have a role in pathogenesis and the initial sensitization might take place in the airways. Also, a high frequency of sensitization to plant-derived food antigens that cross-react with pollens was noted, such as wheat and rye with grass pollens [93]. The most common food allergens involved in pathogenesis of EE are egg, cow's milk, soy, corn, and wheat; other foods have also been recognized as allergens, including beef, pork, chicken, barley, rice, oat, garlic, and legumes [87, 96]. The disease is thought to be a combination of IgE-mediated and non-IgE-mediated food reactions. The symptoms of EE are only partially responsive to acid-controlling medications [87]. In EE speckled exudates, trachealization of esophagus or linear furrows may be found on endoscopy but the endoscopic finding may be normal [88]. Histological analysis of bioptic specimens from the proximal and distal esophagus is important for diagnosis and differentiation from reflux esophagitis [93, 95]. In EE, the inflammation has also often a patchy distribution but is nearly equal throughout the esophagus [92]. More than 15–17 eosinophils per high power field are found in esophageal mucosa; eosinophils may be found deeper than mucosal layer and eosinophilic abscesses may be present [92, 97].

Gallbladder Disease

Cholelithiasis and cholecystitis are relatively uncommon in childhood but may be a cause of the epigastric pain. Factors associated with cholelithiasis in childhood and adolescence are obesity, prolonged total parenteral nutrition (TPN), previous ileal resection, short bowel syndrome, hemolytic disorders, and some neonatal conditions (TPN, bronchopulmonary dysplasia, sepsis, necrotizing enterocolitis) [98, 99]. Black pigment stones are formed in the presence of excess bilirubin in bile and are associated with a hemolytic process or diseases that result in enterohepatic circulation of excess conjugated bilirubin from the large intestine to the liver (Crohn's disease, distal small intestinal resection, cystic fibrosis). Cholesterol stones are associated with hypersecretion of cholesterol into bile and decreased motility of the gallbladder. Biliary sludge may be a precursor of stone formation. Fetal stones predominate in boys and most often resolve spontaneously during the first months of life [100]. Gallstones may lead to biliary colic, a steady intense pain in the upper right quadrant or epigastrium, sometimes radiating to the shoulder and often accompanied with vomiting. The presentation in children in similar although may be atypical in infants and young children [101]. Acute cholecystitis is usually manifested with fever, right upper quadrant pain, and leukocytosis. Gallstone disease can also complicate with pancreatitis, obstruction of the common bile duct, and ascending cholangitis [102].

Chronic acalculous cholecystitis/biliary dyskinesia present with chronic abdominal pain, often in the upper right quadrant, in otherwise healthy children. Routine laboratory investigation and the abdominal ultrasound are normal. Diagnosis is made when reduced ejection fraction (<35%) of the gallbladder is found on hepatobiliary scintigraphy [102].

Recurrent Acute and Chronic Pancreatitis

Recurrent acute pancreatitis is seen in 10% of children after the acute episode of pancreatitis and is associated more often with structural anomalies and familial causes [103]. Chronic pancreatitis is defined by chronic inflammation and fibrosis leading to loss of exocrine and endocrine pancreatic function [104]. Important events in pathogenesis of this inflammatory disorder are acinar cell injury (metabolic disorders) and premature activation of trypsinogen in pancreas due to obstruction of ductal flow (structural causes) or failure in feedback control (hereditary pancreatitis) [103, 104]. Common structural causes of recurrent or chronic pancreatic inflammation are biliary stones, choledochal cyst, and congenital anomalies of pancreas (pancreas divisum) and the most common metabolic disorders are hyperlipidemias, hypercalcemia, and branched chain aminoacidemias [103]. Genetic defects in the cationic trypsinogen gene (*PRSS1*) enhance activation or prevent inactivation of this enzyme within the acinus leading to episodes of acute pancreatitis (autosomal dominant hereditary pancreatitis) [105]. Approximately half of the patients develop chronic pancreatitis with significantly higher risk for development of pancreatic cancer [106]. Mutation of SPINK1 gene acts as a disease modifier and causes pancreatitis in the presence of another genetic or environmental factor, such as malnutrition [107,108]. Several mutations of CFTR (cystic fibrosis transmembrane regulator) gene leading to pancreatic sufficiency were found to be associated with chronic pancreatitis [109, 110].

Recurrent episodes of acute pancreatitis may range from mild abdominal pain to more severe systemic disease. Pain is usually aggravated by food and may be accompanied with vomiting, nausea, and anorexia [103]. Abdominal pain in chronic pancreatitis is most often epigastric, deep or penetrating toward back and may be accompanied by nausea and vomiting. It may be intermittent or continuous but there are individuals who have little or no pain, especially later in the disease process [111]. Steatorrhea and weight loss do not occur until around 98% of pancreatic exocrine function has been lost [112]. The risk of pancreatic carcinoma is significantly higher in all patients, especially in autosomally dominant hereditary pancreatitis where it approaches 40% [113].

Gastroparesis

Gastroparesis is a disorder of impaired emptying of gastric contents into the duodenum in the absence of mechanical obstruction. Patients present with nausea, early satiety, vomiting, postprandial abdominal distension, pain, and weight loss. In gastroparesis, vomiting is postprandial and may occur several hours after ingestion of food. This condition may be caused by drugs (opioids, anticholinergics), metabolic disturbances (hypokalemia, acidosis, hypothyroidism, diabetes mellitus), surgery, eosinophilic gastroenteropathy, and neuromuscular disorders but is most often found in children after viral illness. Postviral gastroparesis is associated with postprandial antral hypomotility and most often resolves within 6–24 months [5, 102].

CONCLUSIONS

Chronic abdominal pain is the most common gastrointestinal symptom in children and in majority of children no clear structural or biochemical pathology can be found. The presence of alarm symptoms and signs suggests a higher probability or prevalence of organic disease and may justify the performance of diagnostic tests. FD probably develops as a result of interaction of biological, psychological, and social factors. Prevalence of *H. pylori* infection in children with and without recurrent abdominal pain is similar and there is no evidence that *H. pylori* gastritis causes symptoms in the absence of duodenal ulcer disease. GERD may usually be distinguished from FD based on clinical grounds. Biliary and pancreatic diseases are relatively uncommon in childhood but may be a cause of the epigastric pain, most often in children with the risk factors. Gastroparesis should also be considered in a differential diagnosis of dyspeptic symptoms in children, especially if occurring after a viral illness.

References

1. Apley J, Naish N. Recurrent abdominal pains: a field survey of 1,000 school children. Arch Dis Child. 1958;33:165–70.
2. Rasquin A, Di Lorenzo C, Forbes D, et al. Childhood functional gastrointestinal disorders: child/adolescent. Gastroenterology. 2006;130:1527–37.
3. Berger MY, Gieteling MJ, Benninga MA. Chronic abdominal pain in children. BMJ. 2007;334:997–1002.
4. Youssef NN, Murphy TG, Langseder AL, Rosh JR. Quality of life for children with functional abdominal pain: a comparison study of patients' and parents' perceptions. Pediatrics. 2006;117:54–9.
5. Sigurdsson L, Flores A, Putnam PE, Hyman PE, Di Lorenzo C. Postviral gastroparesis: presentation, treatment, and outcome. J Pediatr. 1997; 131:751–4.
6. American Academy of Pediatrics Subcommittee on Chronic Abdominal Pain. Chronic abdominal pain in children. Pediatrics. 2005;115:812–5.
7. Miele E, Simeone D, Marino A, et al. Functional gastrointestinal disorders in children: an Italian prospective survey. Pediatrics. 2004;114:73–8.

8. Chitkara DK, Rawat DJ, Talley NJ. The epidemiology of childhood recurrent abdominal pain in Western countries: a systematic review. Am J Gastroenterol. 2005;100:1868–75.

9. Ramchandani PG, Hotopf M, Sandhu B. ALSPAC Study Team. The epidemiology of recurrent abdominal pain from 2 to 6 years of age: results of a large, population-based study. Pediatrics. 2005;116:46–50.

10. Starfield B, Hoekelman RA, McCormick M, et al. Who provides health care to children and adolescents in the United States? Pediatrics. 1984;74:991–7.

11. Stordal K, Nygaard EA, Bentsen B. Organic abnormalities in recurrent abdominal pain in children. Acta Paediatr. 2001;90:638–42.

12. Petersen S, Bergstrom E, Brulin C. High prevalence of tiredness and pain in young schoolchildren. Scand J Public Health. 2003;31:367–74.

13. Saps M, Li BU. Chronic abdominal pain of functional origin in children. Pediatr Ann. 2006;35(246):249–56.

14. Ammoury RF, Pfefferkorn Mdel R, Croffie JM. Functional gastrointestinal disorders: past and present. World J Pediatr. 2009;5:103–12.

15. Perquin CW, Hazebroek-Kampschreur AA, Hunfeld JA, et al. Pain in children and adolescents: a common experience. Pain. 2000;87:51–8.

16. Hyams JS, Davis P, Sylvester FA, Zeiter DK, Justinich CJ, Lerer T. Dyspepsia in children and adolescents: a prospective study. J Pediatr Gastroenterol Nutr. 2000;30:413–8.

17. De Giacomo C, Valdambrini V, Lizzoli F, et al. A population-based survey on gastrointestinal tract symptoms and *Helicobacter pylori* infection in children and adolescents. Helicobacter. 2002;7:356–63.

18. Hyams JS, Burke G, Davis PM, Rzepski B, Andrulonis PA. Abdominal pain and irritable bowel syndrome in adolescents: a community-based study. J Pediatr. 1996;129:220–6.

19. Nelson SP, Chen EH, Syniar GM, Christoffel KK. Prevalence of symptoms of gastroesophageal reflux during childhood: a pediatric practice-based survey. Pediatric Practice Research Group. Arch Pediatr Adolesc Med. 2000;154:150–4.

20. Friesen CA, Lin Z, Singh M, et al. Antral inflammatory cells, gastric emptying, and electrogastrography in pediatric functional dyspepsia. Dig Dis Sci. 2008;53:2634–40.

21. Tack J, Bisschops R, Sarnelli G. Pathophysiology and treatment of functional dyspepsia. Gastroenterology. 2004;127:1239–55.

22. Talley NJ, Vakil NB, Moayyedi P. American Gastroenterological Association technical review on the evaluation of dyspepsia. Gastroenterology. 2005;129:1756–80.

23. Riezzo G, Chiloiro M, Guerra V, Borrelli O, Salvia G, Cucchiara S. Comparison of gastric electrical activity and gastric emptying in healthy and dyspeptic children. Dig Dis Sci. 2000;45:517–24.

24. Friesen CA, Lin Z, Garola R, et al. Chronic gastritis is not associated with gastric dysrhythmia or delayed solid emptying in children with dyspepsia. Dig Dis Sci. 2005;50:1012–8.

25. Friesen CA, Lin Z, Hyman PE, et al. Electrogastrography in pediatric functional dyspepsia: relationship to gastric emptying and symptom severity. J Pediatr Gastroenterol Nutr. 2006;42:265–9.

26. Chitkara DK, Delgado-Aros S, Bredenoord AJ, et al. Functional dyspepsia, upper gastrointestinal symptoms, and transit in children. J Pediatr. 2003;143:609–13.
27. Hoffman I, Vos R, Tack J. Assessment of gastric sensorimotor function in paediatric patients with unexplained dyspeptic symptoms and poor weight gain. Neurogastroenterol Motil. 2007;19:173–9.
28. Chitkara DK, Camilleri M, Zinsmeister AR, et al. Gastric sensory and motor dysfunction in adolescents with functional dyspepsia. J Pediatr. 2005;146:500–5.
29. Lin Z, Chen JD, Parolisi S, Shifflett J, Peura DA, McCallum RW. Prevalence of gastric myoelectrical abnormalities in patients with nonulcer dyspepsia and *H. pylori* infection: resolution after *H. pylori* eradication. Dig Dis Sci. 2001;46:739–45.
30. Perri F, Pastore M, Zicolella A, Annese V, Quitadamo M, Andriulli A. Gastric emptying of solids is delayed in celiac disease and normalizes after gluten withdrawal. Acta Paediatr. 2000;89:921–5.
31. Ravelli AM, Tobanelli P, Volpi S, Ugazio AG. Vomiting and gastric motility in infants with cow's milk allergy. J Pediatr Gastroenterol Nutr. 2001;32:59–64.
32. Colombel JF, Torpier G, Janin A, Klein O, Cortot A, Capron M. Activated eosinophils in adult coeliac disease: evidence for a local release of major basic protein. Gut. 1992;33:1190–4.
33. Tache Y, Perdue MH. Role of peripheral CRF signalling pathways in stress-related alterations of gut motility and mucosal function. Neurogastroenterol Motil. 2004;16 Suppl 1:137–42.
34. Monnikes H, Tebbe JJ, Hildebrandt M, et al. Role of stress in functional gastrointestinal disorders. Evidence for stress-induced alterations in gastrointestinal motility and sensitivity. Dig Dis. 2001;19:201–11.
35. Suerbaum S, Michetti P. *Helicobacter pylori* infection. N Engl J Med. 2002;347:1175–86.
36. Horvitz G, Gold BD. Gastroduodenal diseases of childhood. Curr Opin Gastroenterol. 2006;22:632–40.
37. Drumm B, Day AS, Gold B, et al. *Helicobacter pylori* and peptic ulcer: Working Group Report of the second World Congress of Pediatric Gastroenterology, Hepatology, and Nutrition. J Pediatr Gastroenterol Nutr. 2004;39 Suppl 2:S626–31.
38. Czinn SJ. Helicobacter pylori infection: detection, investigation, and management. J Pediatr. 2005;146 Suppl 3:S21–6.
39. Go MF. Review article: natural history and epidemiology of *Helicobacter pylori* infection. Aliment Pharmacol Ther. 2002;16 Suppl 1:3–15.
40. Logan RP, Walker MM. ABC of the upper gastrointestinal tract: epidemiology and diagnosis of *Helicobacter pylori* infection. BMJ. 2001;323:920–2.
41. Bourke B, Ceponis P, Chiba N, et al. Canadian Helicobacter Study Group Consensus Conference: update on the approach to Helicobacter pylori infection in children and adolescents – an evidence-based evaluation. Can J Gastroenterol. 2005;19:399–408.
42. Everhart JE, Kruszon-Moran D, Perez-Perez GI, Tralka TS, McQuillan G. Seroprevalence and ethnic differences in *Helicobacter pylori* infection among adults in the United States. J Infect Dis. 2000;181:1359–63.

43. Tindberg Y, Bengtsson C, Granath F, Blennow M, Nyren O, Granstrom M. *Helicobacter pylori* infection in Swedish school children: lack of evidence of child-to-child transmission outside the family. Gastroenterology. 2001;121:310–6.

44. Owen RJ, Xerry J. Tracing clonality of *Helicobacter pylori* infecting family members from analysis of DNA sequences of three housekeeping genes (ureI, atpA and ahpC), deduced amino acid sequences, and pathogenicity-associated markers (cagA and vacA). J Med Microbiol. 2003;52:515–24.

45. Drumm B, Perez-Perez GI, Blaser MJ, Sherman PM. Intrafamilial clustering of *Helicobacter pylori* infection. N Engl J Med. 1990;322: 359–63.

46. Rowland M, Daly L, Vaughan M, Higgins A, Bourke B, Drumm B. Age-specific incidence of *Helicobacter pylori*. Gastroenterology. 2006; 130:65–72.

47. Macarthur C, Saunders N, Feldman W. *Helicobacter pylori*, gastroduodenal disease, and recurrent abdominal pain in children. JAMA. 1995;273:729–34.

48. Forman D. The prevalence of *Helicobacter pylori* infection in gastric cancer. Aliment Pharmacol Ther. 1995;9 Suppl 2:71–6.

49. Halitim F, Vincent P, Michaud L, et al. High rate of *Helicobacter pylori* reinfection in children and adolescents. Helicobacter. 2006;11:168–72.

50. Drumm B, Koletzko S, Oderda G. *Helicobacter pylori* infection in children: a consensus statement. European Paediatric Task Force on *Helicobacter pylori*. J Pediatr Gastroenterol Nutr. 2000;30:207–13.

51. Splawski JB. *Helicobacter pylori* and nonulcer dyspepsia: is there a relation? J Pediatr Gastroenterol Nutr. 2002;34:274–7.

52. Gormally SM, Prakash N, Durnin MT, et al. Association of symptoms with *Helicobacter pylori* infection in children. J Pediatr. 1995;126: 753–6.

53. Hassall E, Dimmick JE. Unique features of *Helicobacter pylori* disease in children. Dig Dis Sci. 1991;36:417–23.

54. Guarner J, Bartlett J, Whistler T, et al. Can pre-neoplastic lesions be detected in gastric biopsies of children with *Helicobacter pylori* infection? J Pediatr Gastroenterol Nutr. 2003;37:309–14.

55. Kato S, Nakajima S, Nishino Y, et al. Association between gastric atrophy and *Helicobacter pylori* infection in Japanese children: a retrospective multicenter study. Dig Dis Sci. 2006;51:99–104.

56. Watabe H, Mitsushima T, Yamaji Y, et al. Predicting the development of gastric cancer from combining *Helicobacter pylori* antibodies and serum pepsinogen status: a prospective endoscopic cohort study. Gut. 2005;54:764–8.

57. Graham DY. *Helicobacter pylori* infection in the pathogenesis of duodenal ulcer and gastric cancer: a model. Gastroenterology. 1997;113: 1983–91.

58. Kusters JG, van Vliet AH, Kuipers EJ. Pathogenesis of *Helicobacter pylori* infection. Clin Microbiol Rev. 2006;19:449–90.

59. El-Omar EM. The importance of interleukin 1 beta in *Helicobacter pylori* associated disease. Gut. 2001;48:743–7.

60. Rowland M, Bourke B, Drumm B. *Helicobacter pylori* and peptic ulcer disease. In: Kleinman RE, Sanderson IR, Goulet O, Sherman PM, Mieli-Vergani G, Shneider BL, editors. Walker's pediatric gastrointestinal disease 5th ed. Hamilton, Ontario: BC Decker Inc; 2008. p. 139–52.

61. Baysoy G, Ertem D, Ademoglu E, Kotiloglu E, Keskin S, Pehlivanoglu E. Gastric histopathology, iron status and iron deficiency anemia in children with *Helicobacter pylori* infection. J Pediatr Gastroenterol Nutr. 2004;38:146–51.

62. Annibale B, Capurso G, Lahner E, et al. Concomitant alterations in intragastric pH and ascorbic acid concentration in patients with *Helicobacter pylori* gastritis and associated iron deficiency anaemia. Gut. 2003;52:496–501.

63. Barabino A. *Helicobacter pylori*-related iron deficiency anemia: a review. Helicobacter. 2002;7:71–5.

64. Blecker U, Gold BD. Gastritis and peptic ulcer disease in childhood. Eur J Pediatr. 1999;158:541–6.

65. Boyle JT. Acid secretion from birth to adulthood. J Pediatr Gastroenterol Nutr. 2003;37 Suppl 1:S12–6.

66. Lopes AI, Palha A, Lopes T, Monteiro L, Oleastro M, Fernandes A. Relationship among serum pepsinogens, serum gastrin, gastric mucosal histology and *H. pylori* virulence factors in a paediatric population. Scand J Gastroenterol. 2006;41:524–31.

67. Drumm B, Rhoads JM, Stringer DA, Sherman PM, Ellis LE, Durie PR. Peptic ulcer disease in children: etiology, clinical findings, and clinical course. Pediatrics. 1988;82:410–4.

68. Tam YH, Lee KH, To KF, Chan KW, Cheung ST. *Helicobacter pylori*-positive versus *Helicobacter pylori*-negative idiopathic peptic ulcers in children with their long-term outcomes. J Pediatr Gastroenterol Nutr. 2009;48:299–305.

69. Demir H, Gurakan F, Ozen H, et al. Peptic ulcer disease in children without *Helicobacter pylori* infection. Helicobacter. 2002;7:111.

70. Drumm B, Sherman P, Cutz E, Karmali M. Association of *Campylobacter pylori* on the gastric mucosa with antral gastritis in children. N Engl J Med. 1987;316:1557–61.

71. Goggin N, Rowland M, Imrie C, Walsh D, Clyne M, Drumm B. Effect of *Helicobacter pylori* eradication on the natural history of duodenal ulcer disease. Arch Dis Child. 1998;79:502–5.

72. Gormally SM, Kierce BM, Daly LE, et al. Gastric metaplasia and duodenal ulcer disease in children infected by *Helicobacter pylori*. Gut. 1996;38:513–7.

73. Oderda G, Mura S, Valori A, Brustia R. Idiopathic peptic ulcers in children. J Pediatr Gastroenterol Nutr. 2009;48:268–70.

74. Nijevitch AA, Sataev VU, Vakhitov VA, Loguinovskaya VV, Kotsenko TM. Childhood peptic ulcer in the Ural area of Russia: clinical status and *Helicobacter pylori*-associated immune response. J Pediatr Gastroenterol Nutr. 2001;33:558–64.

75. Dohil R, Hassall E. Peptic ulcer disease in children. Baillières Best Pract Res Clin Gastroenterol. 2000;14:53–73.

76. Ooi CY, Lemberg DA, Day AS. Other causes of gastritis. In: Kleinman RE, Goulet OJ, Mieli-Vergani G, Sanderson IR, Sherman P, Shneider BL, editors. Walker's pediatric gastrointestinal disease. 5th ed. Hamilton, Ontario: BC Decker Inc; 2008. p. 165–74.

77. Gottrand F. Acid-peptic disease. In: Kleinman RE, Goulet OJ, Mieli-Vergani G, Sanderson IR, Sherman P, Shneider BL, editors. Walker's pediatric gastrointestinal disease. 5th ed. Hamilton, Ontario: BC Decker Inc; 2008. p. 152–64.

78. Hawkey CJ. Nonsteroidal anti-inflammatory drug gastropathy. Gastroenterology. 2000;119:521–35.

79. Lazzaroni M, Bianchi Porro G. Gastrointestinal side-effects of traditional non-steroidal anti- inflammatory drugs and new formulations. Aliment Pharmacol Ther. 2004;20 Suppl 2:48–58.

80. Gallagher TK, Winter DC. Diarrhoea, ascites and eosinophilia: an unusual triad. Scand J Gastroenterol. 2007;42:1509–11.

81. Dohil R, Hassall E, Jevon G, Dimmick J. Gastritis and gastropathy of childhood. J Pediatr Gastroenterol Nutr. 1999;29:378–94.

82. Jevon GP, Dimmick JE, Dohil R, Hassall EG. Spectrum of gastritis in celiac disease in childhood. Pediatr Dev Pathol. 1999;2:221–6.

83. De Giacomo C, Gianatti A, Negrini R, et al. Lymphocytic gastritis: a positive relationship with celiac disease. J Pediatr. 1994;124:57–62.

84. Lowichik A, Weinberg AG. A quantitative evaluation of mucosal eosinophils in the pediatric gastrointestinal tract. Mod Pathol. 1996;9:110–4.

85. Khan S, Orenstein SR. Eosinophilic gastroenteritis: epidemiology, diagnosis and management. Paediatr Drugs. 2002;4:563–70.

86. Lee CM, Changchien CS, Chen PC, et al. Eosinophilic gastroenteritis: 10 years experience. Am J Gastroenterol. 1993;88:70–4.

87. Pratt CA, Demain JG, Rathkopf MM. Food allergy and eosinophilic gastrointestinal disorders: guiding our diagnosis and treatment. Curr Probl Pediatr Adolesc Health Care. 2008;38:170–88.

88. Vandenplas Y, Rudolph CD, Di Lorenzo C, et al. Pediatric gastro-esophageal reflux clinical practice guidelines: joint recommendations of the North American Society for Pediatric Gastroenterology, Hepatology, and Nutrition (NASPGHAN) and the European Society for Pediatric Gastroenterology, Hepatology, and Nutrition (ESPGHAN). J Pediatr Gastroenterol Nutr. 2009;49:498–547.

89. Omari T. Gastro-oesophageal reflux disease in infants and children: new insights, developments and old chestnuts. J Pediatr Gastroenterol Nutr. 2005;41 Suppl 1:S21–3.

90. Sherman PM, Hassall E, Fagundes-Neto U, et al. A global, evidence-based consensus on the definition of gastroesophageal reflux disease in the pediatric population. Am J Gastroenterol. 2009;104:1278–95.

91. Vakil N, van Zanten SV, Kahrilas P, Dent J, Jones R. The Montreal definition and classification of gastroesophageal reflux disease: a global evidence-based consensus. Am J Gastroenterol. 2006;101:1900–20.

92. Liacouras CA. Eosinophilic esophagitis in children and adults. J Pediatr Gastroenterol Nutr. 2003;37 Suppl 1:S23–8.

93. Brown-Whitehorn T, Liacouras CA. Eosinophilic esophagitis. Curr Opin Pediatr. 2007;19:575–80.

94. Sant'Anna AM, Rolland S, Fournet JC, Yazbeck S, Drouin E. Eosinophilic esophagitis in children: symptoms, histology and pH probe results. J Pediatr Gastroenterol Nutr. 2004;39:373–7.

95. Liacouras CA, Spergel JM, Ruchelli E, et al. Eosinophilic esophagitis: a 10-year experience in 381 children. Clin Gastroenterol Hepatol. 2005;3:1198–206.

96. Spergel JM, Andrews T, Brown-Whitehorn TF, Beausoleil JL, Liacouras CA. Treatment of eosinophilic esophagitis with specific food elimination diet directed by a combination of skin prick and patch tests. Ann Allergy Asthma Immunol. 2005;95:336–43.

97. Orenstein SR, Shalaby TM, Di Lorenzo C, et al. The spectrum of pediatric eosinophilic esophagitis beyond infancy: a clinical series of 30 children. Am J Gastroenterol. 2000;95:1422–30.

98. Rescorla FJ. Cholelithiasis, cholecystitis, and common bile duct stones. Curr Opin Pediatr. 1997;9:276–82.

99. Wesdorp I, Bosman D, de Graaff A, Aronson D, van der Blij F, Taminiau J. Clinical presentations and predisposing factors of cholelithiasis and sludge in children. J Pediatr Gastroenterol Nutr. 2000;31:411–7.

100. Broderick A. Gallbladder disease. In: Kleinman RE, Goulet OJ, Mieli-Vergani G, Sanderson IR, Sherman P, Shneider BL, editors. Walker's pediatric gastrointestinal disease. 5th ed. Hamilton, Ontario: BC Decker Inc; 2008. p. 1173–83.

101. Klar A, Branski D, Akerman Y, et al. Sludge ball, pseudolithiasis, cholelithiasis and choledocholithiasis from intrauterine life to 2 years: a 13-year follow-up. J Pediatr Gastroenterol Nutr. 2005;40:477–80.

102. Saps M, Di Lorenzo C. Motility disorders. In: Kleinman RE, Goulet OJ, Mieli-Vergani G, Sanderson IR, Sherman P, Shneider BL, editors. Walker's pediatric gastrointestinal disease. 5th ed. Hamilton, Ontario: BC Decker Inc; 2008. p. 195–207.

103. Nydegger A, Couper RT, Oliver MR. Childhood pancreatitis. J Gastroenterol Hepatol. 2006;21:499–509.

104. Khokhar AS, Seidner DL. The pathophysiology of pancreatitis. Nutr Clin Pract. 2004;19:5–15.

105. Whitcomb DC, Gorry MC, Preston RA, et al. Hereditary pancreatitis is caused by a mutation in the cationic trypsinogen gene. Nat Genet. 1996;14:141–5.

106. Whitcomb DC. Genetic predispositions to acute and chronic pancreatitis. Med Clin North Am. 2000;84:531–47.

107. Pfutzer RH, Barmada MM, Brunskill AP, et al. SPINK1/PSTI polymorphisms act as disease modifiers in familial and idiopathic chronic pancreatitis. Gastroenterology. 2000;119:615–23.

108. Threadgold J, Greenhalf W, Ellis I, et al. The N34S mutation of SPINK1 (PSTI) is associated with a familial pattern of idiopathic chronic pancreatitis but does not cause the disease. Gut. 2002;50:675–81.

109. Sharer N, Schwarz M, Malone G, et al. Mutations of the cystic fibrosis gene in patients with chronic pancreatitis. N Engl J Med. 1998;339:645–52.

110. Cohn JA, Friedman KJ, Noone PG, Knowles MR, Silverman LM, Jowell PS. Relation between mutations of the cystic fibrosis gene and idiopathic pancreatitis. N Engl J Med. 1998;339:653–8.
111. Layer P, Yamamoto H, Kalthoff L, Clain JE, Bakken LJ, DiMagno EP. The different courses of early- and late-onset idiopathic and alcoholic chronic pancreatitis. Gastroenterology. 1994;107:1481–7.
112. Gaskin KJ, Durie PR, Lee L, Hill R, Forstner GG. Colipase and lipase secretion in childhood- onset pancreatic insufficiency. Delineation of patients with steatorrhea secondary to relative colipase deficiency. Gastroenterology. 1984;86:1–7.
113. Lowenfels AB, Maisonneuve P, DiMagno EP, et al. Hereditary pancreatitis and the risk of pancreatic cancer. International Hereditary Pancreatitis Study Group. J Natl Cancer Inst. 1997;89:442–6.

Chapter 16
Diagnostic Tests and Treatment of Dyspepsia in Children

Keywords: Dyspepsia, Childhood, Gastric dysmotility, Food allergy, Endoscopy

INTRODUCTION

Dyspepsia – from the Latin word meaning "difficult (or abnormal) digestion" – is a symptom complex that encompasses, in variable combinations, such complaints as pain or discomfort localized in the upper abdomen, a subjective sense of bloating and/or an objective distension of the upper abdomen, nausea, early satiety and/or loss of appetite, regurgitation and/or vomiting, belching, and occasional heartburn. Children of preschool age usually cannot localize abdominal pain properly and cannot fully understand the concept of "nausea." Small children usually report that they feel "sick" and/or "tummy/belly ache" and/or "butterflies in stomach" and/or other more or less imaginative definitions. Therefore, dyspepsia is more easily – and appropriately – diagnosed in school age children, where it appears to be a relatively common condition [1, 2]. Functional dyspepsia (FD) as defined by the Rome II criteria has a prevalence of 0.3% among children seen by primary care physicians in Italy and 12.5% to 15.9% among schoolchildren referred to tertiary care centers in the USA [3–5]. In any age group (including adulthood),

A. Ravelli (✉)
GI Pathophysiology and Gastroenterology, University Department of Pediatrics, Children's Hospital, Spedali Civili, Brescia, Italy
e-mail: alberto_ravelli@yahoo.com

209
M. Duvnjak (ed.), *Dyspepsia in Clinical Practice*,
DOI 10.1007/978-1-4419-1730-0_16,
© Springer Science+Business Media, LLC 2011

the clinical manifestations of dyspepsia are entirely nonspecific and present a considerable overlap with manifestations related to conditions such as gastroesophageal reflux disease (GERD) (with or without esophagitis), irritable bowel syndrome (IBS), constipation, and gastrointestinal infections including gastritis due to *Helicobacter pylori* (*H. pylori*).

PATHOPHYSIOLOGY OF FUNCTIONAL DYSPEPSIA

Several pathophysiologic mechanisms have been suggested to underlie dyspeptic symptoms. These include delayed gastric emptying, impaired gastric accommodation to a meal, hypersensitivity to gastric distention, *H. pylori* infection, altered response to duodenal lipids or acid, abnormal duodenojejunal motility, or central nervous system dysfunction. A variety of disturbances of gastric and gastroduodenal motor activity – including disordered gastric myoelectrical activity, delayed gastric emptying, altered antroduodenal motility, and reduced gastric volume response to feeding – have been described in children with FD [6–11]. Accelerated gastric emptying associated with slow bowel transit was found in dyspeptic children with bloating as predominant symptom [12]. However, the pathogenetic relevance of gastrointestinal dysmotility and its correlation with clinical symptoms are not entirely clear, since gastric dysmotility is not always demonstrable in dyspeptic children and, conversely, a degree of gastric dysmotility may persist in children whose symptoms have subsided following medical therapy of dyspepsia [6, 9]. More recently, studies using the barostat have demonstrated a decreased threshold for perception in the stomach of children with functional abdominal pain compared to healthy controls [13]. Visceral hypersensitivity seems somewhat site-specific, since the thresholds for perception were decreased in the stomach of children with recurrent abdominal pain but not in those with IBS, whereas the thresholds for visceral perception in the rectum were lower in children with IBS compared to those with recurrent abdominal pain [13]. Therefore, gastric hypersensitivity may play a major pathogenetic role in the generation of symptoms than gastric dysmotility.

CLINICAL APPROACH TO THE CHILD WITH DYSPEPSIA

It is widely accepted that childhood dyspepsia is usually a functional disorder; therefore, no specific investigations are required in most cases. The pediatric Rome criteria, devised and periodically revised by an expert Committee on pediatric functional gastrointestinal disorders, should be applied as a first-line approach to every

TABLE 16.1.   Rome III criteria for functional dyspepsia in childhood.

Must include *all* of the following, fulfilled at least once per week for at
  least 2 months before diagnosis:
  Persistent or recurrent pain or discomfort centered in the upper
    abdomen (above the umbilicus)
  Not relieved by defecation and not associated with the onset of a change
    in stool frequency or stool form (i.e., unlike irritable bowel syndrome)
  No evidence of an inflammatory, anatomic, metabolic, or neoplastic
    process that explains the subject's symptoms

child with dyspepsia. The last version (Rome III) of these criteria
is summarized in Table 16.1. [14]. The duration of the symptoms
of at least 2 months is required to eliminate the likelihood of acute
disease and to establish a reasonable degree of chronicity. These criteria also serve the purpose of distinguishing dyspepsia from other
functional pain syndromes of childhood, such as the irritable bowel
syndrome, abdominal migraine, and functional abdominal pain
[14]. According to the expert Committee, upper gastrointestinal
endoscopy is no longer mandatory in order to make the diagnosis
of functional dyspepsia. In fact, the likelihood of finding mucosal
abnormalities responsible for dyspeptic symptoms is much lower in
children than in adults [1]. The previously identified "ulcer-like" and
"dysmotility-like" subtypes of functional dyspepsia have been eliminated because most epidemiological studies suggest that young
children do not fall into either category [1, 4, 5]. Furthermore, it is
clearly difficult if not impossible to distinguish between discomfort
and pain in young children, and there is no clear evidence that
symptoms of dysmotility-like dyspepsia (mostly upper abdominal
bloating/distension/discomfort, early satiety/anorexia, and regurgi-
tation/vomiting) originate from disordered foregut motility [4, 5].
According to the Rome III criteria, there should be no evidence of
an inflammatory process likely to explain the subject's symptoms.
Nonetheless, some children with functional abdominal pain syndromes may have evidence of mild, chronic inflammatory changes
on mucosal biopsies. Since functional gastrointestinal disorders
such as IBS and dyspepsia may follow an acute inflammatory event
(typically, a bacterial or viral gastroenteritis) in up to 30% of cases,
such changes should not impede the diagnosis of FD [15–17].

   In a minority of patients, however, the clinical history and physical examination may suggest the presence of an organic disease [14,
18, 19]. Factors suggesting the presence of organic disease are listed
in Table 15.2. According to the expert Committee of the Rome III
criteria, an upper gastrointestinal endoscopy is warranted in the
presence of dysphagia in patients with persistent symptoms despite

the use of anti-acid medications (proton pump inhibitors or H_2-blockers) and in patients who have recurrent symptoms following cessation of such medications. The current ESPGHAN and NASPGHAN guidelines 2000 both recommend upper gastrointestinal endoscopy with biopsy as the first-line investigation in suspected *H. pylori*-related disease [20,21]. According to the NASPGHAN, endoscopy is indicated only in children with severe symptoms, which suggest the possibility of an ulcer (Fig. 16.1), especially if they also have a positive family history of *H. pylori*-related disease and gastric cancer [20]. The ESPGHAN guidelines are less stringent, as they consider that presenting symptoms are nonspecific for *H. pylori*, and upper gastrointestinal endoscopy with biopsy is probably the single investigation with the highest diagnostic yield [20, 21]. However, gastric or duodenal ulcers are uncommon in children infected by *H. pylori*, so if *H. pylori* infection is suspected, a noninvasive investigation such as the ^{13}C-urea breath test or *H. pylori* stool antigen (see below) could be used instead of endoscopy [20–22]. Studies in animal models suggest that *H. pylori* infection may induce dyspeptic symptoms via a sensory-motor dysfunction of the enteric nervous system [23]. A somewhat similar neuroimmune interaction could underlie the symptoms of dyspepsia in patients with food

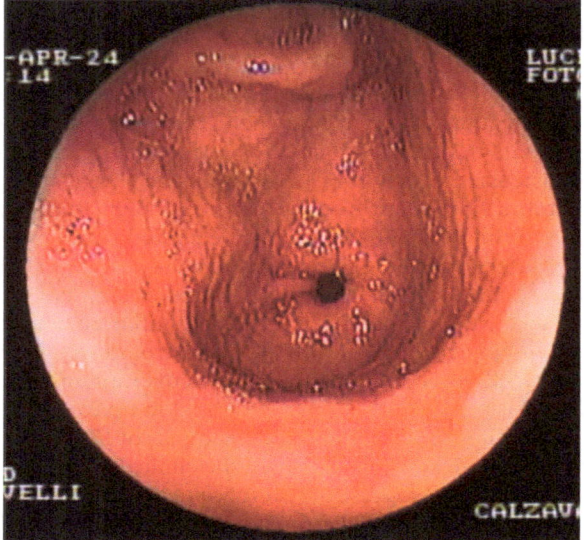

FIG. 16.1 Endoscopic view of a nodular antral gastritis and linear prepyloric ulcer in a child with *H. pylori* infection.

allergy and other inflammatory processes [24]. In recent studies, an increased number of degranulating mast cells and eosinophils were found in the gastric mucosa of dyspeptic children with cow's milk allergy and in the duodenal mucosa of adults with dyspepsia and IBS [25, 26]. Dyspepsia can also be a manifestation of celiac disease, and the prevalence of celiac disease in adult dyspeptic subjects is slightly higher than in the general population [27–29]. Thus it seems reasonable to perform a serological screening for celiac disease with antibodies to tissue transglutaminase (tTG) in a child with dyspepsia, especially if there are other known risk factors for celiac disease such as a first degree relative with celiac disease [30]. If tTG are positive, the diagnosis has to be confirmed by a small bowel biopsy, which should demonstrate the typical features of gluten-sensitive enteropathy: increased intraepithelial lymphocyte count, crypt hyperplasia, and villous atrophy [31, 32] (Fig. 16.2). In most patients, macroscopic features suggestive of villous atrophy such as a nodular pattern of the bulb (Fig. 16.3), a cobblestone or "mosaic" mucosa, and coarse segmented folds ("scalloping") (Fig. 16.4) can also be noted in the duodenum during endoscopy [33].

The demonstration of a food hypersensitivity other than celiac disease is less straightforward, as most chronic gastrointestinal

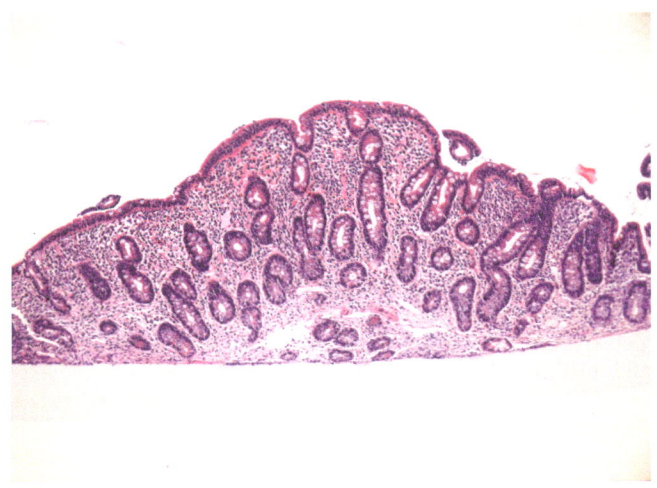

FIG. 16.2 Duodenal biopsy from a child with celiac disease, showing the typical histological features of gluten-sensitive enteropathy: villous atrophy, crypt hyperplasia, and increased number of intraepithelial lymphocytes (H&E, 10×).

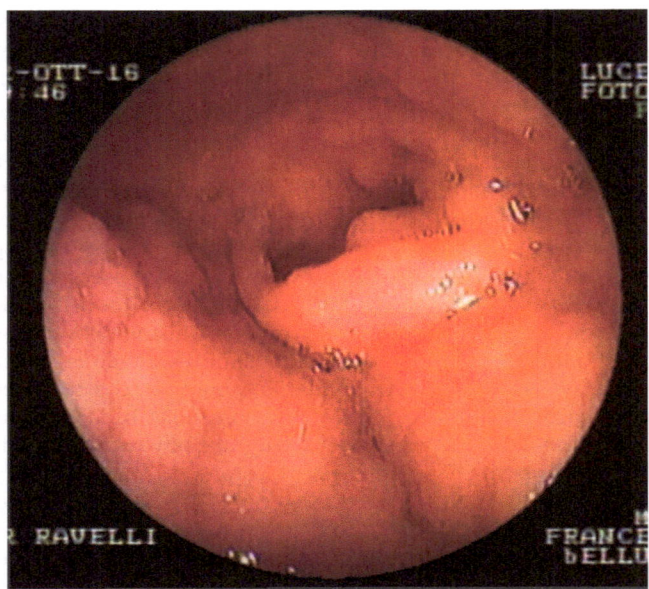

Fig. 16.3 A nodular appearance of the duodenal bulb is a common endoscopic finding in children with gastrointestinal food allergy. It can be related to villous atrophy in celiac disease, or to lymphoid nodular hyperplasia in children with hypersensitivity to cow's milk protein.

manifestations of food allergy are non-IgE mediated, so the serum levels of IgE as well as the skin prick test for specific food allergens are usually negative [34]. A positive family history of atopy and a past personal history of other gastrointestinal or extraintestinal manifestations of allergy (e.g., atopic dermatitis, wheezing, infantile colitis, etc.) should raise the suspicion that dyspeptic symptoms may be due to an immune-mediated reaction to food [34, 35]. If an endoscopy with biopsy is carried out, the presence of lymphoid nodular hyperplasia (Figs. 16.3 and 16.5) and a prominent eosinophilic infiltrate (Fig. 16.6) in the lamina propria of the gastric or duodenal mucosa may suggest an allergic reaction, provided that other causes of eosinophilia (parasites, drugs, inflammatory bowel disease, etc.) can be excluded [34–36]. According to the guidelines of the Pediatric Section of the European Academy of Allergy and Clinical Immunology (EAACI), however, a diagnosis of food hypersensitivity can be established only when symptoms subside on a strict exclusion diet and relapse upon challenge with the specific food [37]. For late and mild reactions such as dyspepsia and other

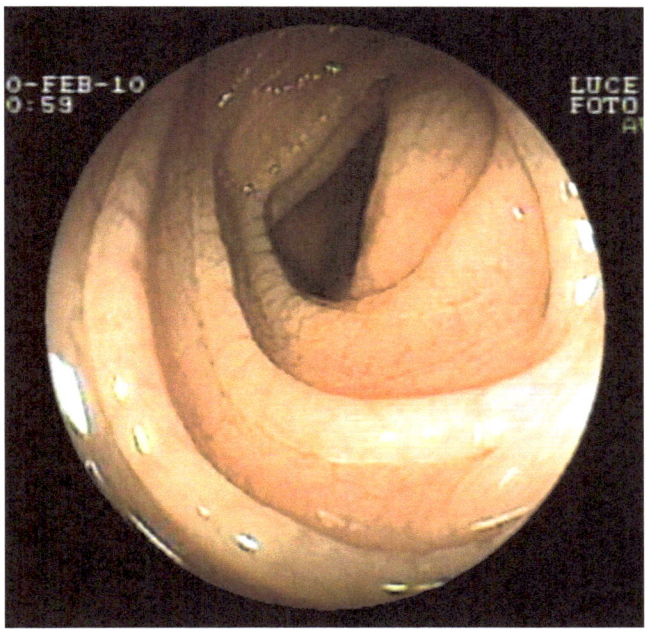

FIG. 16.4 Endoscopic view of cobblestone or mosaic mucosa and coarse, scalloped folds in the duodenum of a child with celiac disease, and total villous atrophy.

functional abdominal pain syndromes, the food challenge should be carried out in a double-blind, placebo-controlled fashion [37, 38].

Lactose intolerance due to lactase deficiency is the best known and commonest food hypersensitivity not due to an immunological mechanism [39]. Lactose malabsorption can sometimes cause dyspepsia, although in most patients bloating and pain are usually localized to the lower abdomen, and flatulence and diarrhea also commonly occur [39]. The presence of lactose malabsorption can be suggested by a good clinical history, which usually reveals the relationship between lactose ingestion and clinical symptoms. In these cases, a strict lactose-free diet can be prescribed, and symptom resolution followed by recurrence upon reintroduction of dairy foods confirms the diagnosis [39]. In dubious cases, lactose malabsorption can be demonstrated by the hydrogen breath test (see below), which shows an early peak of hydrogen excretion following the ingestion of a lactose solution [39]. In patients who report dyspeptic symptoms following ingestion of milk and dairy products, a challenge using a

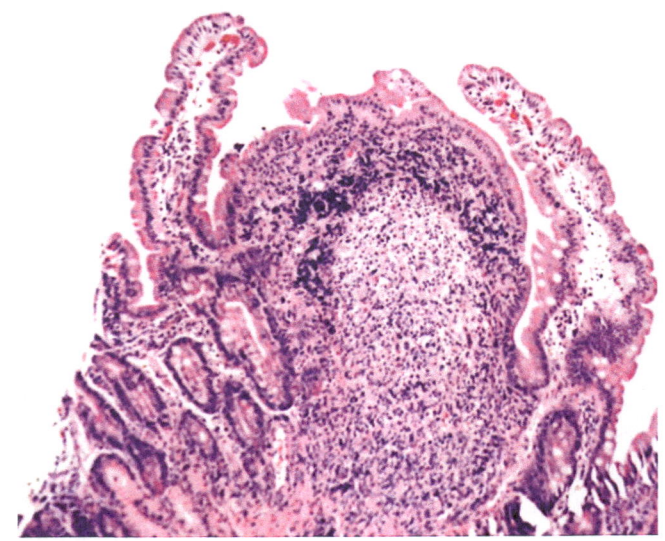

FIG. 16.5 Lymphoid follicle hyperplasia in a child with gastrointestinal food allergy (H&E, 10×).

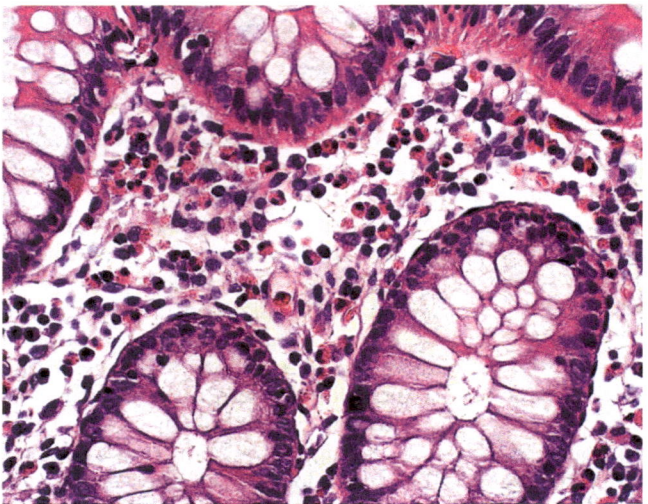

FIG. 16.6 A significant number of eosinophils are present in the lamina propria of the duodenal mucosa in a child with dyspepsia due to food allergy (H&E, 40×).

lactose-free milk can be used to distinguish between lactose intolerance and allergy to cow's milk protein. Obviously, underlying causes
of secondary lactose malabsorption (e.g., celiac disease, infestation
by *Giardia lamblia*) should be excluded.

Dyspeptic symptoms such as nausea, anorexia, and upper
abdominal discomfort or pain are not uncommon in children and
adolescents with Crohn's disease [40, 41]. Although the commonest
localization of pediatric Crohn's disease is to the terminal ileum
and right colon, the upper gastrointestinal tract is involved in about
50% of patients (in 5% to 6% as the sole localization), and indeed
an upper gastrointestinal inflammation can be present in pediatric
Crohn's disease, affecting with seemingly decreasing frequency
the stomach, esophagus, and/or duodenum [40, 41]. Therefore, all
patients in whom Crohn's disease is suspected should undergo an
upper gastrointestinal endoscopy and endoscopic as well as histological features compatible with Crohn's disease – e.g., linear or
aphtous ulcers (Fig. 16.7) and active inflammation with or without
granulomata (Fig. 16.8) – should be sought for.

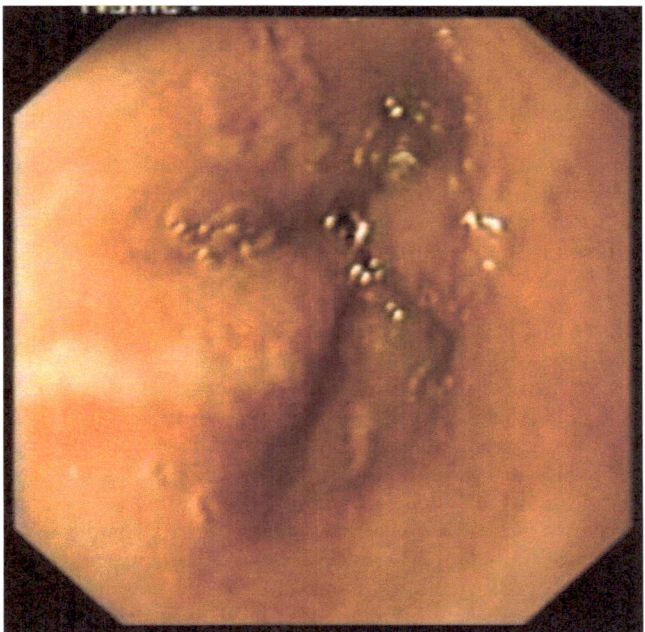

FIG. 16.7 Multiple linear ulcers converging to the pylorus in the gastric
antrum of a child with active Crohn's disease.

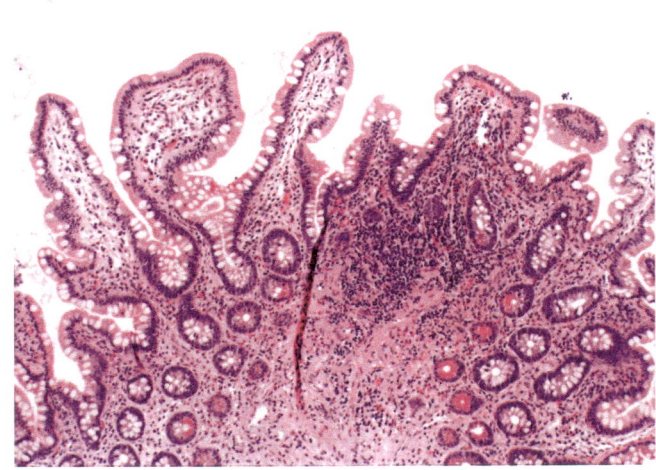

Fig. 16.8 Focal inflammatory infiltrate with partial villous atrophy and a small granuloma in the duodenal mucosa of a child with Crohn's disease (H&E, 10×).

Thus, it could be argued that if an organic disease is suspected, upper gastrointestinal endoscopy (with biopsies) should be the first-line investigation, since it can demonstrate the presence of most organic causes of dyspepsia and thereby allows to address the most appropriate treatment more quickly. A simplified diagnostic algorithm for dyspepsia in children is proposed in Fig. 16.9.

DIAGNOSTIC TESTS FOR CHILDHOOD DYSPEPSIA

A description of the most important tests that can be used in the diagnostic work-up of children with dyspepsia is given below. Even if dyspepsia is a functional disorder in most patients, investigations on gastrointestinal motility and gastric sensitivity are of limited use in the clinical setting, for several reasons. Some of these investigations (e.g., manometry, barostat) are technically difficult, invasive, time consuming, and require considerably experienced and skilled operators. Others (e.g., electrogastrography) are easier to perform, but their results can be easily overlooked or misinterpreted. Radionuclide scan, which is the gold standard for the measurement of gastric emptying, requires very expensive equipment and is not widely available. Essentially, these tests serve to investigate the pathophysiology of functional dyspepsia, and as

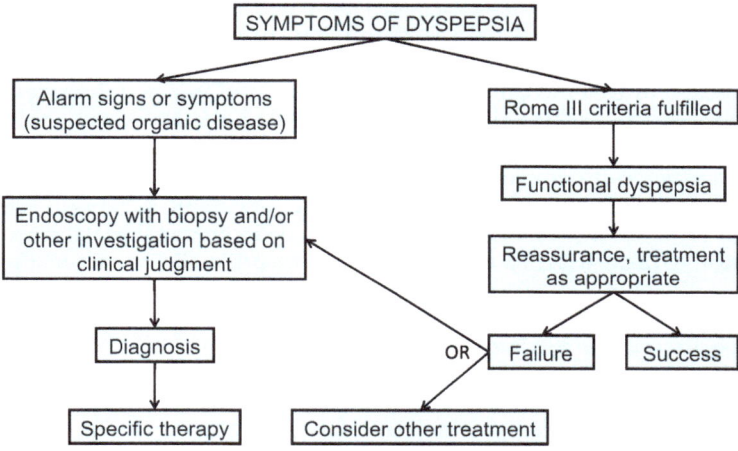

FIG. 16.9 A simplified diagnostic algorithm for dyspepsia in children.

such, they are more useful for research than clinical purposes. Only the measurements of gastric emptying and, to a lesser extent, electrogastrography have found an application in clinical practice and therefore will be considered in this section. The situation is clearly different if the history and clinical examination of the child with dyspepsia elicit features that suggest the possibility of an underlying organic disorder (Table 15.2). The presence of one or more of these "red flags" can raise the suspicion of conditions such as peptic disease, celiac disease, inflammatory bowel disease (IBD), etc., which should be ruled out by appropriate investigation.

LABORATORY INVESTIGATIONS

Routine biochemistry. Laboratory tests should not be carried out in a child with dyspepsia unless an organic disease is suspected. If this is the case, "routine" blood tests make little sense, and tests should be chosen according to the specific suspicion. For instance, a full blood count may reveal the presence of anemia and/or leucocytosis, but even these are nonspecific findings, since they may be due to very different conditions such as *H. pylori* infection, celiac disease, or IBD. If the patient's history or clinical examination suggests the possibility of a hepatic or biliary disorder – e.g., pain or discomfort referred to the upper right quadrant of the abdomen – liver function tests such as serum aspartate and alanine aminotransferases and g-glutamyl transpeptidase should be carried out.

Pancreatic function tests may be considered only in selected cases. If abdominal pain is prominent, recurrent, and localized in the central abdomen, and/or there is a family history of pancreatic disease, serum amylase may be helpful to detect recurrent pancreatitis [42]. However, in this case, pancreatic function testing should be carried out during acute attacks, since pancreatic enzymes can completely revert to normal during periods of well being [42]. A screening test for exocrine pancreatic function such as fecal elastase determination [43] can be indicated if malabsorption with steatorrhea is suspected but the celiac disease screening (see below) is negative. If Crohn's disease is suspected, a positive fecal calprotectin [44] can strengthen the suspicion and thus support more specific investigation (e.g., endoscopy).

Fecal calprotectin is highly sensitive and specific for intestinal inflammation, and being totally noninvasive, it is certainly better accepted by a child than a blood test for ESR, CRP, fibrinogen, mucoproteins, etc. [44, 45]. Serological tests such as anti-*Saccharomyces cerevisiae* antibodies (ASCA) and perinuclear anticytoplasmic antibodies (p-ANCA) are more specific for IBD, but their sensitivity is not high enough to recommend them as a screening test for IBD [45].

TESTS FOR *H. PYLORI* INFECTION

Chronic infection by the Gram-negative, microaerophilic bacterium *H. pylori* is a relatively common organic cause of dyspepsia [2, 20, 21, 46]. Noninvasive laboratory tests for the detection of *H. pylori* should be used during the follow-up of patients with proven *H. pylori*-related disease, in order to demonstrate eradication of the bacteria after an appropriate treatment [20–22].

The *13C-urea breath test* is the gold standard as it has a sensitivity and specificity of nearly 100% for *H. pylori* infection [20–22, 45]. Children aged <6 years do not usually offer enough cooperation to make the breath sampling adequate, so the test is not fully reliable in preschool children. However, since dyspepsia can be reliably diagnosed only in school children and adolescents, this is only a minor limitation. In order to avoid a false positivity, patients should be tested at least one month after the end of treatment [20–22].

The Helicobacter pylori stool antigen (HpSA), usually measured by enzyme immunoassay on frozen stools, has a sensitivity and specificity of 95% to 98% in most studies and is less expensive than the ^{13}C-urea breath test, so it can be reliably used to diagnose *H. pylori* infection as well as to monitor the eradication of the bacterium following treatment [22, 47, 48].

Serum IgG antibodies to H. pylori have a good sensitivity and specificity and are cheaper. However, given the persistence of the serological IgG antibody response after spontaneous healing or eradication, they are more suited for epidemiological studies on large population samples and are not recommended for the diagnosis and posttreatment monitoring of *H. pylori* infection [20–22].

CELIAC DISEASE SCREENING

Screening for celiac disease in a child with dyspepsia can be recommended if there are:

1. Signs or symptoms suggesting an enteropathy (e.g., poor growth, chronic diarrhea, anemia, etc.)
2. Extraintestinal manifestations compatible with celiac disease (such as iron deficiency anemia, dermatitis herpetiformis, etc.)
3. Other autoimmune diseases (especially diabetes mellitus and thyroiditis)
4. First degree relative affected by celiac disease [49].

As in adults, the most sensitive and specific test for celiac disease is the determination of anti-tissue transglutaminase (tTG) IgA antibodies [30, 49]. Anti-endomysial (EMA) IgA antibodies assayed by immunofluorescence are almost as sensitive and specific as tTG IgA, whereas the anti-gliadin IgA antibodies (AGA) are less sensitive and specific, although they may be the only antibody to test positive in celiac children aged 2 years or less [49–51]. Serum tTG, EMA, and AGA IgG antibodies are less sensitive and less specific, so they are mostly useful as a screening test in children with IgA deficiency, where tTG, EMA, and AGA IgA are usually negative [52]. Since selective IgA deficiency occurs in about 1:600 children and the prevalence of celiac disease in children with IgA deficiency is higher than in the general population, total serum IgA should always be tested together with tTG or EMA IgA when screening a child with suspected celiac disease [53]. In case of a positive screening test, the diagnosis should obviously be confirmed by duodenal biopsy.

LACTOSE HYDROGEN BREATH TEST

This test is performed by administering to the patient a standardized amount of lactose (2 g/kg, up to a maximum of 25 g) after an overnight fast, and then measuring the concentration of H_2 in the exhaled air at 15–30 min intervals over a 2–3 h period. A significant increase of the H_2 expired (>20 ppm) after approximately 1 h is consistent with lactose malabsorption [39]. It should be remembered that the lactose hydrogen breath test may give false-negative and false-positive results due to several factors, the most relevant being the recent use of antibiotics (which affect the intestinal flora), lack of hydrogen-producing bacteria (in 10% to 15% of the general population), ingestion of diets containing a high amount of fiber, or the presence of other as yet undiagnosed conditions such as intestinal motility disorders or small bowel bacterial overgrowth [39].

ABDOMINAL ULTRASONOGRAPHY

Abdominal ultrasonography is not recommended in the routine evaluation of childhood recurrent abdominal pain, because its diagnostic yield is very low in this condition [19]. However, an abdominal ultrasound examination may be helpful if liver, biliary, or pancreatic disease is suspected (e.g., abdominal pain or discomfort localized in the right upper abdominal quadrant, positive family history of pancreatitis, raised liver or pancreatic enzymes, etc.).

UPPER GASTROINTESTINAL ENDOSCOPY

From a technical point of view, there are no major differences between adult and child upper gastrointestinal endoscopy. In most children, esophagogastroduodenoscopy with biopsy can be carried out quickly and safely as an outpatient procedure following conscious sedation with i.v. midazolam at a mean dose of 0.1 mg/kg an i.v. opioid analgesic such as meperidine/pethidine at a mean dose of 1 mg/kg [54]. In cooperative children, a local anesthetic (e.g., mepivacaine) can be sprayed onto the back of the throat before sedation, in order to minimize the discomfort of the endoscopes passage through the hypopharinx and the upper esophageal sphincter. Prior to the sedation, however, it is usually advisable to explain the procedure to the child using simple words and keeping a friendly, reassuring attitude. Older children and adolescents, who are usually more curious and cooperative, may wish to follow the procedure on the video as it goes on and thus may require only a minimum sedation (although they may not remember the details of the exam afterwards, due to the amnesic effect of midazolam). In small children, the dose of midazolam should be titrated according to the patient's response (and the endoscopists need), up to 0.5 mg/kg. For uncooperative or agitated children, propofol at incremental doses of 0.5/kg or in a 2–3 mg/kg bolus can be used effectively and safely, remembering that in most countries, this drug can be administered only by anesthesiologists [55]. The size of the endoscope should be chosen according to the patients' age and size. Esophagogastroduodenoscopes with an outer diameter of 7.5 mm are suitable for most children, whereas adult gastroduodenoscopes (outer diameter of about 9 mm) can be safely used in older children and adolescents. In any case, oxygen saturation and heart rate should be continuously monitored during the endoscopy, and for 1–2 h afterwards or until the child wakes up [54, 55]. Even when neonatal endoscopes (outer diameter 5–6 mm) are used, the size of the biopsies can be adequate for histological examination, provided biopsies are carefully orientated. The site and number of biopsies obviously depends on the clinical indication and the macroscopic findings. For instance, if *H. pylori* infection is suspected, two biopsies from different areas of the gastric antrum and one from the gastric corpus should be taken [20–22]. If celiac disease is suspected, multiple biopsies should be taken from different sites of the duodenum, from the duodenojejunal flexure or distal duodenum to the duodenal bulb [56, 57]. If there are no overt endoscopic abnormalities, we suggest taking multiple biopsies from duodenum, stomach, and esophagus, since several disorders including celiac disease, eosinophilic gastroenteropathy, Crohn's disease, etc. may not always cause obvious macroscopic alterations. In any case, biopsies should be carefully orientated before fixation, in order to maximize the diagnostic yield of histology and avoid misdiagnosis (Fig. 16.10) [56, 57]. Eating and drinking can usually be safely resumed once the child is fully awake.

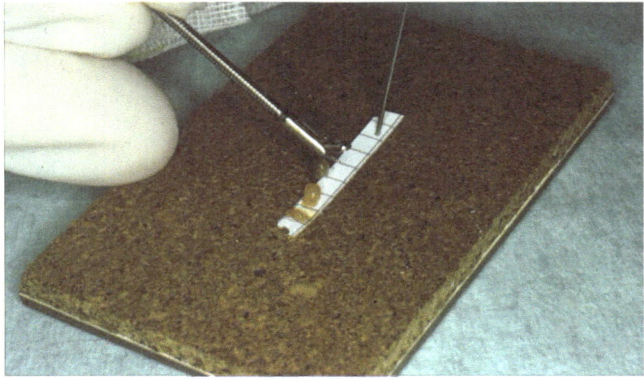

FIG. 16.10 Before fixation, endoscopic biopsies should be carefully orientated with the luminal side uppermost and placed on a strip of filter paper, where some conventional signs (e.g., "A" or "↑") should indicate the beginning of the biopsy sequence.

MOTILITY STUDIES

Invasive investigations are usually required to study gut contractile activity and transit. Such invasive investigations are less acceptable and poorly tolerated by infants and children, and therefore systematic studies are severely limited. The constraints imposed by such poor acceptability of extensive motility studies in childhood are the main reasons why pediatric gastroenterologists have become increasingly interested in noninvasive means of assessing gastrointestinal motility and transit. Such techniques include ultrasonography, breath test, and electrical impedance tomography for the study of gastric emptying, and the recording of gastric electrical control activity by surface electrodes, i.e., electrogastrography.

Electrogastrography

The electrical control activity that underlies gastric antral contractions and acts as the "pacemaker" of the human stomach emanates from the interstitial cells of Cajal and occurs at 0.05 Hz, i.e., about 3 cycles per minute (cpm) [58]. The technique of recording gastric electrical control activity with surface electrodes is called electrogastrography (EGG). The use of bipolar electrodes, adequate amplifiers, and band-pass filters usually allows the recording of a clear signal, whereas the digital conversion of the raw analog signal at frequencies of 1–5 Hz provides a mathematical representation of the signal that is suitable for subsequent computerized analysis (Fig. 16.11). The technique of running spectral analysis

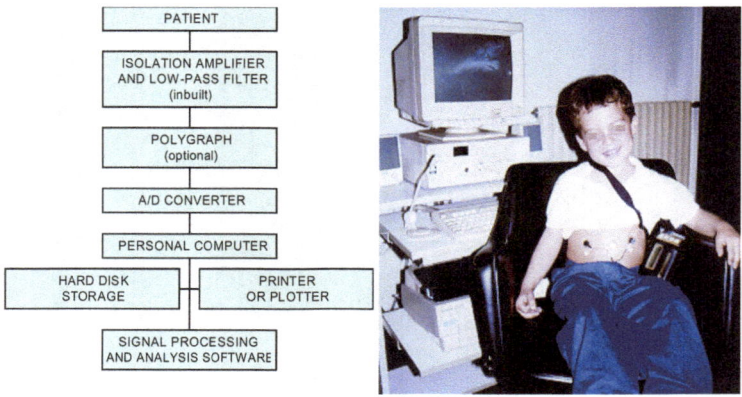

FIG. 16.11 Schematic representation of a standard electrogastrography (EGG) equipment and a child undergoing surface EGG with an ambulatory system.

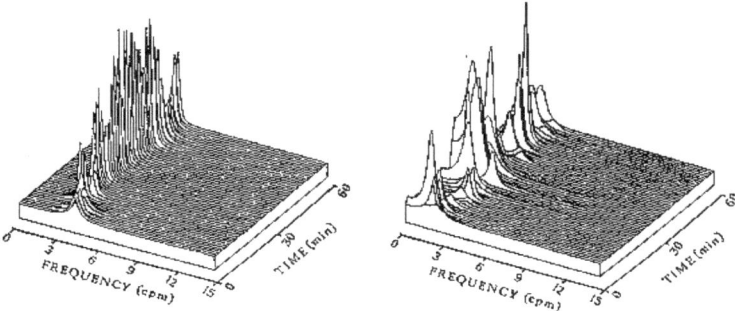

FIG. 16.12 Running spectral 1-h pseudo-three-dimensional plots of the postprandial EGG from a healthy child (*left*), and from a child with functional dyspepsia (*right*). The tracing on the *left* shows a regular high-amplitude 3 cpm activity throughout the recording. The EGG on the *right* shows an unstable electrical activity with a significant degree of bradygastria.

(by Fast Fourier Transform, autoregressive modeling, or exponential distribution) allows the frequency and power of the signal to be assessed in a more objective fashion than the simple visual inspection [59]. In normal healthy children, gastric electrical activity is similar to that of adults in terms of both frequency and response to a meal (Fig. 16.12, left). Relevant abnormalities (gastric dysrhythmias) have been detected and characterized by EGG in several conditions where the different control levels of gastric motor activity are affected [60]. Gastric dysrhythmias, often associated with delayed gastric emptying of a mixed solid–liquid meal, have been reported in a high proportion of children with functional dyspepsia, some of whom responded to a prokinetic therapy (Fig. 16.12, right) [6, 7, 60, 61]. Therefore, EGG (and gastric emptying studies) may provide a means to explore the pathophysiological basis of functional dyspepsia, but it should be remembered that the correlation between gastric dysrhythmias and the patients' symptoms remains controversial.

Gastric Emptying Study

Different methodologies have been applied for the measurement of gastric emptying in children and adults: dye dilution, epigastric impedance, ultrasonography, breath hydrogen test, etc [62]. Radionuclide scan (scintigraphy), however, remains undoubtedly the gold standard for the measurement of gastric emptying and will be briefly described here. Different types of caloric liquid or solid meal can be given, depending on the patient's age.

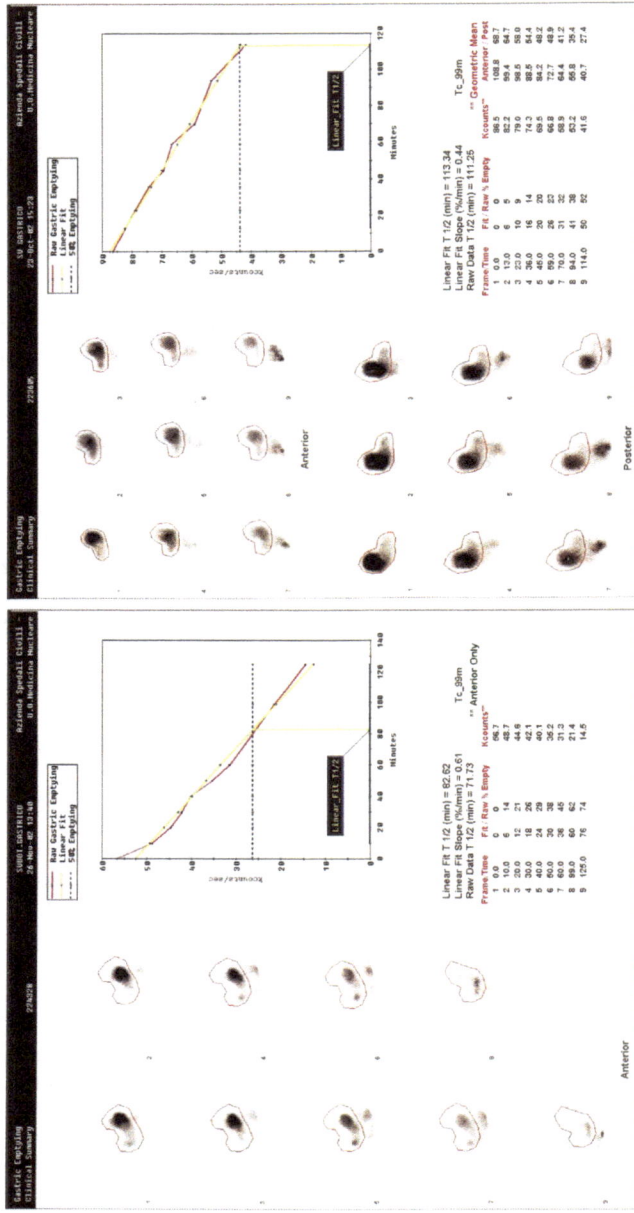

Fig. 16.13 Sequential images and gastric emptying curves from two radionuclide gastric emptying studies showing normal (*left*) and delayed (*right*) gastric emptying.

In children, scrambled egg with toasts are commonly used as test meal, and usually labeled with 99m technetium. After the ingestion of the radio-labeled test meal, the patient is given a small portion of the unlabeled meal to wash out all previously ingested radioactivity from the esophagus. A gamma camera equipped with an adequate collimator is placed in front of the recumbent patient, and a dynamic study of the esophagogastric region is carried out for a few minutes. A few hundred (e.g., 360) successive planar anteroposterior images of a few (e.g., 10) seconds each are collected during the first hour and subsequently integrated by further images collected during the next hour. The images collected during the first hour are elaborated to obtain 1-min frames, which, together with the images collected during the second hour, allow for the evaluation of radioactivity within an area of interest corresponding to the gastric region [62]. The time needed for a 50% reduction of radioactivity within this area at the end of the meal is expressed as time to gastric half-emptying (T½), and this can be generally considered delayed when >90 min (Fig. 16.13). During the study, gastroesophageal reflux episodes and pulmonary aspiration can also be identified [63].

TREATMENT OF CHILDHOOD DYSPEPSIA

The treatment of dyspepsia due to a demonstrable organic cause (e.g., *H. pylori* infection, food allergy, etc.) obviously corresponds to the treatment of the underlying disease, which is beyond the scope of this chapter. In the majority of cases, however, childhood dyspepsia appears to be a functional disorder, and pediatric studies have shown that functional disorders characterized by chronic or recurrent abdominal pain are associated with higher depression and anxiety scores and poor quality of life [64, 65]. The patients but especially the parents are often worried by the absence of a known and easily understandable cause of their child's symptoms, and this is probably the main reason why a confident diagnosis, which includes explanation of pain experience and reassurance, can by itself be therapeutic [18]. The role of stressors and the importance of the brain-gut axis in the generation of symptoms should be explained, avoiding the technical jargon. The child should be an active participant in the management process. It is important to set realistic and achievable goals, such as decrease the pain and improve the quality of life. If the patient is currently missing school, the return to school should be encouraged. It should be explained that school attendance, as well as social and sport activities, may be helpful because they provide distraction so that the child is less focused on pain. The therapy of pediatric functional gastrointestinal disorders is best done within the context of a multidisciplinary biopsychosocial approach [14, 64]. Specific goals of therapy include modifying severity and developing strategies for dealing with symptoms. However, despite the high frequency of functional abdominal pain syndromes and their significant impact on children's quality of life, there is only limited evidence to support most of the treatments that are commonly used to treat these conditions in childhood [66].

Anti-secretory Drugs
The H_2 receptor-antagonist famotidine was used in a double-blinded, placebo-controlled trial for a small group of children with abdominal pain and dyspepsia. This study showed that famotidine provided subjective improvement of symptoms but was equally effective as placebo when an objective score was applied [67].

Peppermint Oil
The efficacy of pH-dependent, enteric-coated peppermint oil capsules was evaluated in a randomized, double-blinded controlled trial on 42 children with irritable bowel syndrome (IBS) [68]. The patients were randomized to 1–2 capsules of a commercial preparation or placebo (1 capsule tid if body weight was <45 kg, 2 capsules tid if body weight was >45 kg). The severity of abdominal pain was reduced in 75% of those children receiving peppermint oil for 2 weeks. The exact mechanism of action of peppermint oil is unknown but is probably related to its spasmolytic and antiflatulent effect [69]. Although enteric-coated peppermint oil is generally safe (the most common side effects are heartburn and perianal pain) and probably associated with a positive benefit-risk ratio, it is relatively expensive, not easily available in many countries, and usually not covered by the National Health Service policy. Even more importantly, the fact that it proved effective in IBS does not imply that it should be effective also in functional dyspepsia. In view of these data, a Cochrane's review concluded that the use of drugs or herbal preparations for treatment of functional abdominal pain disorders in childhood should not be recommended outside of clinical trials [19].

Tricyclic Antidepressants
The efficacy of tricyclic antidepressants in the treatment of childhood functional abdominal pain syndromes – though not specifically in functional dyspepsia – has been evaluated in two recent

studies. A randomized trial in California showed a beneficial effect of amitriptyline therapy in adolescents with IBS [70]. The patients were randomized to 10, 20, or 30 mg dose of amitriptyline depending on their weight or placebo for a period of 8 weeks, and were evaluated after 4 weeks, 8 weeks, and at the end of a 3-week washout period. Patients receiving amitriptyline reported an improvement in their pain and quality of life. However, children in the drug or placebo groups had different quality of life scores at baseline, and the improvement of pain was present only in certain areas of the abdomen and at certain times of follow-up and was not sustained at other times. Furthermore, placebo had a negative effect on pain, and this could have been partially responsible for the statistical difference found between the two groups. A multicenter, randomized placebo-controlled trial in North America tested the efficacy of amitriptyline on 90 children with irritable bowel syndrome, functional abdominal pain, or functional dyspepsia [71]. This study showed an improvement in 59% of the children receiving amitriptyline in intention-to-treat analysis, but 75% of children in the placebo group also reported a fair to excellent pain relief in per-protocol analysis. Patients with mild to moderate intensity of pain responded better to treatment, whereas both patient groups reported a similar improvement in pain, disability, depression, and somatization scores during treatment.

Another antidepressant, the selective serotonin reuptake inhibitor citalopram, was evaluated in an exploratory 12-week open label, flexible-dose trial in children with recurrent abdominal pain [72]. The initial daily dose of 10 mg citalopram was progressively increased to 40 mg by week 4 if no clinical response was obtained. At the end of the trial, there was a significant improvement in abdominal pain index by both parental and child's report, and the study also showed a reduction of anxiety and depression. However, methodological limitations such as the absence of blinding, randomization, and placebo group make it difficult to conclude that the observed improvements were due to citalopram.

Serotoninergic and Anti-serotoninergic Agents

In view of their known effects on gastric motility and gastric emptying, several drugs acting as agonist or antagonist on different 5-HT receptors have been used for the treatment of dyspepsia and other functional gastrointestinal disorders [64]. A double-blinded placebo-controlled trial evaluated the efficacy of the 5-HT$_2$ receptor-antagonist cyproheptadine for 2 weeks in 29 children with functional abdominal pain [73]. Primary outcome measure was the self-reported change in frequency and duration of abdominal pain and parental assessment of children's improvement. At the end of the study, 86% of children in the cyproheptadine group vs. 36% of those in the placebo group reported significant improvement or resolution of abdominal pain. The 5-HT$_4$ receptor-agonist tegaserod combined with an osmotic laxative was found effective in alleviating abdominal pain in adolescents with constipation-predominant IBS [74]. However, tegaserod has been recently removed from the market in several countries due to an increase in cerebrovascular accidents in adults taking the drug. Once again, there are no published experiences of either drug in functional dyspepsia.

ALTERNATIVE THERAPIES

Psychosocial factors can be heavily involved in the development and evolutionary changes of functional gastrointestinal disorders, and there is increasing evidence that selected alternative treatments, including hypnotherapy and cognitive-behavioral therapy, may be effective [75]. Fifty-three children with functional abdominal pain or irritable bowel syndrome were randomized to six sessions of either hypnotherapy or supportive conventional medical care over a 3-month period, and they were followed up at 6 and 12 months after the discontinuation of therapy. Hypnotherapy proved superior to the conventional therapy by significantly reducing pain intensity and frequency as compared with the controlled group at all times even after discontinuation of therapy [76].

A recent Cochrane meta-analysis concluded that cognitive behavioral therapy may be a useful intervention for children with functional abdominal pain [75]. Cognitive behavioral therapy is mostly based on the technique of guided imagery [77]. Guided imagery is a simple, noninvasive procedure that uses progressive muscle relaxation to bring the subject to a state of deep mental relaxation. Then the subject is guided to actively create images that achieve self-regulation, behavioral changes, and ultimately improvement of symptoms. Indeed, three studies showed benefit of guided imagery for the treatment of functional abdominal pain in children [77–79].

DIETARY MODIFICATIONS

Since high fiber and lactose-free diet have been reported as somewhat beneficial in some adult patients with IBS, modifications of dietary habits such as fiber supplementation and lactose restriction have been suggested as a means of improving symptoms in children with recurrent abdominal pain syndromes. Neither of the two randomized controlled trials of fiber supplements in children found a significant beneficial effect of this intervention, and the pooled odds ratio for improvement with treatment was 1.26 with wide confidence intervals [80–82]. Similarly, two old trials with lactose-restricted diets in children with recurrent abdominal pain could not find any convincing relationship between lactose intolerance and symptoms [83, 84].

Changes of gut flora, intestinal inflammation, and alterations of gastrointestinal motility and sensitivity have been implicated in the pathogenesis of functional gastrointestinal disorders in general and IBS in particular [24, 64]. Probiotics such as lactobacilli and bifidobacteria may modulate the mucosal immune response, as well as gastrointestinal motility and sensitivity, and these effects could support a beneficial effect in patients with functional gastrointestinal disorders [85]. Indeed the administration of some probiotic strains has resulted in significant symptom improvement in adult patients with IBS [86]. However, the two pediatric studies published so far, both using *Lactobacillus rhamnosus GG* at doses of 10^{10} or 3×10^9 tid for 4–6 weeks, failed to show any significant effect in children with functional abdominal pain syndromes, including functional dyspepsia [87, 88]. Therefore, at present, there is no clear evidence of efficacy for any form of dietary manipulation, and dietary interventions cannot be recommended to clinicians or families [82].

CONCLUSIONS

Dyspepsia is a common problem among school children in western countries. Although several organic causes can lead to dyspeptic symptoms (e.g., *H. pylori* infection and food allergy), in most cases, dyspepsia is a functional disorder, most likely related to disturbances of gastric motor activity and increased gastric sensitivity. The rigorous and meticulous application of the Rome criteria can reliably identify functional dyspepsia without the need of specific investigations, which can be expensive and often stressful for the child and the parents. However, if the patient's history and clinical examination highlight alarm signs and symptoms, an organic disorder should be accurately sought for by adequate tests, and therapy should be aimed at the underlying disease. A number of therapeutic options exist for functional dyspepsia – including antisecretory drugs, prokinetic agents, low dose antidepressants, and probiotics. As with other functional disorders, a multidisciplinary biopsychosocial approach is always advisable, and cognitive-behavioral therapy can be very helpful.

References

1. Hyams JS, Davis P, Sylvester FA, Zeiter DK, Justinich CJ, Lerer T. Dyspepsia in children and adolescents: a prospective study. J Pediatr Gastroenterol Nutr. 2000;30:413–8.
2. De Giacomo C, Valdambrini V, Lizzoli F, et al. A population-based survey on gastrointestinal tract symptoms and *Helicobacter pylori* infection in children and adolescents. Helicobacter. 2002;7:356–63.
3. Miele E, Simeone D, Marino A, et al. Functional gastrointestinal disorders in children: an Italian prospective survey. Pediatrics. 2004;114:73–8.
4. Walker LS, Lipani TA, Greene JW, et al. Recurrent abdominal pain: symptom subtypes based on the Rome II criteria for pediatric functional gastrointestinal disorders. J Pediatr Gastroenterol Nutr. 2004;38:187–91.
5. Caplan A, Walker L, Rasquin A. Validation of the pediatric Rome II criteria for functional gastrointestinal disorders using the questionnaire on pediatric gastrointestinal symptoms. J Pediatr Gastroenterol Nutr. 2005;41:305–16.
6. Cucchiara S, Riezzo G, Minella R, Pezzolla F, Giorgio I, Auricchio S. Electrogastrography in non-ulcer dyspepsia. Arch Dis Child. 1992;67:613–7.
7. Chen JD, Lin X, Zhang M, Torres-Pinedo RB, Orr WC. Gastric myoelectrical activity in healthy children and children with functional dyspepsia. Dig Dis Sci. 1998;43:2384–91.
8. Barbar M, Steffen R, Wyllie R, Goske M. Electrogastrography versus gastric emptying scintigraphy in children with symptoms suggestive of gastric motility disorders. J Pediatr Gastroenterol Nutr. 2000;30:193–7.
9. Riezzo G, Chiloiro M, Guerra V, Borrelli O, Salvia G, Cucchiara S. Comparison of gastric electrical activity and gastric emptying in healthy and dyspeptic children. Dig Dis Sci. 2000;45:517–24.
10. Di Lorenzo C, Hyman PE, Flores AF, et al. Antroduodenal manometry in children and adults with severe non-ulcer dyspepsia. Scand J Gastroenterol. 1994;29:799–806.
11. Chitkara DK, Camilleri M, Zinsmeister AR, et al. Gastric sensory and motor dysfunction in adolescents with functional dyspepsia. J Pediatr. 2005;146:500–5.
12. Chitkara DK, Delgado-Aros S, Bredenoord AJ, et al. Functional dyspepsia, upper gastrointestinal symptoms, and transit in children. J Pediatr. 2003;143:609–13.
13. Di Lorenzo C, Youssef NN, Sigurdsson L, Scharff L, Griffiths J, Wald A. Visceral hyperalgesia in children with functional abdominal pain. J Pediatr. 2001;139:838–43.
14. Rasquin A, Di Lorenzo C, Forbes D, et al. Childhood functional gastrointestinal disorders: child/adolescent. Gastroenterology. 2006;130:1527–37.
15. Sigurdsson L, Flores A, Putnam PE, Hyman PE, Di Lorenzo C. Postviral gastroparesis: presentation, treatment, and outcome. J Pediatr. 1997;131:751–4.

16. Saps M, Pensabene L, Di Martino L, et al. Post-infectious functional gastrointestinal disorders in children. J Pediatr. 2008;152:812–6.
17. Saps M, Pensabene L, Turco R, Staiano A, Cupuro D, Di Lorenzo C. Rotavirus gastroenteritis: precursor of functional gastrointestinal disorders? J Pediatr Gastroenterol Nutr. 2009;49:580–3.
18. Hyams JS. Irritable bowel syndrome, functional dyspepsia, and functional abdominal pain syndrome. Adolesc Med Clin. 2004;15:1–15.
19. Di Lorenzo C, Colletti RB, Lehmann HP, et al. Chronic abdominal pain in children: a clinical report of the American Academy of Pediatrics and the North American Society for Pediatric Gastroenterology, Hepatology and Nutrition. J Pediatr Gastroenterol Nutr. 2005;40: 245–61.
20. Gold BD, Colletti RB, Abbott M, et al. *Helicobacter pylori* infection in children: recommendations for diagnosis and treatment. J Pediatr Gastroenterol Nutr. 2000;31:490–7.
21. Drumm B, Koletzko S, Oderda G. *Helicobacter pylori* infection in children: a consensus statement of the European Paediatric Task Force on *Helicobacter pylori*. J Pediatr Gastroenterol Nutr. 2000;30:207–13.
22. Oderda G, Rapa A, Bona G. Diagnostic tests for childhood *Helicobacter pylori* infection: invasive, noninvasive or both? J Pediatr Gastroenterol Nutr. 2004;39:482–4.
23. Berčík P, De Giorgio R, Blennerhassett P, Verdú E, Barbara G, Collins SM. Immune-mediated neural dysfunction in a murine model of chronic *Helicobacter pylori* infection. Gastroenterology. 2002;123:1205–15.
24. Mayer EA, Collins SM. Evolving pathophysiologic models of functional gastrointestinal disorders. Gastroenterology. 2002;122:2032–48.
25. Schäppi M, Borrelli O, Knafelz D, et al. Mast cell-nerve interactions in children with functional dyspepsia. J Pediatr Gastroenterol Nutr. 2008;47:472–80.
26. Walker MM, Talley NJ, Prabhakar M, et al. Duodenal mastocytosis, eosinophilia and intraepithelial lymphocytosis as possible disease markers in the irritable syndrome and functional dyspepsia. Aliment Pharmacol Ther. 2009;29:765–73.
27. Zipser RD, Patel S, Yahya KZ, Baisch D, Monarch E. Presentations of adult celiac disease in a nationwide patient support group. Dig Dis Sci. 2003;48:761–4.
28. Incarbone S, Aprile G, Puzzo L, et al. Bioptic evaluation of duodenal mucosa in adult dyspeptic patients: high prevalence of celiac disease. A prospective study. Gut. 2006;55 Suppl 5:A97.
29. Ford AC, Ching E, Moayyedi P. Meta-analysis: yield of diagnostic tests for celiac disease in dyspepsia. Aliment Pharmacol Ther. 2009;30:28–36.
30. Dieterich W, Laag E, Schopper H, et al. Autoantibodies to tissue transglutaminase as predictor of celiac disease. Gastroenterology. 1998;115:1317–21.
31. Marsh MN. Grains of truth: evolutionary changes in small intestinal mucosa in response to environmental antigen challenge. Gut. 1990;31:111–4.

32. Oberhuber G, Granditsch G, Vogelsang H. The histopathology of coeliac disease: time for a standardized report scheme for pathologists. Eur J Gastroenterol Hepatol. 1999;11:1185–94.

33. Ravelli AM, Tobanelli P, Minelli L, Villanacci V, Cestari R. Endoscopic features of celiac disease in children. Gastrointest Endosc. 2001;54:736–42.

34. Rothenberg ME. Eosinophilic gastrointestinal disorders (EGID). J Allergy Clin Immunol. 2004;113:11–28.

35. Guajardo JR, Rothenberg ME. Eosinophilic esophagitis, gastroenteritis, gastroenterocolitis, and colitis. In: Metcalfe DD, Sampson HA, Simon RA, editors. Food allergy: adverse reactions to foods and additives. 3rd ed. Malden, MA: Blackwell Publishing; 2003. p. 217–26.

36. Kokkonen J. Lymphonodular hyperplasia of the duodenal bulb indicates food allergy in children. Endoscopy. 1999;31:464–8.

37. Muraro A, Dreborg S, Halken S, et al. Dietary prevention of allergic diseases in infants and small children. Part III – evaluation of methods in allergy prevention studies and sensitization markers. Definitions and diagnostic criteria of allergic diseases. Pediatr Allergy Immunol. 2004;15:196–205.

38. Niggemann B, Rolinck-Werninghaus C, Mehl A, Binder C, Ziegert M, Beyer K. Controlled oral food challenges in childen – when indicated, when superfluous? Allergy. 2005;60:865–70.

39. Heyman MB, American Academy of Pediatrics Committee on Nutrition. Lactose intolerance in infants, children, and adolescents. Pediatrics. 2006;118:1279–86.

40. Dubinsky M. Special issues in pediatric inflammatory bowel disease. World J Gastroenterol. 2008;14:413–20.

41. Castellaneta SP, Afzal NA, Greenberg M, et al. Diagnostic role of upper gastrointestinal endoscopy in pediatric inflammatory bowel disease. J Pediatr Gastroenterol Nutr. 2004;39:257–61.

42. Keim V. Role of genetic disorders in acute recurrent pancreatitis. World J Gastroenterol. 2008;14:1011–5.

43. Beharry S, Ellis L, Corey M, Marcon M, Durie P. How useful is fecal pancreatic elastase 1 as a marker of exocrine pancreatic disease? J Pediatr. 2002;141:84–90.

44. Bunn SK, Bisset WM, Main MJC, Gray ES, Olson S, Golden BE. Fecal calprotectin: validation as a noninvasive measure of bowel inflammation in childhood inflammatory bowel disease. J Pediatr Gastroenterol Nutr. 2001;33:14–22.

45. Berni Canani R, DeHoratio Tanturri L, Romano MT, et al. Clinical utility of non invasive diagnostic tools in children with suspected inflammatory bowel disease. J Pediatr Gastroenterol Nutr. 2004; 39:s324.

46. Kalach N, Mention K, Guimber D, Michaud L, Spyckerelle C, Gottrand F. Helicobacter pylori infection is not associated with specific symptoms in nonulcer-dyspeptic children. Pediatrics. 2005;115:17–21.

47. Megraud F. European Paediatric Task Force on *Helicobacter pylori*. Comparison of non-invasive tests to detect *Helicobacter pylori* infection in children and adolescents: results of a multicenter European study. J Pediatr. 2005;146:198–203.

48. Sabbi T, De Angelis P, Colostro F, Dall'Oglio L, Federici di Abriola G, Castro M. Efficacy of noninvasive tests in the diagnosis of *Helicobacter pylori* infection in pediatric patients. Arch Pediatr Adolesc Med. 2005;159:238–41.

49. Fasano A, Catassi C. Current approaches to diagnosis and treatment of celiac disease: an evolving spectrum. Gastroenterology. 2001;120: 636–51.

50. Bürgin-Wolff A, Gaze H, Hadziselimovic F, et al. Antigliadin and antiendomysium antibody determination for coeliac disease. Arch Dis Child. 1991;66:941–7.

51. Howdle PD, Robins GG. Advances in celiac disease. Curr Opin Gastroenterol. 2005;21:152–61.

52. Villalta D, Alessio MG, Tampoia M, et al. Testing for IgG class antibodies in celiac disease patients with selective IgA deficiency. A comparison of the diagnostic accuracy of 9 IgG anti-tissue transglutaminase, 1 IgG anti-gliadin and 1 IgG anti-deaminated gliadin peptide antibody assays. Clin Chim Acta. 2007;382:95–9.

53. Collin P, Mäki M, Keyriläinen O, Hällström O, Reunala T, Pasternack A. Selective IgA deficiency and coeliac disease. Scand J Gastroenterol. 1992;27:367–71.

54. Fredette ME, Lightdale JR. Endoscopic sedation in pediatric practice. Gastrointest Endosc Clin N Am. 2008;18:739–51.

55. Lightdale JR, Valim C, Newburg AR, Mahoney LB, Zgleszewski S, Fox VL. Efficiency of propofol versus midazolam and fentanyl sedation at a pediatric teaching hospital: a prospective study. Gastrointest Endosc. 2008;67:1067–75.

56. Ravelli A, Bolognini S, Gambarotti M, Villanacci V, Consolati V, Ravelli A. Variability of histologic lesions in relation to biopsy site in celiac disease. Am J Gastroenterol. 2005;100:177–85.

57. Ravelli A, Villanacci V, Monfredini C, Martinazzi S, Grassi V, Manenti S. How patchy is patchy villous atrophy: distribution pattern of histological lesions in the duodenum of children with celiac disease. Am J Gastroenterol. 2010;105:2103–10.

58. Hinder RA, Kelly KA. Human gastric pacesetter potential. Site of origin, spread, and response to gastric transection and proximal gastric vagotomy. Am J Surg. 1977;133:29–33.

59. Lin Z, Chen JZ. Comparison of three running spectral analysis methods. In: Chen JZ, McCallum RW, editors. Electrogastrography: principles and applications. New York, NY: Raven Press; 1994. p. 75–99.

60. Ravelli AM. Electrogastrography in childhood. NeUroGastroenterologia. 2001;7:71–9.

61. Cucchiara S, Minella R, Riezzo G, et al. Reversal of gastric electrical dysrhythmias by cisapride in children with functional dyspepsia. Dig Dis Sci. 1992;37:1136–40.

62. Smout AJPM, Akkermans LMA. Methods of measurement of gastric motility and emptying. Motility. 1989;5:4–9.

63. Ravelli AM, Panarotto MB, Consolati V, Verdoni L, Bolognini S. Pulmonary aspiration detected by scintigraphy in gastroesophageal reflux-related respiratory disease. Chest. 2006;130:1520–6.

64. Perez ME, Youssef NN. Dyspepsia in childhood and adolescence: insights and treatment considerations. Curr Gastroenterol Rep. 2007;9:447–55.
65. Youssef NN, Murphy TG, Langseder AL, Rosh JR. Quality of life for children with functional abdominal pain: a comparison study of patients' and parents' perceptions. Pediatrics. 2006;117:54–9.
66. Saps M, Di Lorenzo C. Pharmacotherapy for functional gastrointestinal disorders in children. J Pediatr Gastroenterol Nutr. 2009;48: S101–3.
67. See MC, Birnbaum AH, Schechter CB, Goldenberg MM, Benkov KJ. Double-blind, placebo-controlled trial of famotidine in children with abdominal pain and dyspepsia: global and quantitative assessment. Dig Dis Sci. 2001;46:985–92.
68. Kline RM, Kline JJ, Di Palma J, Barbero GJ. Enteric-coated, pH-dependent peppermint oil capsules for the treatment of irritable bowel syndrome in children. J Pediatr. 2001;138:125–8.
69. Grigoleit HG, Grigoleit P. Peppermint oil in irritable bowel syndrome. Phytomedicine. 2005;12:601–6.
70. Bahar RJ, Collins BS, Steinmetz B, Ament ME. Double-blind placebo-controlled trial of amitriptyline for the treatment of irritable bowel syndrome in adolescents. J Pediatr. 2008;152:685–9.
71. Saps M, Youssef N, Miranda A, et al. Multicentre, randomized, placebo-controlled trial of amitriptyline in children with functional gastrointestinal disorders. Gastroenterology. 2009;137:1261–9.
72. Campo JV, Perel J, Lucas A, et al. Citalopram treatment of pediatric recurrent abdominal pain and comorbid internalizing disorders: an exploratory study. J Am Acad Child Adolesc Psychiatry. 2004;43: 1234–42.
73. Sadeghian M, Farahmand F, Fallahi GH, Abbasi A. Cyproheptadine for the treatment of functional abdominal pain in childhood: a double blinded randomized placebo-controlled trial. Minerva Pediatr. 2008;60:1367–74.
74. Khoshoo V, Armstead C, Landry L. Effect of a laxative with and without tegaserod in adolescents with constipation predominant irritable bowel syndrome. Aliment Pharmacol Ther. 2006;23:191–6.
75. Huertas-Ceballos A, Logan S, Bennett C, Macarthur C. Psychosocial interventions for recurrent abdominal pain (RAP) and irritable bowel syndrome (IBS) in childhood. Cochrane Database Syst Rev. 2008;CD003014.
76. Vlieger AM, Menko-Frankenhuis C, Wolfkamp SC, Tromp E, Benninga MA. Hypnotherapy for children with functional abdominal pain or irritable bowel syndrome: a randomized controlled trial. Gastroenterology. 2007;133:1430–6.
77. Ball TM, Shapiro DE, Monheim CJ, Weydert JA. A pilot study of the use of guided imagery for the treatment of recurrent abdominal pain in children. Clin Pediatr (Phila). 2003;42:527–32.
78. Youssef NN, Rosh JR, Loughran M, et al. Treatment of functional abdominal pain in childhood with cognitive behavioral strategies. J Pediatr Gastroenterol Nutr. 2004;39:192–6.
79. Weydert JA, Shapiro DE, Acra SA, Monheim CJ, Chambers AS, Ball TM. Evaluation of guided imagery as treatment for recurrent abdominal pain in children: a randomized controlled trial. BMC Pediatr. 2006;6:29.

80. Christensen MF. Do bulk preparations help in cases of recurrent abdominal pain in children? A controlled study [Hjaelper fyld praeparater pa recidiverende mavesmerter hos born? En kontrolleret study]. Ugeskr Laeger. 1982;144:714–5.

81. Feldman W, McGrath P, Hodgson C, Ritter H, Shipman R. The use of dietary fibre in the management of simple childhood idiopathic recurrent abdominal pain. Results in a prospective, double-blind, randomized, controlled trial. Am J Dis Child. 1985;139:1216–8.

82. Huertas-Ceballos AA, Logan S, Bennett C, Macarthur C. Dietary interventions for recurrent abdominal pain (RAP) and irritable bowel syndrome (IBS) in childhood. Cochrane Database Syst Rev. 2009;CD003019.

83. Lebenthal E, Rossi TM, Nord KS, Branski D. Recurrent abdominal pain and lactose absorption in children. Pediatrics. 1981;67:828–32.

84. Dearlove J, Dearlove B, Pearl K, Parmavesi R. Dietary lactose and the child with abdominal pain. Br Med J. 1983;286:1936.

85. Picard C, Fioramonti J, Francois A, Robinson T, Neant F, Matuchansky C. Bifidobacteria as probiotic agents – physiological effects and clinical benefits. Aliment Pharmacol Ther. 2005;33:495–512.

86. Brenner DM, Moeller MJ, Chey WD, Schoenfeld PS. The utility of probiotics in the treatment of irritable bowel syndrome: a systematic review. Am J Gastroenterol. 2009;104:1033–49.

87. Bausserman M, Michail S. The use of Lactobacillus GG in irritable bowel syndrome in children: a double-blind randomized control trial. J Pediatr. 2005;147:197–201.

88. Gawrońska A, Dziechciarz P, Horvath A, Szajewska H. A randomized double-blind placebo-controlled trial of Lactobacillus GG for abdominal pain disorders in children. Aliment Pharmacol Ther. 2007;25:177–84.

Chapter 17
Dyspepsia in the Elderly

Bojan Tepeš

Keywords: Dyspepsia, Elderly, Organic dyspepsia, Functional dyspepsia, Subgroups, Diagnostic tests, Treatment

INTRODUCTION

Dyspepsia is a chronic disease characterized by one or more of the following symptoms: postprandial fullness, early satiation (meaning inability to finish a normal size meal or postprandial fullness), and epigastric pain or burning [1]. One quarter of affected patients consult their general practitioner [2]. The factors that determine whether a patient consults a physician may include symptom severity, older age, lower social class, fear of serious disease, psychological comorbidity, and insurance status [3–6]. Epidemiologic data on dyspepsia in the elderly vary among studies. Williams et al. reported that the proportion of patients with dyspepsia was 38% in those aged under 25 years compared to 20% in those over 60 years [7]. On the contrary, Heikkinen et al. found that the proportion of patients with dyspepsia rose slightly with age: 31, 33, and 37% for age groups 15–44, 45–64, and >64 years, respectively [8].

The pathophysiology of dyspepsia in the elderly is almost the same as in other age groups, but some differences exist. In the elderly, malignant diseases and the use of concomitant medication are more prevalent [9]. Apart from that, aging per se can have some influence on organic function. However, because of the large functional reserve of the gastrointestinal tract, aging per se has a

B. Tepeš (✉)
ABAKUS MEDICO d.o.o., Diagnostični center Rogaška,
Rogaška Slatina, Slovenia
e-mail: bojan.tepes@siol.net

239

M. Duvnjak (ed.), *Dyspepsia in Clinical Practice*,
DOI 10.1007/978-1-4419-1730-0_17,
© Springer Science+Business Media, LLC 2011

less direct effect on most gastrointestinal functions. In functional gastrointestinal disorders, irritable bowel symptoms decrease with aging, but dysphagia, anorexia, dyspepsia, and disorders of colonic function become more prevalent [10].

In the absence of chronic atrophic gastritis, gastric secretion is well preserved in the elderly. Because of motor changes in gastric function, a delay in gastric emptying of liquids and solids can be seen in the elderly [11]. In addition, significant adverse motor effects on the gastrointestinal tract are produced by coexisting diabetes mellitus, Parkinson's disease, systemic sclerosis, hypothyroidism, and some other conditions. Concomitant use of medicines such as acetylsalicylic acid, nonsteroidal anti-inflammatory agents, calcium channel blockers, methylxanthines, alendronate, orlistat, potassium supplements, acarbose, and certain antibiotics, including erythromycin and metronidazole, can cause dyspepsia [12]. Symptoms of dyspepsia are in the elderly more frequently associated with lower gastrointestinal symptoms and signs, such as constipation and diverticular disease than in younger age groups. The proportion of individuals with frequent abdominal pain increases with age from 24% at 65 years to 30% at 80 years [13].

DIAGNOSTIC TESTS IN DYSPEPSIA IN THE ELDERLY
When a patient presents with dyspeptic symptoms, a careful clinical evaluation and history are essential features to make a correct diagnosis of dyspepsia and to distinguish it from gastroesophageal reflux disease (GERD), irritable bowel syndrome (IBS), or other serious diseases of the upper gastrointestinal tract. If no alarm symptoms are present (see Table 6.1) and patients' age is under the age threshold of country (depending on geographical region between 45 and 55 years), no diagnostic investigation is performed [1]. In the elderly patient with recent onset of dyspepsia with or without alarm symptoms, upper gastrointestinal endoscopy should be performed.

UPPER GASTROINTESTINAL ENDOSCOPY
A review of pooled data from 3,667 patients undergoing endoscopy for dyspepsia showed that 33.6% had normal findings, 23% gastroesophageal reflux, 20% gastritis, 19% ulcers, and 2% cancers [14]. In a more recent study from Canada, 1,040 dyspeptic patients from 49 primary care practices underwent esophagogastroduodenoscopy (EGD). Clinically significant findings were reported in 58% of the population. Esophagitis was found in 43% of the patients (LA A 51%, LA B 37.5%, LA C 10%, and LA D 3%), peptic ulcer disease

(PUD) in 5% of the patients, and nobody had malignant disease. The study did not find differences between the younger group of patients and those over 50 years of age. The study overrepresents the number of patients with esophagitis because the definition of dyspepsia in the Canadian study allowed the inclusion of patients with typical reflux symptoms under the banner of dyspepsia [15].

One third of patients referred for open-access endoscopy due to dyspepsia had high levels of health-related anxiety, preoccupation with illness, and fear of death. Following a normal EGD or demonstration of minor abnormalities, and reassurance by the endoscopist, scales for preoccupation with health and fear of illness and death showed significant improvement and the effects were preserved for 6 months [16]. Another potential benefit is that *Helicobacter pylori* (*H. pylori*) infection can be diagnosed during EGD with rapid urea test, which has a sensitivity of 95% and a specificity of 95%. Two biopsies should be taken, from antrum and corpus of the stomach [17, 18].

OTHER DIAGNOSTIC TESTS

Routine blood counts and biochemistry are usually included in the diagnostic workup, but the clinical value of this has never been formally validated.

Ultrasonography (US) of the gallbladder in dyspepsia has a yield of 1% to 3%, but the finding of gallstones is most often incidental [19, 20]. In contrast with younger patients, abdominal US should be performed as a routine investigation in the elderly because of the increased incidence of malignancy. In case of persistent symptoms, recent history of dyspepsia, especially in association with body weight loss and negative US, computed tomography scanning should be done to detect small pancreatic lesions.

Consistent postprandial symptoms in patients with extensive atheromatous vascular disease should raise the suspicion of mesenteric ischemia. Magnetic angiography or selective angiography with stenting or balloon angioplasty should be done in these circumstances.

DIFFERENTIAL DIAGNOSIS OF DYSPEPSIA
AND TREATMENT

Elderly patients with uninvestigated dyspepsia should undergo diagnostic investigations (Fig. 17.1). The patient has organic dyspepsia when structural or metabolic diseases are found. Most frequent organic causes are listed in Table 2.1. Patients with symptoms of

Uninvestigated dyspepsia in the elderly

(Diagnostic tests: upper gastrointestinal endoscopy, ultrasound, laboratory tests, X-ray tests)

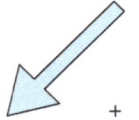 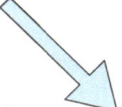

+   −

Organic dyspepsia

Functional dyspepsia

- Postprandial distress syndrome (PDS)
- Epigastric pain syndrome (EPS)

FIG. 17.1 Dyspepsia in the elderly.

dyspepsia without a systemic or metabolic disease have functional dyspepsia (FD). The Rome III Classification System subdivides patients with FD to patients with meal-induced dyspeptic symptoms – postprandial distress syndrome (PDS) – and patients with epigastric pain syndrome (EPS), which is meal-unrelated [1].

ORGANIC DYSPEPSIA IN THE ELDERLY

GERD is the most frequent organic cause of dyspepsia. When GERD is present in the elderly patients, it tends to be more severe with increased frequency of erosive esophagitis and complications [21, 22]. Several physiological and environmental factors may contribute to the higher incidence of complications in elderly patients. These include reduced salivary bicarbonate secretion, sedentary lifestyle, delayed gastric emptying in diabetic patients, and increased use of medication predisposing to GERD. Xerostomia occurs in 16% of elderly men and in 25% of elderly women [23]. The prevalence of hiatal hernia increases with age, reaching a prevalence of 60% in patients 60 years or older [24]. The severity of symptoms in the elderly is significantly lower than in young GERD patients and may contribute to delayed recognition of the disease and increased prevalence of complications in elderly GERD patients [25]. The diagnostic approach and treatment of GERD are the same in elderly and young patients. No dosing adjustments are needed for proton pump inhibitors (PPIs) due to age-related reductions in hepatic or renal function [26].

The second most common cause of organic dyspepsia is PUD. The main etiologic cause is infection with *H. pylori*. *H. pylori* infection is the most common chronic bacterial infection in humans (50% of the world population is infected). The infection causes active chronic gastritis in all infected patients. Clinically, important diseases (gastric and duodenal ulcers, MALT lymphoma, and gastric cancer) are the end result of infection in only 20% of infected carriers [27, 28]. In developing countries, the prevalence rate of infection is over 80% in the 10-year-old age group, while in the developed world it is only 10%. However, in the elderly, the prevalence of the infection is over 50% in developed countries as well [29, 30].

The lifetime prevalence of PUD is also higher in *H. pylori*-positive subjects (approximately 10% to 20% compared to 5% to 10% in the general population) [31].

All patients with *H. pylori* infection found at endoscopy should be treated with triple therapy. The recommended duration of therapy is 1 week in Europe and 10–14 days in the USA. The eradication success should be controlled 1 month after therapy with noninvasive tests (urea breath test or stool antigen test) (see Chap. 9) [32, 33].

The second most common cause of PUD is the use of nonsteroidal anti-inflammatory drugs (NSAID) and salicylates. These drugs cause symptoms of dyspepsia in 15% to 40% of the patients: 10% of the patients quit their medication because of this side effect [34]. There is little correlation between the dyspeptic symptoms sometimes seen with these drugs and the presence or absence of erosive/ulcerative lesions in the stomach and duodenum. Ulcer complications induced by an NSAID can appear with no preceding dyspeptic "warning" symptoms, and dyspeptic symptoms can be present in patients without mucosal damage [35–37]. According to ACCF/ACG/AHA 2008 Expert Consensus Document, all elderly people (>60 years) should be treated with PPIs whenever on NSAIDs or salicylates [38].

FUNCTIONAL DYSPEPSIA IN THE ELDERLY

According to Rome III criteria, FD is defined as the presence of symptoms thought to originate in the gastroduodenal region (early satiety, postprandial fullness, epigastric pain, and epigastric burning) in the absence of organic, systemic, or metabolic disease that is likely to explain the symptoms [1]. Several pathophysiological mechanisms have been suggested to underlie dyspeptic symptoms. These include delayed gastric emptying, impaired gastric accommodation to meals, hypersensitivity to gastric distension, altered duodenal sensitivity to lipids or acid, abnormal intestinal motility, and central nervous system dysfunction. The cause of FD symptoms has not been established. We have evidence of contributions of genetic susceptibility, infectious factors, and psychological factors.

Abnormal accommodation of the gastric fundus and antrum to food is present in up to 40% of dyspeptic patients [39–43]. Studies in patients with postinfectious dyspepsia suggest that impaired accommodation is attributable to impaired function of nitrergic nerves in the stomach [44].

In a meta-analysis of 17 studies, significant delay of solid gastric emptying was present in almost 40% of patients with FD [45].

In one third of FD patients, visceral hypersensitivity is present. Patients may have a lower pain threshold or increased sensitivity even to normal intestinal function (allodynia) or increased sensitivity via central sensitization [46–48].

In some studies, increased sensitivity to duodenal infusion of lipids and increased duodenal acid exposure were found in patients with FD, but the patient numbers in those studies were small [49, 50].

The most common psychiatric comorbidities in FD patients are anxiety disorders, depressive disorders, and somatoform disorders. In clinical studies, 87% of patients with FD had psychiatric diagnoses, compared with 25% of patients with organic dyspepsia [51–53]. A recent or remote history of abuse is a nonspecific risk factor for symptoms of FD [53].

ASSOCIATION BETWEEN SYMPTOMS AND PATHOPHYSIOLOGY IN DYSPEPSIA

Available evidence suggests that the symptom profile is not specific for a particular physiological disturbance. Early fullness, nausea, bloating, and upper abdominal discomfort may be associated with delayed gastric emptying, accelerated gastric emptying, or gastric dysaccommodation [41, 54–56]. Gastric dysaccommodation may be associated with accelerated emptying of liquids or delayed emptying of solids and may reflect impaired vagal function in dyspeptic patients [57–59]. Meal-evoked symptoms are present in 60% of patients with FD [60, 61]. The ability to address the mechanisms causing dyspeptic symptoms is hindered by the limited repertoire of symptoms and by the relatively large number of underlying physiological and psychological disturbances in FD.

TREATMENT OF FUNCTIONAL DYSPEPSIA IN THE ELDERLY

Upper gastrointestinal endoscopy is the investigation that should be done in all elderly patients with dyspepsia with or without alarm symptoms (Fig. 17.2). Reassurance and education after normal upper gastrointestinal endoscopy are the first step in management.

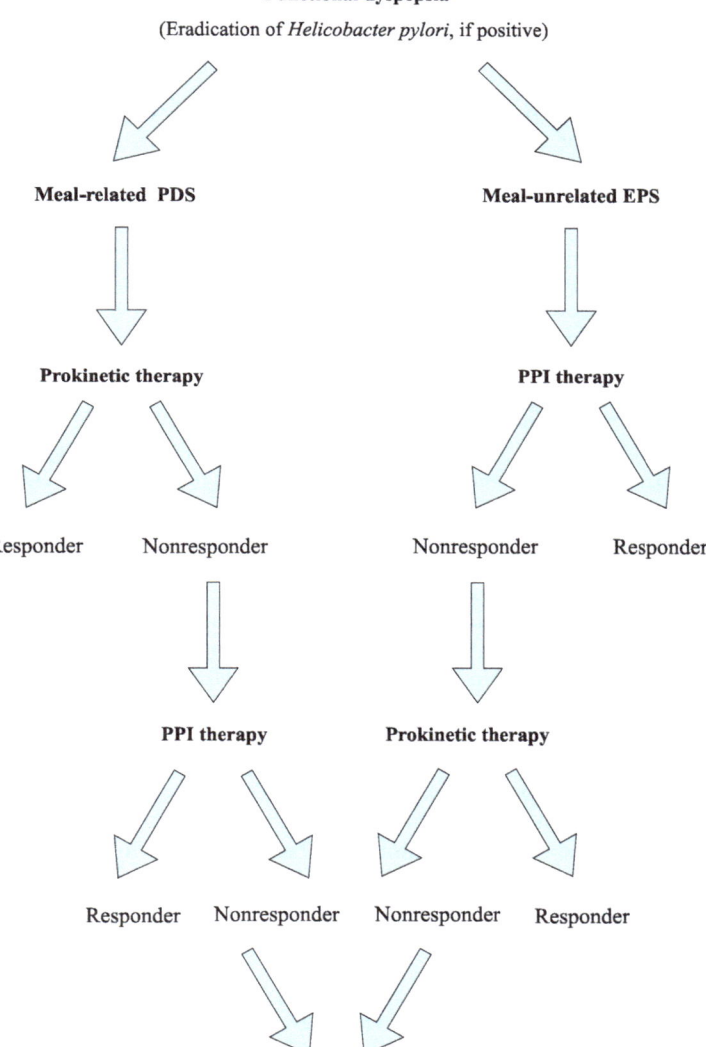

Fɪɢ. 17.2   Treatment algorithm for the management of functional dyspepsia in the elderly.

H. pylori Treatment

During endoscopy, two biopsies (from antrum and corpus) should be taken for rapid urease test. Each *H. pylori*-positive patient should be treated with antimicrobial treatment and treatment success should be confirmed with a noninvasive diagnostic test (urea breath test and stool antibody test) 1 month after therapy [32, 33]. The prevalence of *H. pylori* in FD patients appears to be higher than in healthy asymptomatic controls, but the role of testing and treating the infection with eradication therapy is a subject of debate [62].

Two systemic meta-analyses were performed in an attempt to clarify these uncertainties. Moayyedi et al. found a small but statistically significant benefit of eradication of *H. pylori* in patients with FD. The number needed to treat (NNT) to cure one patient's symptoms was 15 [63]. The second review reported a trend toward a reduction in symptoms in those patients assigned to eradication therapy, but without statistical significance [64]. The last Cochrane systematic review showed that *H. pylori* eradication therapy has a statistically significant effect in reducing symptoms in FD [65]. *H. pylori* eradication also has other potential beneficial effects in patients with PUD and in cancer prevention [32, 66, 67].

Acid Suppressive Treatment

Large prospective studies have shown that treatment with PPIs was approximately 10% to 15% better than placebo in patients with FD [68]. A Cochrane Collaboration systematic review examined the role of PPIs in the management of FD. Ten randomized controlled trials of PPIs in FD showed that this therapy is superior to placebo. The NNT was ten [69]. PPI treatment is more effective in subgroups of patients with reflux-type symptoms and epigastric pain-type symptoms [70].

Treatment with a PPI should be recommended in FD patients with PDS and in patients with EPS after failure of prokinetic therapy.

Prokinetic Agents

Metoclopramide, domperidone, cisapride, and tegaserod are effective in patients with FD who have delayed gastric emptying. Metoclopramide can cross the blood–brain barrier; the use of cisapride is restricted because of cardiac safety issues; and the effects of tegaserod in dyspepsia remain unclear [71]. A meta-analysis suggests that prokinetics may be superior to placebo in the so-called dysmotility-like dyspepsia, but publication bias may also account at least in part for some of the meta-analysis data in the literature [69, 72].

Antidepressants and Behavioral Approaches
Tricyclic antidepressants affect gastric sensitivity, but large control trials have not been conducted [73]. Antidepressants can be useful in patients with functional abdominal pain syndromes, including EPS. Control trials of antidepressants and behavioral therapy have shown benefit in FD patients. To be able to answer the question which are the specific subgroups that benefit and about cost-effectiveness requires further studies [74, 75]. Hypnotherapy is effective in specialized centers [76].

FUTURE PERSPECTIVES
New drugs that affect gastric dysaccommodation and gastric hypersensitivity are awaited. Tailored therapy in specialized tertiary centers that can first determine which dysmotility type (gastric fundic accommodation impairment and delayed or rapid gastric emptying) is present in individual patients and then direct therapy according to the underlying pathophysiological cause are the future of the treatment in FD patients.

CONCLUSIONS
Dyspepsia is a common gastrointestinal disease that affects 20% to 40% of adult population in the Western world. One quarter of affected patients consult their general practitioner. The pathophysiology of dyspepsia in the elderly is almost the same as in other age groups, but some differences exist. In the elderly, malignant diseases and the use of concomitant medication are more prevalent. Elderly patients with uninvestigated dyspepsia should undergo diagnostic investigations (upper gastrointestinal endoscopy, laboratory tests, and ultrasonography). *H. pylori* infection should be treated if present; PPIs are recommended in all elderly patients whenever on NSAIDs or salicylates and in case of patients with meal-unrelated EPS. Prokinetics are the drug of first choice in dyspeptic patients with meal-related PDS. In case of therapeutic failure, we can try with prokinetics in meal-unrelated EPS and with PPI in meal-related PDS form of dyspepsia. Antidepressants and behavioral approaches are the ultimate choice in nonresponders. Tailored therapy in specialized centers that can first determine which dysmotility type is present in individual elderly patients and then direct therapy according to the underlying pathophysiological cause are the future of the treatment in FD.

References

1. Tack J, Talley NJ, Camilleri M, et al. Functional gastroduodenal disorders. Gastroenterology. 2006;130:1466–79.
2. Talley NJ, Weaver AL, Zinsmeister AR, Melton III LJ. Onset and disappearance of gastrointestinal symptoms and functional gastrointestinal disorders. Am J Epidemiol. 1992;136:165–77.
3. Talley NJ, Silverstein MD, Agréus L, Nyrén O, Sonnenberg A, Holtmann G. AGA technical review: evaluation of dyspepsia. American Gastroenterological Association. Gastroenterology. 1998;114:582–95.
4. Talley NJ, Boyce P, Jones M. Dyspepsia and health care seeking in a community: how important are psychological factors? Dig Dis Sci. 1998;43:1016–22.
5. Koloski NA, Talley NJ, Boyce PM. Predictors of health care seeking for irritable bowel syndrome and nonulcer dyspepsia: a critical review of the literature on symptom and psychosocial factors. Am J Gastroenterol. 2001;96:1340–9.
6. Koloski NA, Talley NJ, Huskic SS, Boyce PM. Predictors of conventional and alternative health care seeking for irritable bowel syndrome and functional dyspepsia. Aliment Pharmacol Ther. 2003;17:841–51.
7. Williams B, Luckas M, Ellingham JH, Dain A, Wicks AC. Do young patients with dyspepsia need investigation? Lancet. 1988;2:1349–51.
8. Heikkinen M, Pikkarainen P, Takala J, Rasanen H, Julkunen R. Etiology of dyspepsia: four hundred unselected consecutive patients in general practice. Scand J Gastroenterol. 1995;30:519–23.
9. Talley NJ, Evans JM, Fleming KC, Harmsen WS, Zinsmeister AR, Melton III LJ. Nonsteroidal antiinflammatory drugs and dyspepsia in elderly. Dig Dis Sci. 1995;40:1345–50.
10. Firth M, Prather CM. Gastrointestinal motility problems in the elderly patient. Gastroenterology. 2002;122:1688–700.
11. Clarkston WK, Pantano MM, Morley JE, Horowitz M, Littlefield JM, Burton FR. Evidence for the anorexia of aging: gastrointestinal transit and hunger in healthy elderly vs. young adults. Am J Physiol. 1997;272:R243–8.
12. Hallas J, Bytzer P. Screening for drug related dyspepsia: an analysis of prescription symmetry. Eur J Gastroenterol Hepatol. 1998;10:27–32.
13. Talley NJ, Zinsmeister AR, Schleck CD, Melton III LJ. Dyspepsia and dyspepsia subgroups: a population-based study. Gastroenterology. 1992;102:1259–68.
14. Richter JE. Dyspepsia: organic causes and differential characteristics from functional dyspepsia. Scand J Gastroenterol Suppl. 1991;182:11–6.
15. Thompson ABR, Barkun AN, Armstrong D, et al. The prevalence of clinically significant endoscopic findings in primary care patients with uninvestigated dyspepsia: the Canadian Adult Dyspepsia Empiric Treatment-Promt Endoscopy (CADET-PE) study. Aliment Pharmacol Ther. 2003;17:1481–91.
16. Quadri A, Vakil N. Health-related anxiety and the effect of open-access endoscopy in US patients with dyspepsia. Aliment Pharmacol Ther. 2003;17:835–40.

17. Graham DY, Opekun AR, Hammoud F, et al. Studies regarding the mechanism of false negative urea breath tests with proton pump inhibitors. Am J Gastroenterol. 2003;98:1005–9.
18. Tepeš B. Comparison of two invasive diagnostic tests for *Helicobacter pylori* after antimicrobial therapy. Scand J Gastroenterol. 2007;42:330–2.
19. Kraag N, Thijs C, Knipschild P. Dyspepsia: how noisy are gallstones? A meta-analysis of epidemiologic studies of biliary pain, dyspeptic symptoms, and food intolerance. Scand J Gastroenterol. 1995;30:411–21.
20. Berger MY, van der Velden JJ, Lijmer JG, de Kort H, Prins A, Behnen AM. Abdominal symptoms: do they predict gallstones? A systemic review. Scand J Gastroenterol. 2000;35:70–6.
21. Collen MJ, Abdulian JD, Chen YK. Gastroesophageal reflux disease in the elderly: more severe disease that requires aggressive therapy. Am J Gastroenterol. 1995;90:1053–7.
22. Waring J, Hunter J, Davis L, Kim S. GERD symptoms, medication use and endoscopic findings in elderly patients with strictures. Am J Gastroenterol. 1997;92:1606.
23. Osterberg T, Landahl S, Hedegard B. Salivary flow, saliva, pH and buffering capacity in 70-year-old men and women. Correlation to dental health, dryness in the mouth, disease and drug treatment. J Oral Rehabil. 1984;11:157–70.
24. Stilson WL, Sanders I, Gardiner GA, Gorman HC, Lodge DF. Hiatal hernia and gastroesophageal reflux. A clinicoradiological analysis of more than 1000 cases. Radiology. 1996;93:1323–7.
25. Triadafilopolous G, Sharma R. Features of symptomatic gastroesophageal reflux disease in elderly patients. Am J Gastroenterol. 1997;92:2007–11.
26. Kahrilas PJ, Shaheen NJ, American Gastroenterological Association Institute, Clinical Practice and Quality Management Committee. American Gastroenterological Association Institute technical review on the management of gastroesophageal reflux disease. Gastroenterology. 2008;135:1392–413.
27. Bardhan PK. Epidemiological features of *Helicobacter pylori* infection in developing countries. Clin Infect Dis. 1997;25:973–8.
28. Gubina M, Tepeš B, Vidmar G, et al. *Helicobacter pylori* prevalence in Slovenia in 2005. Zdrav Vestn. 2006;75:169–73.
29. Pounder RE, Ng D. The prevalence of *Helicobacter pylori* infection in different countries. Aliment Pharmacol Ther. 1995;9 Suppl 2:33–9.
30. Everhart JE, Kruszon-Moran D, Perez-Perez GI, Tralka TS, McQuillan G. Seroprevalence and ethnic differences in *Helicobacter pylori* infection among adults in the United States. J Infect Dis. 2000;181:1359–63.
31. Kuipers EJ, Thijs JC, Festen HP. The prevalence of *Helicobacter pylori* in peptic ulcer disease. Aliment Pharmacol Ther. 1995;9 Suppl 2:59–69.
32. Malfertheiner P, Megraud F, O'Morain C, et al. Current concepts in the management of *Helicobacter pylori* infection: the Maastricht III Consensus Report. Gut. 2007;56:772–81.
33. Chey WD, Wong BC, Practice Parameters Committee of the American College of Gastroenterology. American College of Gastroenterology

guideline on the management of *Helicobacter pylori* infection. Am J Gastroenterol. 2007;102:1808–25.

34. Tseng CC, Wolfe MM. Nonsteroidal anti-inflammatory drugs. Med Clin North Am. 2000;84:1329–44.

35. Cryer B, Goldschmiedt M, Redfern JS, Feldman M. Comparison of salsalate and aspirin on mucosal injury and gastroduodenal mucosal prostaglandins. Gastroenterology. 1990;99:1616–21.

36. Lanza FL, Codispoti JR, Nelson EB. An endoscopic comparison of gastroduodenal injury with over-the-counter doses of ketoprofen and acetaminophen. Am J Gastroenterol. 1998;93:1051–4.

37. Cryer B, Feldman M. Cyclooxygenase-1 and cyclooxygenase-2 selectivity of widely used nonsteroidal anti-inflammatory drugs. Am J Med. 1998;104:413–21.

38. Bhatt DL, Scheiman J, Abraham NS, American College of Cardiology Foundation, American College of Gastroenterology, American Heart Association, et al. ACCF/ACG/AHA 2008 expert consensus document on reducing the gastrointestinal risks of antiplatelet therapy and NSAID use. Am J Gastroenterol. 2008;103:2890–907.

39. Kindt S, Tack J. Impaired gastric accommodation and its role in dyspepsia. Gut. 2006;55:1685–91.

40. Troncon LE, Bennett RJ, Ahluwalia NK, Thompson DG. Abnormal intragastric distribution of food during gastric emptying in functional dyspepsia patients. Gut. 1994;35:327–32.

41. Tack J, Piessevaux H, Coulie B, Caenepeel P, Janssens J. Role of impaired gastric accommodation to meal in functional dyspepsia. Gastroenterology. 1998;115:1346–52.

42. Boeckxstaens GE, Hirsch DP, Kuiken SD, Heisterkamp SH, Tytgat GN. The proximal stomach and postprandial symptoms in functional dyspeptics. Am J Gastroenterol. 2002;97:40–8.

43. Bredenoord AJ, Chial HJ, Camilleri M, Mullan BP, Murray JA. Gastric accommodation and emptying in evaluation of patients with upper gastrointestinal symptoms. Clin Gastroenterol Hepatol. 2003;1:264–72.

44. Tack J, Demedts I, Dehondt G, et al. Clinical and pathophysiological characteristics of acute-onset functional dyspepsia. Gastroenterology. 2002;122:1738–47.

45. Perri F, Clemente R, Festa V, et al. Patterns of symptoms in functional dyspepsia: role of *Helicobacter pylori* infection and delayed gastric emptying. Am J Gastroenterol. 1998;93:2082–8.

46. Tack J, Caenepeel P, Fischler B, Piessevaux H, Janssens J. Symptoms associated with hypersensitivity to gastric distension in functional dyspepsia. Gastroenterology. 2001;121:526–35.

47. Vandenberghe J, Vos R, Persoons P, Demyttenaere K, Janssens J, Tack L. Dyspeptic patients with visceral hypersensitivity: sensitisation of pain specific or multimodal pathways? Gut. 2005;54:914–9.

48. Mayer EA, Collins SM. Evolving pathophysiologic models of functional gastrointestinal disorders. Gastroenterology. 2002;122:2032–48.

49. Demarchi B, Vos R, Deprez P, Janssens J, Tack J. Influence of a lipase inhibitor on gastric sensitivity and accommodation to an orally ingested meal. Aliment Pharmacol Ther. 2004;19:1261–8.

50. Lee KJ, Demarchi B, Demedts I, Sifrim D, Raeymaekers P, Tack J. A pilot study on duodenal acid exposure and its relationship to symptoms in functional dyspepsia with prominent nausea. Am J Gastroenterol. 2004;99:1765–73.

51. Locke III GR, Weaver AL, Melton III LJ, Talley NJ. Psychosocial factors are linked to functional gastrointestinal disorders: a population based nested case–control study. Am J Gastroenterol. 2004;99:350–7.

52. Magni G, di Mario F, Bernasconi G, Mastropaolo G. DSM-III diagnoses associated with dyspepsia of unknown cause. Am J Psychiatry. 1987;144:1222–3.

53. Haug TT, Svebak S, Wilhelmsen I, Berstad A, Ursin H. Psychological factors and somatic symptoms in functional dyspepsia. A comparison with duodenal ulcer and healthy controls. J Psychosom Res. 1994;38:281–91.

54. Sarnelli G, Caenepeel P, Geypens B, Janssens J, Tack J. Symptoms associated with impaired gastric emptying of solids and liquids in functional dyspepsia. Am J Gastroenterol. 2003;98:783–8.

55. Stanghellini V, Tosetti C, Paternico A, et al. Risk indicators of delayed gastric emptying of solids in patients with functional dyspepsia. Gastroenterology. 1996;110:1036–42.

56. Delqado-Aros S, Camilleri M, Cremonini F, Ferber I, Stephens D, Burton DD. Contributions of gastric volumes and gastric emptying to meal size and postmeal symptoms in functional dyspepsia. Gastroenterology. 2004;127:1685–94.

57. Greydanus MP, Vassallo M, Camilleri M, Nelson DK, Hanson RB, Thomforde GM. Neurohormonal factors in functional dyspepsia: insights on pathophysiological mechanisms. Gastroenterology. 1991;100:1311–8.

58. Hjelland IE, Hausken T, Svebak S, Olafsson S, Berstad A. Vagal tone and meal-induced abdominal symptoms in healthy subjects. Digestion. 2002;65:172–6.

59. Holtmann G, Goebell H, Jockenhoevel F, Talley NJ. Altered vagal and intestinal mechanosensory function in chronic unexplained dyspepsia. Gut. 1998;42:501–6.

60. Camilleri M, Dubois D, Coulie B, et al. Prevalence and socioeconomic impact of upper gastrointestinal disorders in the United States: results of the US Upper Gastrointestinal Study. Clin Gastroenterol Hepatol. 2005;3:543–52.

61. Castillo EJ, Camilleri M, Locke GR, et al. A community-based, controlled study of the epidemiology and pathophysiology of dyspepsia. Clin Gastroenterol Hepatol. 2004;2:985–96.

62. Rauws EA, Langenberg W, Houthoff HJ, Zanen HC, Tytgat GN. Campylobacter pyloridis-associated chronic active antral gastritis. A prospective study of its prevalence and the effects of antibacterial and antiulcer treatment. Gastroenterology. 1988;94:33–40.

63. Moayyedi P, Soo S, Deeks JJ, et al. Systemic review and economic evaluation of *Helicobacter pylori* treatment for non-ulcer dyspepsia. BMJ. 2000;321:659–64.

64. Laine L, Schoenfeld P, Fennerty MB. Therapy for *Helicobacter pylori* in patients with nonulcer dyspepsia. A meta-analysis of randomized, control trials. Ann Intern Med. 2001;134:361–9.

65. Moayyedi P, Soo S, Deeks J, et al. Eradication of *Helicobacter pylori* for non-ulcer dyspepsia. Cochrane Database Syst Rev. 2006;2:CD002096.
66. Fukase K, Kato M, Kikuchi S, Japan Gast Study Group, et al. Effect of eradication of Helicobacter pylori on incidence of metachronous gastric carcinoma after endoscopic resection of early gastric cancer: an open-label, randomised controlled trial. Lancet. 2008;372:392–7.
67. Tepeš B. Can gastric cancer be prevented? J Physiol Pharmacol. 2009;60:71–7.
68. Talley NJ, Meineche-Schmidt V, Pare P, et al. Efficacy of omeprazole in functional dyspepsia: double-blind, randomized, placebo-controlled trials (the Bond and Opera studies). Aliment Pharmacol Ther. 1998;12:1055–65.
69. Moayyedi P, Soo S, Deeks J, Delaney B, Innes M, Forman D. Pharmacological intervention for non-ulcer dyspepsia. Cochrane Database Syst Rev. 2006;4:CD001960.
70. Moayyedi P, Delaney BC, Vakil N, Forman D, Talley NJ. The efficacy of proton pump inhibitors in nonulcer dyspepsia: a systematic review and economic analysis. Gastroenterology. 2004;127:1329–37.
71. Degen L, Matzinger D, Mertz M, et al. Tegaserod, a 5-HT4 receptor partial agonist, accelerates gastric emptying and gastrointestinal transit in healthy male subjects. Aliment Pharmacol Ther. 2001;15:1745–51.
72. Hiyama T, Yoshihara M, Matsuo K, et al. Meta-analysis of the effects of prokinetic agents in patients with functional dyspepsia. J Gastroenterol Hepatol. 2007;22:304–10.
73. Mertz H, Fass R, Kodner A, Yan-Go F, Fullerton S, Mayer EA. Effect of amitriptyline on symptoms, sleep, and visceral perception in patients with functional dyspepsia. Am J Gastroenterol. 1998;93:160–5.
74. Hamilton J, Guthrie E, Creed F, et al. A randomized controlled trial of psychotherapy in patients with chronic functional dyspepsia. Gastroenterology. 2000;119:661–9.
75. Creed F, Fernandes L, Guthrie E, et al. The cost-effectiveness of psychotherapy and paroxetine for severe irritable bowel syndrome. Gastroenterology. 2003;124:303–17.
76. Calvert EL, Houghton LA, Cooper P, Morris J, Whorwell PJ. Long-term improvement in functional dyspepsia using hypnotherapy. Gastroenterology. 2002;123:1778–85.

Chapter 18
Diabetes Mellitus and Dyspepsia

Lea Smirčić-Duvnjak

Keywords: Dyspepsia, Diabetes mellitus, Glycemic control, Autonomic neuropathy

INTRODUCTION

The term dyspepsia has been widely used by health care professionals to describe different upper gastrointestinal symptoms related to organic disease or presumed to be functional if such causal pathology could not be identified [1]. The lack of clarity in terminology creates a lot of problems in everyday clinical practice as a large proportion of the population complains of symptoms that might be related to dyspepsia. As the prevalence of diabetes mellitus is estimated to be around 246 million people worldwide and is rapidly rising, diabetic patients represent a significant percentage of the affected population [2].

DEFINITION

Diabetes is a severe and life-threatening disease, associated with macrovascular and specific microvascular complications. It carries an increased cardiovascular risk and often leads to blindness, end-stage renal disease, and leg amputation. It is also very closely related to other cardiovascular risk factors such as obesity, hypertension, and dyslipidemia [3]. This picture of multiple vascular risk factors

L. Smirčić-Duvnjak (✉)
Vuk Vrhovac University Clinic for Diabetes,
Endocrinology and Metabolic Diseases, University of Zagreb,
School of Medicine, Dugidol 4a, Zagreb, Croatia
e-mail: lduvnjak@idb.hr

253

M. Duvnjak (ed.), *Dyspepsia in Clinical Practice*,
DOI 10.1007/978-1-4419-1730-0_18,
© Springer Science+Business Media, LLC 2011

and wide-ranging complications makes the approach to individual diabetic patient complaining of dyspeptic symptoms very complex. Furthermore, there is still no agreement about the symptoms that should be included in the definition of functional dyspepsia [1, 4]. The most widely used definition is the International Committee of Clinical Investigators revised definition (Rome III criteria) that includes one or more of the following symptoms: bothersome post-prandial fullness, early satiation, epigastric pain, and epigastric burning with at least a 3-month history in the last year [1].

It appears that at some point in any diabetic patient's life, the chances of presenting with dyspeptic symptoms are extremely high.

EPIDEMIOLOGY

Literature data reporting on the prevalence of dyspepsia in diabetic patients are limited and conflicting. While some studies have confirmed the increased incidence of gastrointestinal (GI) symptoms in diabetic population compared with the nondiabetic one, others have failed to detect a difference in the prevalence rate of GI symptoms between the two groups [5–9]. The conflicting results can be explained by different populations and ethnic groups studied. In fact, investigations differed in study population comprising patients attending diabetes clinics who were unrepresentative of diabetic population in general or focused on selected subgroups of diabetic patients [6–8]. GI symptoms were also inconsistently defined, and some studies lacked an appropriately defined control group [7]. A large population-based survey has identified increased prevalence of both upper and lower GI symptoms in type 1 and type 2 diabetic patients compared with community controls. The authors have suggested that the effect may be associated with poor glycemic control but not with the duration of diabetes or the type of treatment. The study included a representative population of diabetic patients of all ages and grades of severity [10]. Recently published data documented an increased prevalence of upper GI symptoms in type 2 diabetic patients compared with age- and gender-matched nondiabetic controls, which are also associated with poor glycemic control [11].

CLINICAL PRESENTATION

Diabetes can affect the entire gastrointestinal tract, from the oral cavity to the anorectal region resulting in various symptoms whose severity and specificity depend not only on the composite of dysfunctional elements but also on diabetes itself [4,12].

Approximately 75% of patients referred to diabetes clinics have at least one gastrointestinal symptom. The most common symptoms related to dyspepsia are: heartburn, nausea, early satiety, bloating, and vomiting, while gastroesophageal reflux and gastroparesis represent the most frequent conditions associated with these symptoms [12].

Gastroparesis denotes delayed gastric emptying in the absence of mechanical obstruction of the stomach [1, 4, 12].

In type 1 diabetes, delayed emptying has been identified in 27% to 58% of cases, while in long standing type 2 diabetes, the prevalence rate is about 30% [13, 14]. A meta-analysis has documented delayed gastric emptying in 40% of patients with functional dyspepsia [15].

However, the presentations vary in individual patient and can often be clinically silent [16]. According to literature data, symptoms associated with gastroparesis occur only in 5% to 12% of diabetic patients [10]. It appears that in diabetic patients with delayed gastric emptying, a particular pattern of characteristic symptoms is missing [17].

Although a large spectrum of dyspeptic symptoms is strongly suggestive of slow gastric emptying, a significant correlation between the severity of these symptoms and the rate of gastric emptying has not been documented [17].

In diabetic patients, gastroparesis often develops after at least 10 years of diabetes duration and is typically associated with other microvascular complications – nephropathy, retinopathy, and neuropathy. Apart from suffering from impaired quality of life and glucose control, patients with gastroparesis are at risk of malnutrition, weight loss, and impaired drug absorption [12, 16].

PATHOGENESIS

To maintain a normal process of food digestion, absorption, and elimination, an interaction between the nerve endings embedding the muscle wall, neurotransmitters, hormones, and the muscle fibers is required. The natural history of dyspepsia and its pathogenesis in patients with diabetes remains poorly understood. Several mechanisms have been implicated in its development including autonomic neuropathy, microangiopathy, altered production of insulin and glucagon, increased susceptibility to gastrointestinal infections, and poor glycemic control. Diabetic autonomic neuropathy (DAN), involving the entire autonomic nervous system (ANS), has significant impact on morbidity and mortality in diabetic patients. Gastrointestinal dysfunction represents only one of its numerous manifestations, including cardiovascular, genitourinary, sudomotor, or ocular complications. The widespread effects of DAN can be explained by ANS vasomotor, visceromotor, and sensory fibers innervating every organ in our body [16]. The pathogenesis of DAN is complex and includes metabolic, vascular, autoimmune, and neurohormonal factors. Hyperglycemia can cause direct neuronal damage activating the polyol pathway with subsequent sorbitol accumulation [18]. Formation of advanced glycosylation end products, reduction in neurotrophic growth factors, and increased oxidative stress have also been implicated in the process. These factors decrease nerve blood flow and damage the vascular endothelium and neurons [19–22]. An involvement of sympathetic and parasympathetic nerve antibodies in the pathogenesis of both types of diabetic patients has also been documented [23, 24]. GI manifestations of DAN have been classified, according to the affected section of the GI tract, into esophageal enteropathy, gastroparesis diabeticorum, diarrhea, constipation, fecal incontinence, gallbladder atony, and enlargement [17]. Besides gastroparesis, esophageal enteropathy can also be associated with dyspeptic symptoms. It includes disordered peristalsis and abnormal lower esophageal sphincter function, results at least in part from vagal neuropathy, and presents as heartburn and dysphagia for solids [17].

In diabetic gastroparesis, disturbances of the nervous system and of muscular and hormonal activities of the digestive system have been recognized [12, 16, 25].

DAN damages the vagus nerve, leads to reduction in the number of intrinsic inhibitory neurons critical for motor coordination and in the number of the interstitial cells of Cajal [26, 27]. Neurohormonal changes in diabetes such as increased glucagon levels retard gastric emptying and reduce the frequency of antral contractions [28].

Delayed gastric emptying can further worsen glycemic control by impairing the delivery of food to the intestines and the relation between glucose absorption and exogenous insulin administration. It can also alter the pharmacokinetics of orally administered hypoglycemic agents [12, 17].

It has to be emphasized that, although GI symptoms are commonly attributed to DAN, they may be caused by other factors as well. Studies have demonstrated an increased prevalence of GI symptoms in diabetic patients without signs of DAN, although in some of them, DAN was diagnosed using cardiovascular reflex test instead of specific test of GI autonomic function [10, 12, 25].

Poor glycemic control may in itself promote GI symptoms. Variations in blood glucose concentrations affect neuromuscular function throughout the gut and perception of sensations arising from the gut [29–32].

Acute hyperglycemia can affect motor function and cause proximal gastric distension, leading to increased perception of nausea. Slow gastric emptying and reduced lower esophageal sphincter pressure have been described during acute hyperglycemia episodes in diabetic patients [10]. Many studies have confirmed the association of poor glycemic control and GI symptoms by comparing self-reported glycemic profile and the presence of GI symptoms [10]. In type 1 diabetic patients, the sensation of postprandial fullness was associated with blood glucose concentration [29]. Upper dysmotility-like symptoms were significantly more prevalent in individuals with self-reported poor glycemic control than in those reporting good or average glycemic control [10].

A significant correlation between higher glycated hemoglobin levels and the increased rate of GI symptoms has also been documented [16].

Evidently, the association between DAN, glycemic control, and GI symptoms is complex. Whether DAN or poor glycemic control **per se** represent a key player in the pathogenesis of dyspepsia remains unclarified, these factors obviously being interrelated. As they progress with time, it is not possible to determine which factor precedes the other.

Coexisting psychiatric disorders, alcohol intake, use of drugs apart from insulin, and oral hypoglycemic agents such as anticholinergics, antidepressants, and calcium-channel blockers may also contribute to dyspepsia [12, 16, 25].

As the prevalence of the metabolic syndrome in type 2 diabetic patients is increased, abdominal discomfort or pain can also be caused by nonalcoholic fatty liver disease (NAFLD). NAFLD represents a spectrum of several nonalcoholic-related steatotic liver diseases, ranging from benign fatty liver to nonalcoholic steatohepatitis (NASH), associated with cirrhosis and hepatocellular carcinoma. Increased prevalence of obesity, diabetes, hyperlipidemia, and insulin resistance in patients with NAFLD implicates a close link with the metabolic syndrome. The diagnosis can be confirmed with elevated liver enzyme tests, abdominal ultrasonography, and liver biopsy [32].

Dyspeptic symptoms associated with the use of diabetes medications represent a very important issue from the clinical point of view. Metformin and acarbose are often prescribed for type 2 diabetes.

Metformin is widely accepted as a first-line therapy in type 2 diabetes and a very effective insulin sensitizer. It also has some side-effects, including gastrointestinal symptoms, among which nausea and diarrhea are the most prominent ones. About 10% to 15% of people taking metformin have significant gastrointestinal side effects and are unable to tolerate the drug [1, 4, 12, 25].

Glucagon-like peptide 1 (GLP-1) analogs, the recently introduced agents for type 2 diabetes treatment, have raised considerable interest because of their additional favorable effects [33]. GLP-1 agonists augment insulin secretion from the beta cells and inhibit glucagon secretion, leading to reduced hepatic glucose production, lower fasting glucose, and improved postprandial glucose profile. Binding to certain receptors in the appetite-regulating centers in the hypothalamus and the hindbrain, GLP-1 agonists lead to a decreased appetite and promote weight loss. There is evidence that on a long-term basis, these agents can preserve the beta-cell function [33].

Another important effect refers to the inhibition of gastrointestinal motility and delayed gastric emptying that slow the entry of carbohydrates into the systemic circulation, thus decreasing the rise in postprandial glucose [34–36].

Nausea represents the major side-effect, occurring in 20% to 30% of patients, which can be minimized by starting with lower doses of GLP-1 analogs. The fact that this inhibitory action contributes to dyspeptic symptoms had raised concerns that it could represent a problem in patients with gastroparesis. However, so far, not a single case has been reported [33].

DIAGNOSTIC APPROACH

Data concerning the duration of diabetes, glycemic control, and current diabetic medications should be obtained by careful history taking. Medication history includes the use of other agents, anticholinergic agents, ganglion blockers, and psychotropic drugs associated with dyspeptic symptoms. The presence of other related diabetic complications – retinopathy, nephropathy, and neuropathy should also be evaluated. History of pancreatitis and biliary stone disease should be considered. If celiac disease is suspected, laboratory tests including serum levels of celiac disease, gliadin, endomysial, gluten, and reticulin antibodies should be performed. Based on clinical signs, some of the alternative causes such as pregnancy and uremia can be easily excluded [12, 37, 38].

Physical examination findings might suggest autonomic dysfunction (abnormal pupil responses, abnormal sweating, urinary retention, or impotence) and reveal signs of peripheral neuropathy and epigastric distention. The absence of a splashing sound on

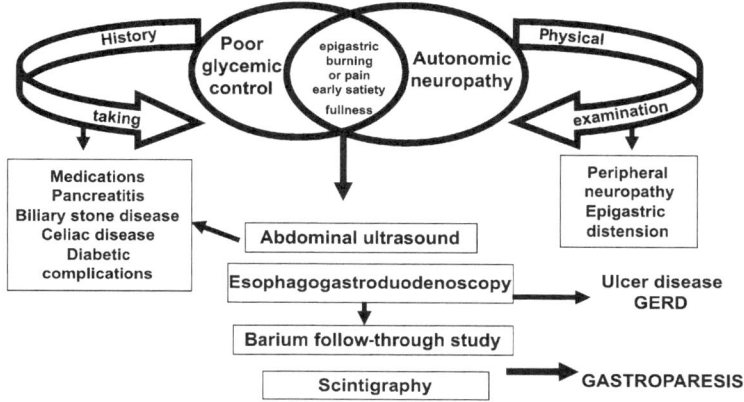

FIG. 18.1 Diagnostic approach to diabetic patients with dyspepsia.

abdominal succussion 1 hour after a meal suggests normal gastric emptying of liquids [17].

While patients complain of unexplained troublesome abdominal symptoms, diagnostic approach usually begins with a hepatobiliary ultrasound. Obstruction of the GI tract should be ruled out by esophagogastroduodenoscopy or a barium follow-through examination.

Endoscopy often reveals reflux esophagitis, ulcers, or food debris in severe gastroparesis. In the majority of patients with delayed gastric emptying, endoscopy findings are normal. To assess disorders of storage, grinding, and propulsion caused by gastric pump failure, it is essential to perform a summative measurement of these functions. Scintigraphy represents the gold standard for measuring gastric emptying. The test is not widely available, requiring special equipment and expertise, and involving exposure to radiation. Other specialized evaluations for the assessment of gastroparesis include manometry to detect antral hypomotility and/or pylorospasm and electrogastrography to detect abnormalities in GI pacemaking (Fig. 18.1) [12, 17, 38].

THERAPEUTIC APPROACH

Because of an incompletely understood and multifactorial pathogenesis, the management of dyspepsia in diabetes is less than optimal. Treatment strategies focus on normalization of glucose regulation and control of symptoms [38]. Dyspeptic symptoms can alter food intake, delivery, and absorption from the intestines, impairing the effects of antidiabetic drugs and insulin administration. This can result in wide variations in 24-h glucose profile with sudden episodes of postprandial hypoglycemia [12, 17]. Consumption of frequent small meals while avoiding high-fiber and fatty foods, smoking cessation, and light postprandial exercise can improve gastric emptying. While consumption of frequent small meals provides symptomatic relief, during an exacerbation of gastroparesis, a liquid diet is recommended. To achieve an optimal glucose profile, insulin therapy is advisable for the majority of patients with severe symptoms. In those with brittle diabetes, the use of insulin pumps might be necessary [17, 25]. Pharmacological approach includes the use of prokinetic and antiemetic agents [16, 38]. As prokinetic drugs stimulate peristalsis and improve gastric pump function, they may be useful in the treatment of diabetic patients with dyspepsia. Metoclopropamide is a dopaminergic antagonist with antiemetic properties that enhances gastric emptying. Unfortunately, it crosses the blood–brain barrier causing neurological side effects that limit its use. Cisapride is a prokinetic agent that efficaciously facilitates gastric emptying. Due to its potential to cause cardiac dysrhythmias by prolonging QT interval, it was withdrawn from the market [16, 25]. A range of antiemetics might be useful in controlling nausea and vomiting, among them prochlorperazine and promethazine, and 5HT3 receptor antagonists such as ondansetron or dolastetron. If pain relief is required, the agents frequently used in clinical practice are low-dose tricyclics and pregabalin. Tramadol and opiates are not agents of choice because of their inhibiting effect on motility [12, 16, 25, 38]. Novel therapies, including implantable gastric pacemaker, are promising in patients with severe gastroparesis but are still subjects of ongoing investigations [16, 37, 38].

CONCLUSIONS

The global diabetes pandemic is likely to result in a heavy burden of diabetes complications that will pose a significant challenge to healthcare systems in the future.

The frequent association between dyspepsia and diabetes is more than a chance finding. Due to a poorly understood pathogenesis and the lack of a specific pattern of symptoms, many diabetic patients with dyspepsia remain undiagnosed and undertreated. Diagnostic strategies should be directed at excluding other disorders, particularly peptic ulcer and gastroesophageal reflux disease, and medication use. Strong consideration should be given to glucose regulation and ANS evaluation. Treatment strategies focus on the normalization of blood glucose profile and the control of symptoms. It is important not only to diagnose and treat patients with diabetes and its comorbidities but also to prevent their development by promoting healthy lifestyle. In patients with diabetes and dyspepsia, a multitarget approach based on the assessment of the overall metabolic risk should be applied. Increased understanding of the mechanisms contributing to dyspepsia in diabetes needs to be obtained in future follow-up studies in order to develop a logical, evidence-based treatment strategy.

References

1. Tack J, Talley NJ, Camilleri M, et al. Functional gastroduodenal disorders. Gastroenterology. 2006;130:1466–79.
2. Wild S, Roglic G, Green A, Sicree R, King H. Global prevalence of diabetes: estimates for the year 2000 and projections for 2030. Diab Care. 2004;27:1047–53.
3. Adeghate E, Saadi H, Adem A, Obinoche E, editors. Diabetes mellitus and its complications: molecular mechanisms, epidemiology, and clinical medicine, The Annals of the New York Academy of Science, vol. 1084. New York: Wiley-Blackwell; 2007.
4. Chandran M, Chu NV, Edelman S. Gastrointestinal disturbances in diabetes. Curr Diab Rep. 2003;3:43–8.
5. Schvarcz E, Palmer M, Ingberg CM, Aman J, Berne C. Increased prevalence of upper gastrointestinal symptoms in long-term type 1 diabetes mellitus. Diabet Med. 1995;13:478–81.
6. Janatuinen E, Pikkarainen P, Laakso M, Pyörälä K. Gastrointestinal symptoms in middle-aged diabetic patients. Scand J Gastroenterol. 1993;28:427–32.
7. Ko GT, Chan WB, Chan JC, Tsang LW, Cockram CS. Gastrointestinal symptoms in Chinese patients with type 2 diabetes mellitus. Diabet Med. 1999;16:670–4.
8. Enck P, Rathmann W, Spiekermann M, et al. Prevalence of gastrointestinal symptoms in diabetic patients and non-diabetic subjects. J Gastroenterol. 1994;32:637–41.
9. Maleki D, Locke III GR, Camilleri M, et al. Gastrointestinal tract symptoms among persons with diabetes mellitus in the community. Arch Intern Med. 2000;160:2808–16.
10. Bytzer P, Talley NJ, Leemon M, Young LJ, Jones MP, Horowitz M. Prevalence of gastrointestinal symptoms associated with diabetes mellitus: a population-based survey of 15, 000 adults. Arch Intern Med. 2001;161:1989–96.
11. Kim JH, Park HS, Ko SY, et al. Diabetic factors associated with gastrointestinal symptoms in patients with type 2 diabetes. World J Gastroenterol. 2010;16:1782–7.
12. Camilleri M. Diabetic gastroparesis. N Engl J Med. 2007;356:820–9.
13. Jones KL, Russ A, Stevens JE, et al. Predictors of delayed gastric emptying in diabetes. Diab Care. 2001;24:1264–9.

14. Horowitz M, Harding PE, Maddox AF, et al. Gastric and oesophageal emptying in patients with type 2 (non-insulin dependent) diabetes mellitus. Diabetologia. 1989;32:151–9.

15. Soykan I, Sivri B, Sarosiek I, et al. Demography, clinical characteristics, psychological and abuse profiles, treatment and long-term follow-up of patients with gastroparesis. Dig Dis Sci. 1998;43:2398–402.

16. Talley NJ. Diabetic gastropathy and prokinetics. Am J Gastroenterol. 2003;98:264–71.

17. Vinik A, Raelene E, Maser E, Mitchell BD, Freeman R. Diabetic autonomic neuropathy. Diab Care. 2003;26:1553–79.

18. Greene DA, Lattimer SA, Sima AA. Are disturbances of sorbitol, phosphoinositide, and Na+-K+-ATPase regulation involved in pathogenesis of diabetic neuropathy? Diabetes. 1988;37:688–93.

19. Veves A, King GL. Can VEGF reverse diabetic neuropathy in human subjects? J Clin Invest. 2001;107:1215–8.

20. Cameron NE, Cotter MA. Metabolic and vascular factors in the pathogenesis of diabetic neuropathy. Diabetes. 1997;46 Suppl 2:31S–7.

21. Duvnjak L, Vučković S, Car N, Metelko Ž. Relationship between autonomic function, 24-h blood pressure and albuminuria in normotensive, normoalbuminuric patients with type 1 diabetes. J Diabet Complications. 2001;15:314–9.

22. Hoeldtke RD, Bryner KD, McNeill DR, et al. Nitrosative stress, uric acid, and peripheral nerve function in early type 1 diabetes. Diabetes. 2002;51:2817–25.

23. Vinik AI, Pittenger GL, Milicevic Z, Knezevic-Cuca J. Autoimmune mechanisms in the pathogenesis of diabetic neuropathy. In: Eisenbarth G, editor. Molecular mechanisms of endocrine and organ specific autoimmunity. Austin, TX: R.G. Landes; 1999. p. 217–51.

24. Sundkvist G, Lind P, Bergstrom B, Lilja B, Rabinowe SL. Autonomic nerve antibodies and autonomic nerve function in type 1 and type 2 diabetic patients. J Intern Med. 1991;229:505–10.

25. Koch CA, Uwaifo G. Are gastrointestinal symptoms related to diabetes mellitus and glycemic control? Eur J Gastroenterol Hepatol. 2008;20:822–5.

26. Watkins CC, Sawa A, Jaffrey S, et al. Insulin restores neuronal nitric oxide synthase expression and function that is lost in diabetic gastropathy. J Clin Invest. 2000;106:373–84.

27. He CL, Soffer EE, Ferris CD, Walsh RM, Szurszewski JH, Farrugia G. Loss of interstitial cells of Cajal and inhibitory innervation in insulin-dependent diabetes. Gastroenterology. 2001;121:427–34.

28. Couturier O, Bodet-Milin C, Querellou S, Carlier T, Turzo A, Bizais Y. Gastric scintigraphy with a liquid-solid radiolabelled meal: performances of solid and liquid parameters. Nucl Med Commun. 2004;25:1143–50.

29. Jones KL, Horowitz M, Wishart J, et al. Gastric emptying and intragastric meal distribution in diabetes mellitus–relationship between gastric emptying and blood glucose concentrations. J Nucl Med. 1995;36:2220–8.

30. Jones KL, Horowitz M, Berry M, et al. Blood glucose concentration influences post-prandial fullness in IDDM. Diab Care. 1997;20:1141–6.
31. Rathmann W, Enck P, Frieling T, Gries FA. Visceral afferent neuropathy in diabetic gastroparesis. Diab Care. 1991;14:1086–9.
32. Kotronen A, Yki-Jarvinen H. Fatty liver: a novel component of the metabolic syndrome. Arterioscler Thromb Vasc Biol. 2008;28:27–38.
33. Holst JJ, Vilsbøll T, Deacon CF. The incretin system and its role in type 2 diabetes mellitus. Mol Cell Endocrinol. 2009;297:127–36.
34. Nauck MA, Niedereichholz U, Niedereichholz U, Ettler R, et al. Glucagon-like peptide 1 inhibition of gastric emptying outweighs its insulinotropic effects in healthy humans. Am J Physiol. 1997;273:E981–8.
35. Wettergren A, Schjoldager B, Mortensen PE, Myhre J, Christiansen J, Holst JJ. Truncated GLP-1 (proglucagon 78–107-amide) inhibits gastric and pancreatic functions in man. Dig Dis Sci. 1993;38:665–73.
36. Willms B, Werner J, Holst JJ, Orskov C, Creutzfeldt W, Nauck MA. Gastric emptying, glucose responses and insulin secretion after a liquid test meal: effects of exogenous glucagon-like peptide-1 (GLP-1)-(7–36) amide in type 2 (noninsulin-dependent) diabetic patients. J Clin Endocrino Metab. 1996;81:327–32.
37. Patrick A, Epstein O. Review article: gastroparesis. Aliment Pharmacol Ther. 2008;27:724–40.
38. Ma J, Rayner CK, Jones KL, Horowitz M. Diabetic gastroparesis: diagnosis and management. Drugs. 2009;69:971–86.

Index

M. Duvnjak (ed.), *Dyspepsia in Clinical Practice*,
DOI 10.1007/978-1-4419-1730-0,
© Springer Science+Business Media, LLC 2011

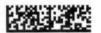